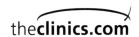

CLINICS IN PODIATRIC MEDICINE AND SURGERY

Medical Management of the Podiatric Patient

GUEST EDITOR
Jonathan M. Labovitz, DPM

CONSULTING EDITOR
Vincent J. Mandracchia, DPM, MSHCA

April 2007 • Volume 24 • Number 2

SAUNDERS

An Imprint of Elsevier, Inc.
PHILADELPHIA   LONDON   TORONTO   MONTREAL   SYDNEY   TOKYO

W.B. SAUNDERS COMPANY
A Division of Elsevier Inc.

1600 John F. Kennedy Blvd., Suite 1800, Philadelphia, PA 19103-2899

http://www.theclinics.com

CLINICS IN PODIATRIC MEDICINE   Volume 24, Number 2
AND SURGERY   ISSN 0891-8422
April 2007   ISBN-13: 978-1-4160-4781-0
Editor: Sarah Barth   ISBN-10: 1-4160-4781-6

The ideas and opinion expressed in *Clinics in Podiatric Medicine and Surgery* do not necessarily reflect those of the Publisher. The Publisher does not assume any responsibility for any injury and/or damage to persons or property arising out of or related to any use of the material contained in this periodical. The reader is advised to check the appropriate medical literature and the product information currently provided by the manufacturer of each drug to be administered to verify the dosage, the method and duration of administration, or contraindications. It is the responsibility of the treating physician or other health care professional, relying on independent experience and knowledge of the patient, to determine drug dosages and the best treatment for the patient. Mention of any product in this issue should not be construed as endorsement by the contributors, editors, or the Publisher of the product of manufacturers' claims.

Reprints. For copies of 100 or more of articles in this publication, please contact the Commercial Reprints Department, Elsevier Inc., 360 Park Avenue South, New York, New York 10010-1710 Tel.: (212) 633-3813, Fax: (212) 462-1935, e-mail: reprints@elsevier.com

Clinics in Podiatric Medicine and Surgery (ISSN 0891-8422) is published quarterly by Elsevier Inc., 360 Park Avenue South, New York, NY 10010-1710. Months of publication are January, April, July, and October. Business and Editorial Offices: 1600 John F. Kennedy Blvd., Suite 1800, Philadelphia, PA 191023-2899. Customer Service Office: 6277 Sea Harbor Drive, Orlando, FL 32887-4800. Periodicals postage paid at New York, NY, and additional mailing offices. Subscription prices are $189.00 per year for US individuals, $297.00 per year for US institutions, $97.00 per year for US students and residents, $227.00 per year for Canadian individuals, $360.00 for Canadian institutions, $254.00 for international individuals, $360.00 per year for international institutions and $130.00 per year for Canadian and foreign students/residents. To receive student/resident rate, orders must be accompanied by name of affiliated institution, date of term, and the *signature* of program/residency coordinator on institution letterhead. Orders will be billed at individual rate until proof of status is received. Foreign air speed delivery is included in all *Clinics* subscription prices. All prices are subject to change without notice. POSTMASTER: Send address changes to *Clinics in Podiatric Medicine and Surgery,* Elsevier Periodicals Customer Service, 6277 Sea Harbor Drive, Orlando, FL 32887-4800. **Customer Service: 1-800-654-2452 (US). From outside of the US, call 1-407-345-1000.**

Clinics in Podiatric Medicine and Surgery is covered in *Index Medicus* and *EMBASE/Excerpta Medica.*

Printed in the United States of America.

CONSULTING EDITOR

VINCENT J. MANDRACCHIA, DPM, MSHCA, Chief Medical Officer; Staff Podiatrist, Section of Podiatric Surgery, Department of Surgery, Broadlawns Medical Center; Clinical Professor, Department of Podiatric Medicine and Surgery, College of Podiatric Medicine and Surgery, Des Moines University-Osteopathic Medicine Center, Des Moines, Iowa

GUEST EDITOR

JONATHAN M. LABOVITZ, DPM, FACFAS, Private Practice, Torrance, California; Attending Staff, West Los Angeles-Veterans Administration Medical Center, Los Angeles, California; Baja Project for Crippled Children, Torrance, California

CONTRIBUTORS

MARK R. ABBRUZZESE, MD, Clinical Instructor, Georgetown University School of Medicine, Washington, DC

MARTIN A. ACQUADRO, MD, DMD, FACP, FACPM, Associate Clinical Professor of Anesthesia, Tufts University School of Medicine; Director, Department of Anesthesiology and Pain Services; Perioperative Medical Director, Caritas Carney Hospital, Dorchester, Massachusetts

DAVID AUNGST, DPM, Attending, Podiatric Medicine and Surgery, Olive View-UCLA Medical Center, VA Greater Los Angeles Healthcare System, Department of Surgery, Los Angeles, California

EMILY A. COOK, DPM, Clinical Fellow in Surgery, Harvard Medical School, Boston; Division of Podiatric Surgery, Department of Surgery, Beth Israel Deaconess Medical Center, Boston, Massachusetts

JEREMY J. COOK, DPM, Clinical Fellow in Surgery, Harvard Medical School, Boston; Division of Podiatric Surgery, Department of Surgery, Beth Israel Deaconess Medical Center, Boston, Massachusetts

JEFFREY G. CRAMBLETT, DPM, FACFAS, PGY-1 Resident, Botsford General Hospital, Botsford Podiatry Clinic, Farmington Hills, Michigan

JOHN M. GIURINI, DPM, Associate Professor in Surgery, Harvard Medical School, Boston; Chief, Division of Podiatric Surgery, Department of Surgery, Beth Israel Deaconess Medical Center, Boston, Massachusetts

PADMA GULUR, MD, Assistant in Anesthesia, Massachusetts General Hospital, Boston, Massachusetts; Instructor in Anaesthesia, Harvard Medical School, Massachusetts General Hospital Pain Center, Boston, Massachusetts

BRUCE I. KACZANDER, DPM, FACFAS, Chief of Podiatry, William Beaumont Hospital, Royal Oak, Michigan; and Vice Chief of Staff, Botsford General Hospital, Botsford Podiatry Clinic, Farmington Hills, Michigan

PAUL J. KIM, DPM, Assistant Professor, Arizona Podiatric Medicine Program, Midwestern University Division of Dental and Medical Education, Midwestern University College of Health Sciences, Glendale, Arizona

JONATHAN M. LABOVITZ, DPM, FACFAS, Private Practice, Torrance, California; Attending Staff, West Los Angeles-Veterans Administration Medical Center, Los Angeles, California; Baja Project for Crippled Children, Torrance, California

GURBIR S. MANN, DPM, PGY-1 Resident, Botsford General Hospital, Botsford Podiatry Clinic, Farmington Hills, Michigan

AKSONE NOUVONG, DPM, FACFAS, Assistant Clinical Professor of General Surgery, David Geffen School of Medicine-UCLA, VA Greater Los Angeles Healthcare System, Department of Surgery, Los Angeles, California

NEIL M. PAIGE, MD, MSHS, Associate Clinical Professor of Medicine, David Geffen School of Medicine-UCLA, VA Greater Los Angeles Healthcare System, Department of Medicine, Los Angeles, California

DAVID H. RAHM, MD, President, VitaMedica Corporation, Manhattan Beach, California

KATE REVILL, Samuel Merritt College of Podiatric Medicine, Oakland, California

SIMON MAURICE SOLDINGER, MD, Assistant Clinical Professor, University of California Los Angeles, Sherman Oaks, California

JOHN S. STEINBERG, DPM, Assistant Professor, Department of Plastic Surgery, Georgetown University School of Medicine, Washington, DC

AILEEN M. TAKAHASHI, MD, Association of South Bay Surgeons, Torrance, California

JAMES H. TING, MD, Faculty, Family and Sports Medicine, Northridge Family Medicine Residency Program, Northridge, California; Volunteer Team Physician, California State University Northridge, Northridge, California; Team Physician, James Monroe High School, North Hills, California

SONDRA VAZIRANI, MD, MPH, Associate Clinical Professor of Medicine, David Geffen School of Medicine-UCLA, VA Greater Los Angeles Healthcare System, Department of Medicine, Los Angeles, California

DAVID H. WALLIS, MD, Private Practice, Family and Sports Medicine, South Bay Family Medical Group, Torrance, California; Team Physician, Chivas USA, Major League Soccer; Associate Team Physician, United States Soccer Women's National Team

CONTENTS

Providing care to athletes involves much more than simply treating musculoskeletal injuries. Many of the illnesses and disease processes that affect the general population are also seen in competitive athletes. Medical management of these conditions, however, can be challenging. Treatment plans need to be tailored to the individual athlete and take into consideration the rigors and demands of his or her particular sport. Important conditions that all physicians who provide care for athletes should be familiar with are sudden cardiac death, hypertension, concussion, methicillin-resistant *Staphylococcus aureus* infections, the female athlete triad, diabetes mellitus, and asthma.

The increasing pervasiveness of diabetes mellitus on a global stage has been well documented. Many groundbreaking studies have detailed the consequences of inadequate glycemic control, but only recently have data supported evidence that demonstrates benefits in the acute setting. Consensus is lacking with regard to how to achieve glycemic control in the hospital setting. This article discusses glycemic control, with special emphasis on the perioperative patient. Emerging therapeutic treatments and less frequently encountered protocols such as insulin pump management and insulin infusion are considered.

Morbid obesity is a worldwide pandemic. Medical problems associated with being obese include hypertension, diabetes, pulmonary restrictive disease, obstructive sleep apnea, and increased risk of cancer. In addition, there is a tremendous financial burden on society and the health care system to take care of these individuals. Bariatric surgery has proved to be a safe, effective means of sustained weight loss, which can lead to improvement or resolution of obesity-related medical conditions. Individuals who are morbidly obese represent a unique population requiring special consideration when presenting for medical care.

Advanced thought and planning are required when preparing for podiatric surgery. In addition to appropriate procedure selection and follow-up, perioperative management has a key role in patient and physician satisfaction. Neglect of this aspect of podiatric care can also be a source of malpractice. This article analyzes many of the common medical treatments currently employed and makes recommendations for treatment before, during, and after surgery.

The poor dietary habits and aging of the US population have caused a steady increase in the incidence of chronic disease. The prevalence of these diseases, such as obesity, diabetes, and heart disease, may have a significant effect on perioperative management, surgical outcome, and complication rates in these patients. Nutritional intervention and supplementation may help curb some of these potential adverse affects of poor nutrition by promoting wound healing; enhancing immunity; reducing swelling, bruising, and inflammation; and reducing oxidation caused by anesthetic agents and surgery. Although a perioperative regimen of dietary supplements may enhance surgical outcomes, it is equally important to know the popular herbal products that are contraindicated in the perioperative period.

FORTHCOMING ISSUES

July 2007
Advances in the Treatment of the Diabetic Foot
Thomas Zgonis, DPM, *Guest Editor*

October 2007
Adult Acquired Flatfoot
Adam M. Budny, DPM and Jordan P. Grossman,
DPM, *Guest Editors*

January 2008
Lower Extremity Radiology
Denise Mandi, DPM, *Guest Editor*

RECENT ISSUES

January 2007
Residency Training
George F. Wallace, DPM, MBA, *Guest Editor*

October 2006
Implants in Foot and Ankle Surgery
Jesse B. Burks, DPM, MS, *Guest Editor*

July 2006
Diagnosis and Treatment of Peripheral Nerve Entrapments and Neuropathy
Babak Baravarian, DPM, *Guest Editor*

April 2006
The Management of Lower Extremity Trauma and Complications
Thomas Zgonis, DPM
and Demetrios G. Polyzois, MD, *Guest Editors*

THE CLINICS ARE NOW AVAILABLE ONLINE!

http://www.theclinics.com

ELSEVIER
SAUNDERS

Clin Podiatr Med Surg
24 (2007) xi–xiii

CLINICS IN
PODIATRIC
MEDICINE AND
SURGERY

Foreword

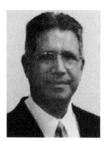

Vincent J. Mandracchia, DPM, MSHCA
Consulting Editor

"Are you a real doctor?"

"No, but I did stay at a Holiday Inn Express last night."
—Commercial paraphrase

I think we have got it all wrong when it comes to our professional image. I don't make that statement lightly, and unfortunately it forces us to take a long, hard look at the product we have made visible to the world.

Recently, I had the immense pleasure of being selected as the Chief Medical Officer (CMO) of our medical center. Through all of the excitement of the challenge of the job, I had lost site of the sheer volume of work that went into being a successful CMO. I find myself juggling the duties of administration with those of being a podiatrist. Although abbreviated in time, I still practice podiatry and feel that it is a necessity to remain connected with my physician brethren at the hospital. After all, it has been my experience that when a practicing physician gives up the practice and becomes "just a suit," other physicians loose confidence in that individual.

When the official announcement was made, there were many accolades, and it was a time to celebrate both a personal and professional

doi:10.1016/j.cpm.2007.02.002

accomplishment, until... We are the County hospital and thus beholden to the County tax payers. Therefore, we are frequently the target of the *Des Moines Register*'s watchdog reporter, and just about anything we do seems to make the paper. The reporter who covers our institution called the day after the announcement was made and asked, "Is he a real doctor?"

This got me thinking about where we are going and what we are trying to accomplish as a profession. I have been involved in meetings in which we argue about who is going to be cutting patients' toenails, who should be physically debriding ulcers, should the physical therapist be recommending or making inserts, and so forth—and we fight vehemently about these items. I have seen the profession become exclusionary to its own members, almost gleeful that we are not all one brotherhood under podiatry and competing against each other rather than working toward a goal of podiatry for all and all for podiatry (yes, there is a bit of the Three Musketeers in that statement, but why not?)—and all for the benefit of our patients!

Apart from the internal fighting, what have we done to promote ourselves to the world? How does the public see us? How do our colleagues in the allopathic and osteopathic professions see us? If the public and other professionals see us as "less than," then isn't it our fault? How could it not be? No, I don't believe that changing our degree is the answer—I believe changing our image is! And it starts from the get-go. Are colleges of podiatric medicine preparing their students *mentally* to be physicians? I'm not talking about parity in the curriculum with allopathic and osteopathic centers of education; I'm referring to attitude. Are we a "systemically shy" profession that passes that insecurity onto our future podiatrists and focuses on the technical aspects of treatment? I know the answer, and so do many of you. Do we really take the time to learn from the bright students who have chosen our profession, or do we ignore their questions with a perfunctory "That's the way I've always done it" type of attitude? In turn, do we push our students to be physicians in the true sense of the word? By definition, a physician is a person trained in the art of healing. How simple, yet perfect. It doesn't say MD, or DO; it does, however, imply a "healer."

We need to express to the public and professional communities, through a strongly united profession, that we are indeed physicians, doctors, and healers—not show a fragmented bunch of individuals who only care about the individual and not the whole. Mr. Spock of the *Star Trek* movies said it very well: "The needs of the many outweigh the needs of the few or the one." There are many positive ways to satisfy one's ego; just consider the grateful patients we all have the privilege of treating.

A strong professional presence that clearly defines our mission as one of caring for the needs of our patients will go a long way toward answering the question, "Are we real doctors?" This is accomplished by a united effort of the profession to educate the world about our mission and to present ourselves as a desirable profession working toward a common goal. Then we will easily have the numbers of applicants we need to fill our classrooms with quality students, and we will be graduating a future generation of podiatrists that will be clearly recognized as "doctors."

Vincent J. Mandracchia, DPM, MSHCA
Department of Surgery
Broadlawns Medical Center
1801 Hickman Road
Des Moines, IA 50314, USA

E-mail address: vmandracchia@broadlawns.org

ELSEVIER
SAUNDERS

Clin Podiatr Med Surg
24 (2007) xv–xvi

CLINICS IN
PODIATRIC
MEDICINE AND
SURGERY

Preface

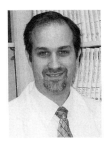

Jonathan M. Labovitz, DPM, FACFAS
Guest Editor

This issue of the *Clinics* was somewhat of a challenge to put together. It struck me as I started to assemble the Table of Contents how difficult and challenging our profession can be. It also dawned on me how rewarding our profession can be. Interestingly, I found that the same common thread makes the challenge and reward one in the same. It leads us to the realization that although we all label ourselves as specialists, we are also primary care doctors, "gatekeepers," and sometimes both. We are the consulting doctor, yet for the next patient, we are likely to be the only doctor.

This dichotomy that we encounter is exciting yet concerning. We treat patients medically and surgically, yet many of us prefer to focus on the surgical education. How many of us read and constantly continue to educate ourselves in podiatric surgery? Many of our colleagues read one or two journals, *Journal of Foot and Ankle Surgery* and *Journal of the American Podiatric Medical Association*, and maybe *Foot and Ankle International* too. Although I don't mean to imply that many of our colleagues neglect the nonsurgical aspect of medicine, there are some who may not place enough emphasis on it.

We like to look at ourselves as surgeons—those who enjoy operating. We are training the next generation of podiatrists to think surgery as we continue to mold our profession as the "specialist of the foot and ankle." That catch phrase usually implies surgeon in our own minds and hopefully in the minds of the public and our colleagues of other medical specialties.

However, I offer you the following: how many people think that to be the "specialist of the foot and ankle" we need to understand the foot, ankle, leg,

0891-8422/07/$ - see front matter © 2007 Elsevier Inc. All rights reserved.
doi:10.1016/j.cpm.2007.02.001

pelvis, and spine? How about understanding the colon and gastrointestinal system as medications are ingested? What about the cardiovascular system and pulmonary system as our patients are under anesthesia? Maybe those systems are important for the athletes we encounter or any patient as they breathe in the office and as their heart beats faster during an injection. What about the diabetic patient whose sugar spikes on a sliding scale, despite being on insulin therapy in the hospital and then they proceed to develop an infection that is limb threatening? Have we truly stayed in tune with the recent changes in antibiotics? Gastric bypass is becoming more and more common and so is the use of psychiatric medications for off-label use. What about the aging baby boomers and the disease processes that affect the elderly patient? Do these affect us? Should we pay attention to this? I mean, we are the foot and ankle specialist...a surgeon after all.

This issue was used to focus attention away from the surgical journals for a moment in time, to make us look at our education. No, not the education in school, or during residency when you live in the hospital managing these patients regularly; this is our everyday life education we do to stay abreast of the latest medical developments (notice I said medical and not surgical developments).

This issue of the *Clinics* is different. This issue is to remind ourselves of the necessity to read, study, and learn all areas of medicine. All areas, medical and surgical, apply to the podiatric physician. This issue attempts to emphasize the importance of medicine because the best surgeons are well versed in medicine. The best surgeons understand their patient. The best surgeons are well trained in all systems and know the implications of all systems. Hopefully the dedicated authors of this issue of *Clinics in Podiatric Medicine and Surgery* will be able to bring us all up to date on the latest in medicine and instill some motivation to stay that way.

"Perfection is not attainable. But if we chase perfection we can catch excellence."

—Vince Lombardi

Jonathan M. Labovitz, DPM, FACFAS
3400 Lomita Boulevard, # 403
Torrance, CA 90505, USA

E-mail address: dr_labovitz@feetandankles.com

ELSEVIER
SAUNDERS

Clin Podiatr Med Surg
24 (2007) 127–158

CLINICS IN
PODIATRIC
MEDICINE AND
SURGERY

Medical Management of the Athlete: Evaluation and Treatment of Important Issues in Sports Medicine

James H. Ting, MD[a,*], David H. Wallis, MD[b,c,d]

[a]Family and Sports Medicine, Northridge Family Medicine Residency Program,
18406 Roscoe Boulevard, Northridge, CA 91325, USA
[b]Family and Sports Medicine, South Bay Family Medical Group,
3701 Skypark Drive #100, Torrance, CA 90505, USA
[c]Chivas USA, Major League Soccer
[d]United States Soccer Women's National Team

Athletes represent a unique subset of the population. These individuals are highly motivated and skilled at their craft; nonetheless, they are subjected to demands and circumstances within their respective sports that can expose them to injuries and illnesses. Although the feats of elite-level competitors may at times appear superhuman, the illnesses and diseases that can affect athletes are no different from those seen in the general population. Management of these conditions, however, can present a unique challenge to the sports medicine physician because treatment plans often need to be individualized to the athlete and to the particular sport in which he or she competes. Comprehensive coverage of the full gamut of disease processes seen in the athletic population is not the intent of this review. Rather, the authors have sought to present a brief but detailed review of several important disease processes that can afflict athletes, ranging from catastrophic conditions such as sudden cardiac death to more chronic illnesses such as hypertension (HTN), the female athlete triad, and diabetes mellitus.

Sudden cardiac death

Sudden cardiac death on the athletic field is a rare but tragic event. Although the exact frequency of these events is not known, it has been estimated at approximately 1 in 200,000 to 1 in 300,000 individual student athletes

---

* Corresponding author. Northridge Family Medicine Residency Program, 18406 Roscoe Boulevard, Northridge, CA 91325.
   E-mail address: james.ting@chw.edu (J.H. Ting).

per academic year [1,2]. There are a variety of conditions associated with sudden cardiac death in athletes. In individuals older than 35 years, most cases (up to 80%) are attributable to atherosclerotic coronary artery disease [3]. Under the age of 35 years, however, previously undetected congenital cardiac abnormalities are the predominant cause of sudden cardiac death. Of these, the two most common etiologies are hypertrophic cardiomyopathy (HCM) and congenital coronary artery anomalies [1,3,4].

Hypertrophic cardiomyopathy

HCM has consistently been implicated as the leading cause of sudden cardiac death in young athletes, accounting for approximately one third of all such events [4]. HCM is an inherited, autosomal dominant condition. It is the most common genetic cardiovascular disease [5], with a prevalence in the general adult population estimated at approximately 1 in 500 [6]. Mutations in any of 10 genes encoding proteins of the cardiac sarcomere can result in HCM [5], and as such, it displays great variability in its genetic, phenotypic, and clinical expression.

The characteristic cardiac finding in HCM is an undilated, asymmetrically hypertrophied left ventricle that cannot be attributed to any other co-existing disorder such as HTN or valvular heart disease. Associated histologic changes seen in HCM include disorganized cardiac myocytes and fibrosis. This change in the normal cardiac architecture is thought to predispose to fatal ventricular arrythmias, which appears to be the primary mechanism by which sudden death occurs in HCM [7]. In addition, the thickening of the myocardium seen in HCM may result in impaired myocardial perfusion or left ventricular (LV) outflow obstruction, both of which can be exacerbated by the stress of exercise, resulting in ischemia, arrhythmias, and syncope [8].

The diagnosis of HCM is often difficult to make on clinical grounds alone because patients are often asymptomatic. The first presentation of HCM may be sudden cardiac death. Given the strong genetic predisposition for the condition, a thorough family history screening for HCM or any unexplained early sudden death is imperative. Concerning symptoms include a history of syncope or near-syncope with exercise (due to LV outflow obstruction or arrythmia), and exertional chest pain or dyspnea (secondary to ischemia). Indeed, the presence of exertional symptoms or a positive family history in a young athlete should prompt consideration of the diagnosis [9]. On physical examination, the classic finding is a loud systolic murmur that is heard best at the left lower sternal border. The intensity of the murmur is accentuated by maneuvers that decrease venous return (thereby increasing the degree of LV outflow obstruction), such as the Valsalva maneuver or standing. Most patients who have HCM do not have LV outflow obstruction [5], however, and the murmur may therefore be absent. Further diagnostic testing in HCM includes ECG and two-dimensional echocardiography.

The vast majority (75%–95%) of patients who have HCM have abnormal ECG findings [5]. No one pattern is considered diagnostic, and findings may vary from normal to marked voltage changes consistent with LV hypertrophy (LVH) [10]. Two-dimensional echocardiography is generally considered to be the most reliable method to establish a diagnosis of HCM. Generally, a LV wall thickness of up to 12 mm is considered normal. Thicknesses greater than 15 mm are abnormal and should strongly raise the index of suspicion for HCM. A milder enlargement of between 13 and 15 mm, however, is often difficult to interpret because it may represent normal physiologic hypertrophy secondary to training (ie, athlete's heart) or a milder form of HCM [11,12]. A trial of deconditioning (cessation of training), along with serial echocardiographic studies, may be useful in making the distinction between the two entities [10]. It should be noted that abnormalities in LV wall thickness may not be notable until adolescence [4,10], so serial examinations and follow-up are prudent for any young symptomatic athlete in whom the diagnosis of HCM is being considered.

The 36th Bethesda Conference on Eligibility Recommendations for Competitive Athletes with Cardiovascular Abnormalities [13] recommended that individuals who have a probable or established diagnosis of HCM be excluded from all competitive athletics, with the possible exception of low-intensity sports such as golf or bowling. No current evidence is available, however, to justify precluding asymptomatic individuals harboring a HCM mutant gene from activity in the absence of morphologic features of the disease or a family history of sudden cardiac death.

Congenital coronary artery anomalies

The second most common cause of sudden cardiac death in young athletes is a group of congenital anomalies involving the coronary arteries [1,3,4]. Examples include the anomalous origin of the left or the right main coronary arteries and congenitally hypoplastic coronary arteries. The prevalence of such abnormalities based on autopsy results has been estimated at roughly 0.3% [14]. Although isolated congenital abnormalities involving the coronary arteries are rare, as a group they account for approximately 14% of the cases of sudden cardiac death in young athletes [7].

The malformation most commonly implicated in sudden cardiac death on the athletic field is the anomalous origin of the left main coronary artery from the right (anterior) sinus of Valsalva [15], whereby the left main coronary artery courses between the pulmonary trunk and the aorta. The aberrant course of the left coronary artery is significant for two reasons. First, the ostium of the anomalous left coronary artery is frequently slitlike and therefore more susceptible to compromised blood flow [16]. Second, the anomalously arising coronary artery frequently leaves its origin at an acute angle [16,17]. These factors, coupled with extrinsic compression of the artery between the expanding aorta and the pulmonary trunk during exertion, are believed to cause decreased myocardial oxygen delivery and, therefore, ischemia, arrythmias, and sudden death. A competing theory regarding the mechanism by which ischemia occurs involves the dynamic flattening of the anomalous coronary artery within the aortic wall during exercise secondary to increased systemic blood pressure and aortic wall tension [18].

Congenital anomalies of the coronary arteries are difficult to diagnose. Just as in HCM, patients are often asymptomatic. Symptoms, if present, may mimic those of myocardial ischemia, ranging from chest pain to exertional syncope [19]. As with HCM, the presence of exertional symptoms in an athlete should prompt consideration of the diagnosis and additional diagnostic work-up. ECG findings are not particularly helpful because they are usually normal at rest and during exertion [13]. Focused echocardiographic images of the coronary arteries using high-quality imaging systems [20] and color Doppler imaging [19] can help identify abnormalities. When echocardiographic findings are not diagnostic, other available imaging modalities include CT imaging, MRI, and ultimately, coronary angiography. When an anomaly is identified, surgical correction can be performed [21].

The 36th Bethesda Conference recommended that any athletes identified as having congenital anomalies of the coronary arteries be excluded from participation in all competitive sports [13] unless they have undergone a successful surgical correction of the malformation. In such cases, an athlete may be allowed to participate in all sports starting 3 months postoperatively, provided there is no demonstrable ischemia, arrhythmia, or dysfunction during maximal exercise testing [13].

Other rare causes of sudden cardiac death

There are multitudes of other less common causes of sudden cardiac death in young athletes that are not covered in this review. Intrinsic cardiac etiologies include myocarditis, aortic dissection secondary to Marfan syndrome, arrythmogenic right ventricular dysplasia, valvular heart disease such as aortic stenosis, atherosclerotic coronary artery disease, dilated cardiomyopathy, and arrhythmias such as the long QT syndrome. Important extrinsic etiologies of sudden cardiac death include commotio cordis and illicit drug abuse [7].

Hypertension

HTN is an increasingly common medical condition, affecting roughly 50 million individuals in the United States and approximately 1 billion individuals worldwide [22]. The diagnosis is based on elevations in an individual's systolic blood pressure (SBP) or diastolic blood pressure (DBP) on at least two separate measurements. The prevalence of HTN in the population increases with age, and it has been cited as an independent risk factor for adverse cardiovascular events such as myocardial infarction and stroke. It is also the most common cardiovascular condition seen in athletes [13].

The "Seventh Report of the Joint National Committee on Prevention, Detection, Evaluation, and Treatment of High Blood Pressure" (JNC 7 report) defines normal blood pressure in individuals 18 years or older as SBP less than 120 mm Hg and DBP less than 80 mm Hg. HTN is defined by a persistent elevation in SBP greater than 140 mm Hg or in DBP greater than 90 mm Hg. The report further subclassified HTN severity into stage 1 HTN (SBP 140–159 mm Hg or DBP 90–99 mm Hg) and stage 2 HTN (SBP ≥ 160 mm Hg or DBP ≥ 100 mm Hg). A new category of pre-HTN (SBP 120–139 mm Hg or DBP 80–89) was also added [22]. Although not hypertensive by definition, individuals who have pre-HTN are at significantly increased risk of developing HTN compared with their normotensive peers.

The diagnostic criteria for HTN differ for adults and children. In children and adolescents, HTN is defined as SBP or DBP greater than or equal to the 95th percentile by sex, age, and height. Measurements between the 90th and 95th percentile are termed "high normal." (For more information see "The Fourth Report on the Diagnosis, Evaluation, and Treatment of High Blood Pressure in Children and Adolescents" [23].)

All athletes should have their blood pressure measured before beginning competition or training. The measurements should be performed by sphygmomanometry using an appropriately sized blood pressure cuff (bladder at least 80% of arm circumference) with the patient quietly seated [24]. Physicians should be wary of diagnosing HTN solely on the basis of an elevated office blood pressure reading because of possible "white-coat" HTN, an anxiety-provoked elevation in blood pressure secondary to the office examination. Repeat ambulatory blood pressure readings should be taken to confirm or refute the abnormal office measurements [22].

Hypertensive patients should have a thorough history and physical examination to assess other cardiovascular disease risk factors (eg, tobacco use, dyslipidemia, diabetes mellitus, family history), target organ damage (eg, LVH, coronary artery disease, heart failure, stroke, peripheral arterial disease, chronic kidney disease, retinopathy), and secondary causes of HTN (eg, sleep apnea, chronic kidney disease, pheochromocytoma, thyroid disease). Diagnostic tests to be obtained before initiating therapy should include ECG, urinalysis, hematocrit, basic metabolic panel (including electrolytes, blood glucose, and creatinine), and lipid profile. (For more information, see the JNC 7 report [22].) If initial test results are abnormal or if BP control is not adequate, then further testing including echocardiography should be obtained in addition to starting therapy [13,22].

With regard to treatment, lifestyle modifications (eg, healthy diet, decreased sodium intake, cessation of tobacco use, increased cardiovascular exercise, avoidance of excessive alcohol intake) should be given to all patients. If necessary, several classes of antihypertensive medications are available for use; however, some may exert a negative effect on exercise capacity and athletic performance. β-adrenergic receptor blocking agents (β-blockers), for example, may be more problematic in this regard than other classes of antihypertensive medications due to their inherent negative chronotropic effects [13,25].

In athletes classified as having pre-HTN or stage 1 HTN (provided no evidence of target organ damage or coexisiting cardiac disease), the 36th Bethesda Conference recommended instituting lifestyle modifications but not precluding athletes from activity. Hypertensive individuals who have documented LVH, however, should be limited from participation until their blood pressure is normalized. Athletes who have stage 2 HTN, even in the absence of target organ damage, should be restricted from all high static sports (eg, weight lifting, rowing, cycling) until their blood pressure is adequately controlled. (For a complete list of classification of sports, see the 36th Bethesda Conference "Eligibility Recommendations for Competitive Athletes with Cardiovascular Abnormalities" [13].) In addition, to avoid potential disqualification, athletes being treated with certain antihypertensive agents may need to obtain permission for the use of these medications from their sport's appropriate governing bodies [13].

Sports-related concussion

Concussive injuries are common occurrences at sporting events. It has been estimated that roughly 300,000 sports-related concussions occur in the United States annually [26], but the actual incidence is likely even higher due to the propensity of athletes to not report their symptoms because of a lack of awareness of their potential severity and/or the fear of being withheld from play [27].

The definition of concussion is still evolving. In 1966, the Congress of Neurological Surgeons [28] proposed that concussion is a "clinical syndrome characterized by immediate and transient impairment of neural function, such as alteration of consciousness, disturbance of vision, equilibrium, etc., due to mechanical forces." In 1997, the American Academy of Neurology (AAN) endorsed its own definition of concussion as "a trauma-induced alteration in mental status that may or may not involve a loss of consciousness" (LOC) [29].

More recently, a revised definition of concussion was proposed by the Concussion in Sport Group (CISG) in 2001 at the first International Conference on Concussion in Sport in Vienna, Austria. This symposium, organized by the International Ice Hockey Federation in conjunction with the Federation Internationale de Football and the International Olympic Committee, brought together a panel of experts with the aim of providing recommendations for improvement in the care and management of sports-related concussion. The CISG's definition, which was subsequently re-endorsed in 2004 at the second International Conference on Concussion in Sport in Prague, Czech Republic, defined concussion as "a

pathophysiological process affecting the brain, induced by traumatic biomechanical forces" [30,31]. A key point regarding the causative traumatic force
is that it may not necessarily involve a direct blow to the head, as concussive
injury can also result from a blow delivered elsewhere on the body that is
subsequently transmitted to the head. As with the AAN, the CISG reiter-
ated that concussion may or may not involve LOC (Fig. 1A) [30,31].

The most commonly reported symptoms of an acute concussion are
headache, dizziness, confusion/disorientation, nausea, LOC, retrograde amnesia, and vomiting [32]. Other important signs may include fatigue, visual
changes such as blurred vision or photosensitivity, difficulties with balance
or coordination, and poor attention or focus. Because of the wide variation
in possible symptoms, the presence of any cognitive deficits in an athlete following a suspected head injury should trigger a closer assessment for
concussion.

Initial on-field assessment of the concussed athlete follows the principles
of basic life support. The athlete's level of consciousness and the stability of
his or her airway, breathing, and circulation must be evaluated first. Cervical spine evaluation, particularly in the case of LOC, should also be performed before the athlete is moved. If intracranial or spinal injury is
suspected, appropriate cervical spine precautions such as immobilization
with a cervical collar and backboard should be implemented. Football hel-
mets, if applicable, should not be removed, and immediate arrangements
should be made for transport to an appropriate facility for definitive evaluation and treatment. When potentially life-threatening injury has been ruled
out, the athlete should be removed from competition and further assessment
of the athlete's mental status should ensue.

Because the detection of cognitive deficits on the sideline can be difficult,
several attempts have been made to develop standardized, objective assessment tools to aid in the rapid assessment of a concussed athlete's mental status. One such tool is the Standardized Assessment of Concussion (SAC),
which grades athletes on measures including orientation, immediate memory, concentration, and delayed recall [33,34]. More recently, the 2004
Prague group developed the Sport Concussion Assessment Tool, which
sought to combine several existing sideline evaluation tools including the
SAC into one standardized tool (see Fig. 1A; Fig. 1B) [31]. With all such
tools, however, comparison with baseline test scores (obtained before injury)
is necessary to maximize detection of acute cognitive deficits. Any concussed
athlete should also have a complete neurologic examination including cra-
nial nerve testing and assessment of strength, sensation, reflexes, coordination, and gait.

Regardless of the tool used for examination, it is imperative that serial
examinations be performed at regular (eg, 5-minute) intervals while on the
sideline to monitor improvement or worsening of the athlete's condition.
Progressive deterioration in mental status or alertness and worsening
of symptoms such as headache or vomiting may indicate potentially

Sport Concussion Assessment Tool (SCAT)

This tool represents a standardized method of evaluating people after concussion in sport. This Tool has been produced as part of the Summary and Agreement Statement of the Second International Symposium on Concussion in Sport, Prague 2004

Sports concussion is defined as a complex pathophysiological process affecting the brain, induced by traumatic biomechanical forces. Several common features that incorporate clinical, pathological and biomechanical injury constructs that may be utilized in defining the nature of a concussive head injury include:

1. Concussion may be caused either by a direct blow to the head, face, neck or elsewhere on the body with an 'impulsive' force transmitted to the head.
2. Concussion typically results in the rapid onset of short-lived impairment of neurological function that resolves spontaneously.
3. Concussion may result in neuropathological changes but the acute clinical symptoms largely reflect a functional disturbance rather than structural injury.
4. Concussion results in a graded set of clinical syndromes that may or may not involve loss of consciousness. Resolution of the clinical and cognitive symptoms typically follows a sequential course.
5. Concussion is typically associated with grossly normal structural neuroimaging studies.

Post Concussion Symptoms

Ask the athlete to score themselves based on how they feel now. It is recognized that a low score may be normal for some athletes, but clinical judgment should be exercised to determine if a change in symptoms has occurred following the suspected concussion event.

It should be recognized that the reporting of symptoms may not be entirely reliable. This may be due to the effects of a concussion or because the athlete's passionate desire to return to competition outweighs their natural inclination to give an honest response.

If possible, ask someone who knows the athlete well about changes in affect, personality, behavior, etc.

Remember, concussion should be suspected in the presence of ANY ONE or more of the following:
- Symptoms (such as headache), or
- Signs (such as loss of consciousness), or
- Memory problems

Any athlete with a suspected concussion should be monitored for deterioration (i.e., should not be left alone) and should not drive a motor vehicle.

For more information see the "Summary and Agreement Statement of the Second International Symposium on Concussion in Sport" in the April, 2005 edition of the Clinical Journal of Sport Medicine (vol 15), British Journal of Sports Medicine (vol 39), Neurosurgery (vol 59) and the Physician and Sportsmedicine (vol 33). This tool may be copied for distribution to teams, groups and organizations. ©2005 Concussion in Sport Group

The SCAT Card
(Sport Concussion Assessment Tool)
Athlete Information

What is a concussion? A concussion is a disturbance in the function of the brain caused by a direct or indirect force to the head. It results in a variety of symptoms (like those listed below) and may, or may not, involve memory problems or loss of consciousness.

How do you feel? You should score yourself on the following symptoms, based on how you feel now.

Post Concussion Symptom Scale

	None		Moderate			Severe	
Headache	0	1	2	3	4	5	6
"Pressure in head"	0	1	2	3	4	5	6
Neck Pain	0	1	2	3	4	5	6
Balance problems or dizzy	0	1	2	3	4	5	6
Nausea or vomiting	0	1	2	3	4	5	6
Vision problems	0	1	2	3	4	5	6
Hearing problems / ringing	0	1	2	3	4	5	6
"Don't feel right"	0	1	2	3	4	5	6
Feeling "dinged" or "dazed"	0	1	2	3	4	5	6
Confusion	0	1	2	3	4	5	6
Feeling slowed down	0	1	2	3	4	5	6
Feeling like "in a fog"	0	1	2	3	4	5	6
Drowsiness	0	1	2	3	4	5	6
Fatigue or low energy	0	1	2	3	4	5	6
More emotional than usual	0	1	2	3	4	5	6
Irritability	0	1	2	3	4	5	6
Difficulty concentrating	0	1	2	3	4	5	6
Difficulty remembering	0	1	2	3	4	5	6

(follow up symptoms only)

	None		Moderate			Severe	
Sadness	0	1	2	3	4	5	6
Nervous or Anxious	0	1	2	3	4	5	6
Trouble falling asleep	0	1	2	3	4	5	6
Sleeping more than usual	0	1	2	3	4	5	6
Sensitivity to light	0	1	2	3	4	5	6
Sensitivity to noise	0	1	2	3	4	5	6
Other: _____	0	1	2	3	4	5	6

What should I do?
Any athlete suspected of having a concussion should be removed from play, and then seek medical evaluation.

Signs to watch for:
Problems could arise over the first 24-48 hours. You should not be left alone and must go to a hospital at once if you:
- Have a headache that gets worse
- Are very drowsy or can't be awakened (woken up)
- Can't recognize people or places
- Have repeated vomiting
- Behave unusually or seem confused; are very irritable
- Have seizures (arms and legs jerk uncontrollably)
- Have weak or numb arms or legs
- Are unsteady on your feet; have slurred speech

Remember, it is better to be safe. Consult your doctor after a suspected concussion.

What can I expect?
Concussion typically results in the rapid onset of short-lived impairment that resolves spontaneously over time. You can expect that you will be told to rest until you are fully recovered (that means resting your body and your mind). Then, your doctor will likely advise that you go through a gradual increase in exercise over several days (or longer) before returning to sport.

Fig. 1. The Sport Concussion Assessment Tool (SCAT). (*From* McCrory P, Johnston K, Meeuwisse W, et al. Summary and agreement statement of the 2nd International Conference on Concussion in Sport, Prague 2004. Clin J Sport Med 2005;15(2):55; with permission; © Concussion in Sport Group.)

Sport Concussion Assessment Tool (SCAT)

The SCAT Card
(Sport Concussion Assessment Tool)
Medical Evaluation

Name: _____   Date _____

Sport/Team: _____   Mouth guard? Y N

1) SIGNS
Was there loss of consciousness or unresponsiveness?   Y   N
Was there seizure or convulsive activity?   Y   N
Was there a balance problem / unsteadiness?   Y   N

2) MEMORY
Modified Maddocks questions (check correct)

At what venue are we? __; Which half is it? __; Who scored last?__

What team did we play last? __; Did we win last game? __?

3) SYMPTOM SCORE
Total number of positive symptoms (from reverse side of the card) = _____

4) COGNITIVE ASSESSMENT

5 word recall		Immediate	Delayed
	(Examples)		(after concentration tasks)
Word 1 _____	cat	___	___
Word 2 _____	pen	___	___
Word 3 _____	shoe	___	___
Word 4 _____	book	___	___
Word 5 _____	car	___	___

Months in reverse order:
Jun-May-Apr-Mar-Feb-Jan-Dec-Nov-Oct-Sep-Aug-Jul   (circle incorrect)
                        or
Digits backwards (check correct)
5-2-8   3-9-1   _____
6-2-9-4   4-3-7-1   _____
8-3-2-7-9   1-4-9-3-6   _____
7-3-9-1-4-2   5-1-8-4-6-8 _____

Ask delayed 5-word recall now

5) NEUROLOGIC SCREENING

	Pass	Fail
Speech	___	___
Eye Motion and Pupils	___	___
Pronator Drift	___	___
Gait Assessment	___	___

Any neurologic screening abnormality necessitates formal neurologic or hospital assessment

6) RETURN TO PLAY
Athletes should not be returned to play the same day of injury.
When returning athletes to play, they should follow a stepwise
symptom-limited program, with stages of progression. For example:
1. rest until asymptomatic (physical and mental rest)
2. light aerobic exercise (e.g. stationary cycle)
3. sport-specific exercise
4. non-contact training drills (start light resistance training)
5. full contact training after medical clearance
6. return to competition (game play)

There should be approximately 24 hours (or longer) for each stage
and the athlete should return to stage 1 if symptoms recur.
Resistance training should only be added in the later stages.
Medical clearance should be given before return to play.

Instructions:
This side of the card is for the use of medical doctors,
physiotherapists or athletic therapists. In order to
maximize the information gathered from the card, it is
strongly suggested that all athletes participating in
contact sports complete a baseline evaluation prior to
the beginning of their competitive season. This card
is a suggested guide only for sports concussion and is
not meant to assess more severe forms of brain
injury. **Please give a COPY of this card to the
athlete for their information and to guide follow-
up assessment.**

Signs:
Assess for each of these items and circle
Y (yes) or N (no).

Memory: If needed, questions can be modified to
make them specific to the sport (e.g. "period" versus "half")

Cognitive Assessment:
Select any 5 words (an example is given). Avoid
choosing related words such as "dark" and "moon"
which can be recalled by means of word association.
Read each word at a rate of one word per second.
The athlete should not be informed of the delayed
testing of memory (to be done after the reverse
months and/or digits). Choose a different set of
words each time you perform a follow-up exam with
the same candidate.
Ask the athlete to recite the months of the year
in reverse order, starting with a random month. Do
not start with December or January. Circle any
months not recited in the correct sequence.
For digits backwards, if correct, go to the next
string length. If incorrect, read trial 2. Stop after
incorrect on both trials.

Neurologic Screening:
Trained medical personnel must administer this
examination. These individuals might include medical
doctors, physiotherapists or athletic therapists.
Speech should be assessed for fluency and lack of
slurring. Eye motion should reveal no diplopia in any
of the 4 planes of movement (vertical, horizontal and
both diagonal planes). The pronator drift is performed
by asking the patient to hold both arms in front of
them, palms up, with eyes closed. A positive test is
pronating the forearm, dropping the arm, or drift away
from midline. For gait assessment, ask the patient to
walk away from you, turn and walk back.

Return to Play:
A structured, graded exertion protocol should be
developed; individualized on the basis of sport, age
and the concussion history of the athlete. Exercise or
training should be commenced only after the athlete is
clearly asymptomatic with physical and cognitive rest.
Final decision for clearance to return to competition
should ideally be made by a medical doctor.

For more information see the "Summary and
Agreement Statement of the Second International
Symposium on Concussion in Sport" in the April, 2005
Clinical Journal of Sport Medicine (vol 15), British
Journal of Sports Medicine (vol 39), Neurosurgery (vol
59) and the Physician and Sportsmedicine (vol 33).
©2005 Concussion in Sport Group

Fig. 1 (*continued*)

life-threatening pathology such as an evolving intracranial hemorrhage or
an epidural/subdural hematoma. Any athlete exhibiting such a decline
should be promptly transported to an appropriate facility for further
evaluation and imaging.

Conventional neuroimaging techniques such as CT or MRI are typically normal and of limited usefulness in evaluating concussions [30,31,35]. These conventional techniques, however, should be used for instances in which severe structural brain injuries or lesions are suspected, such as in cases in which an athlete exhibits focal neurologic deficits or in the case of progressively worsening symptoms as noted earlier [30,31]. Because the pathophysiology behind the cognitive dysfunction following concussive injury has been theorized to be primarily functional or metabolic rather than structural [36,37], functional imaging techniques are being developed to better evaluate concussive injuries. Modalities such as single-photon emission CT, positron emission tomography, and functional MRI, although still largely experimental, may provide clinically useful information in the near future regarding alterations in cerebral metabolism and brain function that occur in concussed athletes [35].

There is currently no universally accepted management guideline in place regarding sports-related concussive injuries, although over 20 have been proposed [38]. Among the more commonly used guidelines are the Cantu [39], modified Cantu [40], Colorado [41], and AAN guidelines [29]. The intent of these various guidelines is to provide an objective method of grading the injury severity to guide an athlete's safe return to play. Of particular concern in young athletes is the second-impact syndrome [42], a condition in which uncontrolled swelling of the brain is thought to result from a second sustained impact while the athlete is recovering from a previous concussive injury.

A comprehensive review of each of the aforementioned guidelines is beyond the scope of this discussion, but a common feature among them is the prominent use of the presence or absence of LOC in determining concussion severity and return-to-play criteria. In each of the scales, a grade 1 (least severe) concussion cannot involve LOC. The presence of LOC, however, constitutes a grade 3 (most severe) concussion by most guidelines. The significance of LOC in regard to concussive severity, however, has been more recently called into question [32,43]. Amnesia, not LOC, may be more predictive of the neurocognitive deficits [44] and the number and duration of symptoms seen in the postinjury period [32]. In returning an athlete to play, each of the guidelines generally allows same-day return to play for grade 1 concussions, provided the athlete is completely asymptomatic within 15 minutes [29] to 20 minutes [41] following the injury, at rest and with exertion. Return to play on the same day of injury is disallowed for grade 2 and 3 concussions in each of the scales. Timelines for return to play after becoming asymptomatic following a grade 2 or 3 injury vary from 1 week [29] to 2 weeks [39] for grade 2 concussions and from 1 to 2 weeks [29] to 1 month [39,40] for grade 3 concussions. For athletes who have suffered multiple concussions, additional recommendations, varying from prolonged periods of rest from activity to termination of the athlete's season, may be considered.

The CISG, in examining each of the concussion guidelines, determined that no one guideline was sufficient to guide concussion management, and as such, it was recommended that concussion grading scales be abandoned [30,31]. Instead, the 2004 Prague group proposed categorizing all concussions as simple ("an injury that progressively resolves without complication over 7–10 days") or complex ("cases where athletes suffer persistent symptoms (including persistent symptom recurrence with exertion), specific sequelae (eg, concussive convulsions), prolonged LOC (>1 minute), or prolonged cognitive impairment following the injury") [31].

In addressing the management of a concussive injury, the CISG advocated a conservative approach such that return to play on the same day of injury in an athlete showing any signs or symptoms of a concussion was not allowed. In regard to a return-to-play protocol for a simple concussion, the 2004 Prague group detailed a stepwise and graded program of exertion that involves a gradual increase in activity from complete rest (physical and cognitive), progressing to resumption of aerobic activity and resistance training, to increasing contact activity, and ultimately to game play (see Fig. 1B) [31]. In implementing this stepwise protocol, the athlete is to progress to the next level of training only if asymptomatic at the current level for 24 hours. If there is any recurrence of symptoms while progressing, then the athlete should drop back to the previous asymptomatic level and try to progress again after a period of 24 hours [31]. In cases of complex concussions or athletes who have suffered multiple concussions, the CISG suggested that other investigations such as formal neuropsychologic testing be considered to help aid return-to-play advice.

Cognitive deficits may persist for several days after a concussive injury [45]. To better assess the recovery of these deficits, the use of neuropsychologic testing and, more recently, computerized neuropsychologic testing, has become increasingly more prominent in concussion management. There are a number of computer-based test batteries available, among them the Automated Neuropsychological Assessment Metrics, CogSport, the Concussion Resolution Index, and Immediate Postconcussion Assessment and Cognitive Testing. Each of these batteries has the potential to allow clinicians to measure more subtle markers of cognitive function such as reaction time, information processing speed, and memory [38,46]. Baseline test scores, however, are still necessary for a more useful interpretation of results in a concussed athlete. Research continues in regard to the validity of these testing batteries and their potential role in the assessment and management of concussion.

The decision to return an athlete to play following a concussive injury is complex and should be individualized to the involved athlete [38]. Several guidelines have been proposed to aid the clinician in this endeavor, each with its own respective strengths and weaknesses. The Cantu, Colorado, and AAN guidelines may be seen by some as restrictive in regard to mandating a specified number of postinjury days before return to play is allowed. Conversely, others may view the CISG guidelines as restrictive in regard to disallowing same-day return to play. There is currently no universally accepted standard for concussion classification or return to play, and until one exists, guidelines in and of themselves should be considered adjuncts to, not substitutes for, experience and sound clinical judgment. The assessment and management of sports-related concussion is an evolving area in sports medicine. As more data and information from research in this area become available, practice guidelines will invariably evolve.

Methicillin-resistant *Staphylococcus aureus* infections

Staphylococcus aureus is a ubiquitous gram-positive bacteria that possesses an impressive ability (by way of intraspecies genetic [ie, DNA] transfer) to acquire means of resistance to multiple antibiotics at once, including methicillin, to which resistance was first noted in 1961 [47]. Today, methicillin-resistant *Staphylococcus aureus* (MRSA) is one of the most common causes of bacterial infections in the nosocomial, or hospital-based, setting [48]. Risk factors for MRSA infection include any history of hospitalization or a chronic underlying illness/disease that predisposes to hospitalization, nursing home admission, outpatient office visits, antibiotic exposure, or close contact with individuals who have these risk factors [49]. The emergence of new and aggressive MRSA infections in the community, however, among young, otherwise-healthy individuals and athletes who do not have identifiable risk factors [49–51] has been the focus of much recent attention and concern within the medical community.

An important aspect of dealing with community-acquired MRSA is determining whether the source of the infection is a nosocomial strain spread from contact with colonized individuals or an entirely new strain, as this may influence treatment. Because individuals can unknowingly be colonized with MRSA [52] (particularly in the nares and skin) for long periods without being actively infected, transmission by contact with colonized persons is plausible in many cases. There is also evidence, however, that some infections are due to new strains of MRSA arising within the community [53]. Genetic analysis [48] has confirmed MRSA isolates within the community that are genetically distinct from typical nosocomial strains [54]. In addition, reports of community-acquired MRSA in young patients who do not have known exposures or risk factors further suggest that new strains of MRSA are emerging [50,55], probably as a result of selection pressures secondary to antibiotic use [56].

The most common clinical presentation of community-acquired MRSA is superficial soft tissue infection, although other less common presentations such as necrotizing pneumonia and septic chock can occur [48]. Direct invasion of the skin by MRSA followed by tissue destruction from the release of bacterial toxins results in necrotic skin lesions that patients often attribute to "spider bites." Lesions are commonly crusted or coalesce into plaques and often progress to abscesses or overt cellulitis [48]. Although the infection tends to stay confined to the skin and soft tissues, it can progress to bacteremia and subsequent systemic disease. Transmission and host-to-host spread of MRSA occurs by close contact with draining lesions and with colonized individuals.

Recent outbreaks of MRSA infections involving groups of competitive athletes and their household contacts have been noted. Clusters of MRSA skin infections have been reported in several sports, including fencing, wrestling, and football [51]. Skin trauma and direct skin-to-skin contact between players, such as occurs frequently in football and wrestling, is the easiest and most likely mode of transmission of infection. In sports that involve limited or no close physical contact among competitors, however, it has been suggested that transmission of infection can occur through the use of shared equipment, such as scoring sensor wires used in fencing. Indeed, following a group of cases seen in a Colorado fencing club in February 2003, no further infections were reported after implementation of MRSA transmission control measures involving increased hygiene and routine cleaning and laundering of shared equipment [51]. The use of contaminated shared equipment was also implicated in the spread of MRSA infections among members of an Indiana high school wrestling team who had never wrestled one another and had no other identifiable common exposures between them [51].

Antibiotic therapy forms the mainstay of treatment for MRSA infections. As alluded to earlier, determining the origin of the infection is important because of possible treatment implications. Nosocomial MRSA strains are typically resistant to multiple antibiotics [48], whereas community-acquired methicillin-resistant strains have been noted to display susceptibilities to a wide spectrum of antibiotics including clindamycin, trimethoprim-sulfamethoxazole, macrolides (to a variable degree), tetracyclines, and fluoroquinolones [48,57,58]. Other factors to consider before initiating antibiotic therapy are the prevalence of MRSA in the particular community, the presence of risk factors for MRSA infection, and the severity of infection [48]. If possible, wound cultures in all patients and blood cultures, if indicated, should be obtained. In areas in which the prevalence of community-acquired MRSA is high, severe infections should be treated empirically with vancomycin, particularly if the patient has a history of MRSA colonization, intravenous drug abuse, or risk factors for MRSA infection [48]. Individuals who have less severe infections and no risk factors may be treated initially with clindamycin or trimethoprim-sulfamethoxazole [48,57]. Individuals who have mild or moderate infections and no risk factors who reside in areas that have a low prevalence of community-acquired MRSA can be treated with a penicillinase-resistant penicillin such as oxacillin or nafcillin or with a first-generation cephalosporin such as cefazolin pending culture results [48].

Just as important as the treatment of community-acquired MRSA is the prevention of its spread. Because this bacteria tends to take up residence in the nares, nasal surveillance cultures and eradication therapy using topical mupirocin may be considered. Trials of decolonization therapy, however, have met with variable success, and its use is somewhat controversial [48]. Within the sporting community, improved education and hygiene may be an effective tool in containing the spread of MRSA. Recommendations such as increased hand-washing with soap, regular showering with soap after each practice or competition, keeping skin wounds covered until healed, laundering towels and equipment after each use, routine scheduled cleaning of shared athletic equipment, and appropriate evaluation of all infected or nonhealing wounds [51] may be the only interventions necessary. The sports medicine physician can be instrumental in this regard in helping to minimize and manage this ongoing public health issue.

Female athlete triad

The female athlete triad is a syndrome described in athletic women characterized by disordered eating, amenorrhea, and osteoporosis. Women usually do not present with all three elements; however, the presence of any one element should prompt a clinical evaluation for the others because they are closely associated and share inter-related pathophysiologies, treatments, and consequences. Physicians familiar with this grouping of symptoms may be able to more appropriately screen for the other elements when caring for athletic women.

Although their underlying psychologic profile may vary widely, women who have the female athlete triad typically share certain behavioral characteristics. These women commonly feel pressure, whether real or perceived, to maximize athletic performance, to achieve a certain body image, or both. This preoccupation with body image and weight often results in pathologic controlling behaviors such as excessive dieting and overexertion. Risk factors for this pressure, and hence the ensuing behaviors, may vary throughout a woman's life cycle. Overzealous parents and demanding coaches put youth at risk. Adolescent girls who have compulsive personalities may also be at risk for these disorders.

The normal changes seen in adolescence with regard to hormones, body composition, and athletic abilities can be dramatic even for teens not predisposed to the triad. Especially when an individual's athletic ability peaks before puberty, there can be great pressure to control or somehow contain the changes involved with physical development. These pressures may also be intensified during adolescence when young women are being considered for athletic scholarships.

In addition to the general risk factors for female athletes, there exist sport-specific risk factors that may further accentuate the problem. Sports that have subjective judging, such as gymnastics, figure skating, and diving, place a particular emphasis on one's physical appearance and can lead to overly controlling or restrictive behaviors. Sports that have weight classifications such as rowing or judo can exert pressure to gain a competitive advantage through unhealthy weight loss. Similar pressures are also visible in other sports such as distance running, ballet dancing, and swimming in which a lean physique is in itself advantageous.

Physicians who provide care for athletic women must be vigilant in screening for this syndrome. The presence of particular warning signs such as stress fractures, weight changes, dehydration, and depression and other behavioral changes should trigger a full evaluation to screen for the female athlete triad. Treatment is difficult and it is essential to take a multidisciplinary approach involving education of the patient, parents, coaches, and trainers. Education regarding a healthy approach to sport should be tailored to the underlying problems and clinical manifestations for the involved individual. Proper treatment should involve attention to nutritional concerns and dietary modification, hormonal and nutritional supplements, and psychologic assessment to address self-esteem and other related issues.

Eating disorders and disordered eating

One percent to 3% of all women may have an eating disorder. In athletic women, however, the prevalence is dramatically increased. Estimates place the rate of disordered eating in this population between 16% and greater than 50%. This wide range in the estimates is due to the differing age groups and varying criteria used in the various studies of disordered eating.

Most athletes do not meet *Diagnostic and Statistical Manual of Mental Disorders* (DSM) [59] criteria for overt anorexia nervosa or bulimia nervosa, but pathologic weight control measures such as fasting, induced vomiting, and use of diet pills, laxatives, enemas, and diuretics are also included in the category of disordered eating. Instead of resulting in the selective loss of adipose tissue and performance improvement, these measures often result in starvation (with subsequent loss of muscle mass), dehydration, and diminished athletic performance.

Anorexia nervosa involves a distortion of one's own body image. Anorectic patients have a prominent fear of becoming fat and generally refuse to maintain at least 85% of ideal body weight. Two variations of anorexia nervosa are common: a restricting type, which exhibits excessive control and limitations over food intake, and a binge and purge type, which may display reliance on laxatives, diuretics, and induced vomiting [59]. Many athletes who have disordered eating, however, do not have a distorted view of their own body image but still rely on the same maladaptive and harmful behaviors to maintain a desired body weight. The term *anorexia athletica* is sometimes used to describe this condition, which is usually characterized by a compulsive or obsessive exercise habit combined with weight control strategies that do not completely fulfill diagnostic criteria for other eating disorders.

Bulimia nervosa is more common than anorexia nervosa but is often harder to detect because these patients commonly have normal body weight. This disorder involves a loss of the sense of control over food intake, with subsequent compensatory behaviors. Compensation may or may not involve purging. Typical nonpurging behaviors involve cycles of excessive exercise, fasting, or both. DSM criteria specify that these cycles occur an average of twice a week for 3 months; however, as with anorexia nervosa, most female athletes who have this type of disordered eating do not fully meet the criteria.

Physical examination of most women who have disordered eating reveals no significant abnormalities. A range of abnormalities such as bradycardia, hypotension, hypothermia, skin changes (edema, dryness, laguno hair), gastrointestinal disturbances, parotid gland swelling, and dental enamel erosion may be present depending on the patient's behaviors. Selective laboratory testing to be considered may include a complete blood count (CBC), glucose, a comprehensive metabolic panel, magnesium, thyroid function testing (TFT), hormone levels (estradiol, insulin-like growth factor-1, urinary free cortisol [60]), an ECG, and bone mineral density (BMD) measurements. None of these tests, however, is diagnostic.

The sequelae of eating disorders are significant and commonly underappreciated by those who have them. Electrolyte abnormalities, cardiac arrhythmias, and other endocrine abnormalities can have serious and life-threatening consequences; mortality in anorectic women is approximately six times higher than in unaffected peers [61,62], ranging from 4% to 15% [61–63].

These disorders should not be taken lightly because patients who have eating disorders also have very high rates of comorbid psychiatric disorders, including problems with self-esteem, major depression, anxiety, obsessive-compulsive disorder, drug abuse, and suicide. Proper treatment requires a multidisciplinary team that has a primary care physician, a nutritionist, and a mental health professional. Open communication optimizes everyone's ability to safely treat any medical abnormalities, alter maladaptive behaviors, and change the pathologic thought processes that lead to these behaviors to minimize the chance of recurrence.

The patient and this team should agree on minimum allowable weight limits, a close follow-up routine, and the use of tools such as food diaries, cognitive behavioral therapy, and medications in the treatment plan. Multivitamins with iron, calcium, and zinc should be prescribed, with weekly follow-up and a slow but closely monitored plan for weight gain (0.5 pounds per week). Failure to maintain agreed levels of body weight may indicate a need for inpatient treatment.

Amenorrhea

Estimates of the prevalence of amenorrhea in athletes are much higher than in the general population (<5%) but vary widely among athletic women, ranging from 10% to 50% depending on the population studied and the degree of oligomenorrhea (or of amenorrhea). Amenorrhea is classified as primary (lacking secondary sexual characteristics by age 14 years or lacking menarche by age 16 years) or as secondary (cessation of established menses for at least 3 consecutive months). Both are seen with increased frequency in female athletes. In addition to screening for these criteria, however, it is important to also consider any recent changes in menstrual patterns because the hormonal axis can be adversely altered long before these criteria are met.

The menstrual cycle is controlled by the hypothalamus and pituitary glands, and irregularities can range from luteal phase defects to anovulation, oligomenorrhea, or amenorrhea. Consequences of even mild, subclinical levels of menstrual dysfunction are reflected in altered concentrations of growth hormone, cortisol, and other hormones as the body tries to adjust to the state of negative energy balance [64]. Amenorrhea is also associated with a worsened lipid profile and endothelial dysfunction [65]; however, this endothelial dysfunction seems to be improved by oral contraceptive administration [66].

Exercise-associated amenorrhea (EAA) is often seen in athletic women in association with weight loss, decreased body fat percentage, high-intensity workouts, abrupt changes in training, and emotional stress. EAA, however, remains a diagnosis of exclusion. A thorough history should include a review of contraceptives and other medications, energy intake and expenditure, and weight changes. A physical examination, including an examination of the pelvis, thyroid, breast, and skin should also be performed. Laboratory tests such as pregnancy testing, CBC, TFT, and prolactin, luteinizing hormone (LH), and follicle stimulating hormone (FSH) levels may be considered. LH and FSH levels are often decreased, with resultant low estrogen and progesterone levels. Cortisol levels may also be elevated, and insulin levels may be suppressed; however, these findings may be nonspecific and are not required to make a diagnosis. Diagnostic imaging such as pelvic ultrasound and MRI of the brain may also be indicated in certain circumstances.

Because EAA functionally represents an adaptive response to starvation by the reproductive system, it is also usually reversible with changes in lifestyle. Nutritional improvement involving increased caloric intake (usually an additional 250–750 kcal/d), reduced training intensity (by 5%–20%), closely monitored weight gain (usually 5–15 lb at a rate of 0.5 to 1 lb/wk), and correction of any suspected vitamin deficiencies is paramount. Many women will resist these measures, so it is important that they be implemented by a cohesive team of nutritionists, counselors, coaching staff, and physicians.

Most athletes are often more receptive to change when asked to reduce their training by a specified proportion or amount rather than to stop altogether. Sports are often a primary source of stress management, self-esteem, and social interaction and friendship; depriving women of these important elements does not foster a therapeutic relationship between the patient and care team and does not teach the athlete to develop and maintain a proper balance of sport and nutrition in her life.

Treatment of EAA also carries implications in other related areas of health care. For example, women who have been infertile for some time may require contraceptive counseling when they start ovulating because they may not be in the habit of protecting themselves from undesired pregnancy. In addition, calcium and vitamin supplementation and BMD testing should be considered. Although many of these women are still young and can increase their bone density with restoration of proper nutrition, irreversible bone loss can still take place even in these early years.

Hormone replacement should also be considered for amenorrheic and oligomenorrheic women. This therapy is often accomplished through oral contraceptives (avoiding progestin-only pills) or more traditional hormone replacement therapy. Common concerns or fears regarding hormone therapy include weight gain, breast tenderness, mood changes, and bloating. Women who wish to avoid menstruation can be prescribed a monophasic combination pill for 3 months at a time, with the placebo pills omitted. The timing for initiation of these therapies varies widely in clinical practice, and the clinician must factor in the athlete's need for contraception. Hormone therapy should be considered after 6 months of amenorrhea because this may reduce the osteoporosis risk and other effects of hypoestrogenemia [67]. It is important for the physician and the patient to recognize, however, that none of these interventions addresses the underlying negative energy balance at the root of the problem. Long-term treatment needs to focus on correcting this deficiency.

Osteoporosis and osteopenia

The density and integrity of an athlete's skeleton is determined by a complex interplay of genetic, nutritional, endocrinologic, and physical factors. The strongest predictor of peak BMD is one's genetic makeup. Exercise and an individual's hormonal environment also alter the formation and breakdown of bone. The hypoestrogenemic state seen in postmenopausal women and those who have the female athlete triad favors resorbtive osteoclastic activity over formative osteoblastic activity [68].

Regular weight-bearing exercise increases bone density and should be encouraged throughout the lifecycle because decreased peak bone density during youth predisposes to disease in adulthood and in advanced age. Postmenopausal women who exercise, however, carry a decreased risk for fractures compared with those who do not (even within a given level of bone density) due to improved strength, balance, and coordination.

Given all the benefits of exercise on BMD, it is counterintuitive to many athletic women that they could be at risk for osteoporosis despite their frequent exercise. The abnormal hormonal milieu that exists in the female athlete triad, however, markedly blunts the protective effects of weight-bearing exercise. Other endocrine changes seen in these athletic women, such as elevated cortisol levels, may also contribute to diminished bone formation, some of which may be irreversible [63].

Osteoporosis and osteopenia, although not rare, are nonetheless relatively uncommon during peak athletic years. Female athletes who have menstrual irregularities or eating disorders demonstrate a lower average BMD than those who do not have these disturbances [69], even when they do not formally meet criteria for osteopenia or osteoporosis. Fracture risk is estimated to increase 50% to 150% for each SD of bone loss. The lack of appropriate bone formation that is seen in these hypoestrogenemic athletes thus predisposes them to future preventable disease throughout their lifespan.

Routine BMD testing is not recommended for young, healthy women. Physicians must therefore be vigilant in identifying patients who have risk factors to undergo early screening for the disease. Because the risk of irreversible bone loss increases with the duration of amenorrhea, bone densitometry should be performed in women who have been amenorrheic for more than 6 months [59,67,70]. Other risk factors for osteoporosis (Box 1) should be factored into the decision of who to screen. All risk factors should also be reviewed to educate the athlete on the bone formation process and to stress the importance of addressing the factors that are modifiable.

Although readily available, peripheral BMD measurements such as calcaneal ultrasound have very significant limitations in this population and should not be used in premenopausal athletes. The highest risk of discordance of bone mass measurements among various skeletal sites is seen in younger women [71]. Variations in impact loading of different sports also alter the interpretation of results. Only serial dual-energy x-ray absorptiometry measurements have been shown to be predictive and useful in assessing the efficacy of therapy.

Treatment guidelines for osteoporosis are generally based on postmenopausal women and are not appropriate for female athletes who are premenopausal. Z scores should be evaluated in addition to T scores for adolescents and young women, and those who are found to have low BMD should generally be referred to a physician who has particular expertise in osteoporosis. Further testing, including CBC, TFT, comprehensive metabolic panel, 25-hydroxylated vitamin D level, and a 24-hour urine calcium, should be done in addition to other laboratory tests as indicated on an individual basis. A differential diagnosis including renal, parathyroid or thyroid disease, malabsorption, osteomalacia, malignancy, and other conditions needs to be considered even in athletic women.

Treatment of low BMD in the female athlete should generally focus on the underlying disorder, with a focus on normalizing the hormonal milieu and restoring a positive energy balance. Appropriate calcium (1500 mg

---

Box 1. Risk factors for osteoporosis

- Female gender
- Family history
- Caucasian or Asian race
- Low weight or body mass index
- Low percentage of body fat
- Sedentary lifestyle
- Immobilization
- Estrogen deficiency
- Androgen deficiency
- Medications
    Anticonvulsants
    Glucocorticoids
- Advanced age
- Low calcium intake
- Low vitamin D intake
- Caffeine intake
- Alcohol intake
- Smoking
- Eating disorders
- Chronic disease
    Diabetes
    Rheumatoid arthritis
    Hyperthyroidisn
    Hyperparathyroidism

---

daily) and vitamin D (400–800 IU daily) intake should be ensured, and other modifiable risk factors such as smoking need to be addressed. Hormonal treatment such as oral contraceptives or hormone replacement therapy, as mentioned earlier, should also be considered.

Diabetes mellitus

Diabetes is a disorder of glucose uptake and regulation. Type 1 diabetes mellitus represents a failure of endogenous insulin production, involving genetic predisposition and environmental components. Although it can present at any age, its incidence peaks in early adolescence. Type 2 diabetes mellitus, in contrast, is a state of relative insulin resistance. It is at least 10 times as prevalent as type 1 diabetes mellitus. Its onset is usually during adulthood; however, there is an increasing prevalence in children. Both types can also be brought on by other medical conditions such as pancreatic insufficiency, pregnancy, medications, and other endocrine disorders. A thorough evaluation of all new diabetics is warranted.

There has been a worldwide increase in diabetes of epidemic proportions over the last 10 to 20 years, a trend that is projected to increase in the years to come. Our society is dramatically less physically active than in years past, with 75% of United States adults not engaging in recommended levels of physical activity [72,73]. Over half of our population is overweight [74]; this national trend continues to worsen annually.

Elevated glucose levels in poorly controlled diabetes may exceed the capacity for renal reabsorption, which results in an osmotic diuresis, with patients noting abnormal urine odor, nocturia, polyuria, or thirst. They also may note blurry vision, weight loss, recurrent infections, or fatigue. Testing should be considered when any of these symptoms are present because early detection and treatment of diabetes can have a dramatic impact on a patient's long-term prognosis. Periodic screening is also recommended for asymptomatic patients older than 45 years who have a body mass index higher than 25 and additional risk factors such as a history of gestational diabetes, HTN, dyslipidemia, vascular disease, family history of diabetes, and so forth. Screening is recommended using a 2-hour 75-g oral glucose tolerance test (≥ 200 mg/dL) or a fasting plasma glucose test (≥ 126 mg/dL). Confirmatory testing should be done if initial values are over these limits. Impaired glucose tolerance, or prediabetes, is diagnosed with these same tests but at lower thresholds (≥ 140 and ≥ 110, respectively).

Studies from around the world have demonstrated that therapeutic lifestyle interventions focusing on diet and exercise can delay and even prevent type 2 diabetes mellitus and its complications [75–77]. Dietary interventions and increased physical activity are particularly important because these changes can result in improved glucose levels, insulin sensitivity, lipid profiles, blood pressure, and self-esteem, in addition to a decreased risk of osteoarthritis, depression, and other comorbidities. Physicians should also be aware that because a disproportionately high number of young women who have type 1 diabetes mellitus may also have eating disturbances [78,79], screening for these problems should take place. Patients should receive individualized counseling and instruction regarding American Diabetes Association (ADA) dietary recommendations and the use of tools such as the glycemic index to increase the effectiveness of and compliance with the therapeutic program.

The exercise component of therapeutic lifestyle changes should similarly be individualized to the patient. Prior to prescribing an exercise program, the ADA recommends stress testing for patients older than 35 years who have had type 2 diabetes mellitus for longer than 10 years, type 1 diabetes mellitus for longer than 15 years, or complications such as neuropathy, retinopathy, known vascular disease, or any additional cardiac risk factors such as HTN, dyslipidemia, or smoking [80].

There are no sports that are specifically prohibited for diabetic athletes. Individualized attention needs to be paid, however, to the unique considerations of the athlete and the sport in question, and adaptations may need to be made to ensure safety. Complications of diabetes must first be identified because these may dictate contraindications for certain sports or activities. Patients who have proliferative retinopathy need to avoid contact sports, heavy weight lifting, scuba diving, or inverted positions in which the head is below the body, such as may routinely be used in yoga and gymnastics. Those who have peripheral neuropathy are best advised to minimize foot trauma and pursue activities such as swimming as opposed to running. Athletes who have nephropathy should be especially cautious about any activities that increase their blood pressure, and those who have autonomic neuropathy should be careful of hypoglycemia, dehydration, hypothermia, and HTN.

After an athlete who has diabetes has found a safe mode of exercise, he or she should embark on a gradual increase in appropriate conditioning. Target levels of activity include at least 150 minutes of cardiovascular exercise with moderate (50%–70% maximum heart rate) or vigorous (>70% maximum heart rate) intensity, divided among at least 3 days of the week [81]. The effect that this exercise has on glucose levels, however, can be highly variable and depends on many factors such as medications, hydration, temperature, nutrition, and others. A gradual and well-planned increase in activity is even more important in diabetics than in nondiabetic patients because the effect of various training regimens on blood glucose levels needs to be monitored carefully.

Despite the great benefits of therapeutic lifestyle interventions in diabetes, many patients also require medications to minimize the risk of morbidity and mortality. Even a cursory review of the many medications used to treat diabetes is beyond the scope of this article; however, a few points should be made. The choice of medication used should take into account the risk of producing hypoglycemia (such as with insulin and certain oral hypoglycemic agents), the effects on lipid profiles or other risk factors, other medications being taken (which may mask symptoms of hypoglycemia), convenience, cost, and effectiveness. Optimizing medical therapy minimizes short- and long-term risks of the disease while optimizing athletic performance. The risk of hypoglycemia is more pronounced in athletes, and particular care and close monitoring is essential for safe participation in sports.

The various forms of insulin on the market have widely varying absorption characteristics, with some used for basal control throughout the day and others used for more immediate action with meals. Insulin, used by type 1 and type 2 diabetics, is now available in injectable and inhalational forms. Whichever insulin is used, patients should be familiar with its use and with the absorption characteristics and onset of action. Exercise should generally be avoided at the time of the peak insulin action, and insulin should not be injected over exercising muscle groups for approximately 1 hour before exertion. Basal insulin is usually reduced by 30% to 50%, and additional monitoring is advised. It is generally recommended that insulin pumps be shut off during prolonged bouts of exercise because there is an increased risk of late hypoglycemia when they are on. Whatever the routine used, it is critical that diabetic athletes practice their routine and try to simulate competitive conditions as closely as possible before actual competition so that all controllable variables (time of day, time and content of meals and hydration, and even weather conditions) are stable, allowing the effects of a particular insulin/medication regimen to be evaluated with respect to the glucose control it produces during an anticipated bout of exercise.

Guidelines for participation for insulin-dependent diabetics rely on close monitoring of glucose levels immediately before, during, and after exercise. Optimal baseline control during days and weeks leading up to competition is especially important because this allows for maximal storage of glycogen in muscle tissue. Immediately before exercise, target glucose levels should generally be in the 100 to 200 mg/dL range. Carbohydrates should be taken beforehand and glucose rechecked 15 minutes later if levels are too low. Extra insulin and a rapidly bioavailable source of carbohydrate should be close at hand, and the athlete and any medical personnel present should be familiar with signs or symptoms of hypoglycemia (shakiness, dizziness, weakness, disorientation) and hyperglycemia. Symptoms of anxiety before a race can mimic hypoglycemia, so checking glucose levels of those individuals who have symptoms and reminding those who do not have hypoglycemia to avoid overeating is useful.

During exercise, glucose levels generally tend to decline. Ongoing monitoring at least every 30 to 45 minutes during competition is advised, with carbohydrate intake adjusted accordingly. If glucose levels before exercise are greater than 250 mg/dL or if they rise to this level during exercise, then ongoing exercise paradoxically tends to drive them higher. In this hyperglycemic state, the cellular machinery actually senses a low glucose level due to a lack of insulin-mediated glucose entry, which then stimulates gluconeogenesis and glycogenolysis, further contributing to the hyperglycemia created by the lack of peripheral uptake. The osmotic diuresis from glucosuria and resultant dehydration further perpetuate the problem. Athletes who have these elevated pre-exercise glucose levels should therefore be checked for urinary ketones, and if they are present, exercise should be stopped. Glucose levels should also be checked regularly for up to 24 hours after prolonged exercise sessions due to increased sensitivity and muscle uptake.

Diabetes is a common condition that has life-threatening implications to an individual's health when not managed well. Through appropriate patient education, lifestyle changes, medication prescription, close monitoring, and careful supervision, however, type 1 and 2 diabetics can lead full and healthy lives that include all the sport-specific goals that nondiabetics have. In assisting patients with this process, clinicians can also help them to build their self-esteem, social support networks, and sense of self-reliance while minimizing the morbidity and mortality otherwise associated with this disease.

Asthma

Mortality rates from asthma have increased over the last decade despite many advances in the understanding, education, and treatment of the condition [82]. While death is uncommon, several thousand people still die from asthma each year in the United States, including some very fit and high-level athletes. Approximately 500,000 people are hospitalized each year and four times this number are seen in emergency rooms for treatment annually. Nearly 20% of athletes may experience signs or symptoms of asthma at some time, so all health care professionals involved with sports should be educated in the recognition and management of this disease.

Asthma is a disease characterized by episodic airflow obstruction. It is generally diagnosed clinically, and objective testing is used to monitor the disease. Common symptoms include episodic wheezing, chest tightness, cough, and difficulty breathing. These may be worse at night or may vary with factors such as exertion, temperature, humidity, infection, menstrual stage, irritants, allergens, emotional states, and other stimuli. Airway hyper-responsiveness leads to local bronchospasm and a hyperinflammatory state. These reversible changes can be quantified by way of pulmonary function tests.

Asthma classification systems are based on symptoms, medications, and pulmonary function test measurements (Table 1). Asthma severity, however, is frequently underestimated, even by the patients themselves [83], and symptoms are variable over time. Lung function can vary greatly as conditions change. In the athletic population in particular, classification may be difficult because exertional variation in symptoms is not currently addressed in standard guidelines.

Many other diseases can masquerade as asthma and need to be considered in the differential diagnosis of a wheezing athlete. Foreign-body aspiration, congenital heart disease, and allergies should be considered for wheezing children, whereas symptomatic adult athletes may have chronic obstructive pulmonary disease, congestive heart failure, side effects from medications, aspiration, vocal cord dysfunction, and other causes of airway obstruction. In addition to treatment of the bronchospastic process, physicians must also look for and treat possible exacerbating conditions such as allergies, gastroesophogeal reflux, sinusitis, and medication side effects. Flu shots are advised annually for asthmatics; allergy testing should be considered for those who have persistent asthma to direct environmental modifications; and immunotherapy is a possibility.

Objective measurements of pulmonary function are used in patients older than 5 years to quantify the symptoms and reversibility of the bronchospasm. An increase of 10% in the forced expiratory volume in 1 second (FEV_1) after bronchodilator administration is usually considered diagnostic for asthma. A decrease in peak expiratory flow and the ratio of FEV_1 to forced vital capacity may also indicate an obstructive process and should improve with bronchodilator administration. A provocative methacholine

Table 1
Asthma classification in adults and children

Asthma classification	Daytime symptom frequency	Nighttime symptom frequency	Lung function
Mild intermittent	≤2 d/wk	≤2 nights per mo	PEF or FEV$_1$: ≥80% of predicted
Mild persistent	>2 d/wk but <1 per d	>2 nights per mo	PEF or FEV$_1$: ≥80% of predicted
Moderate persistent	Daily	>1 night per wk	PEF or FEV$_1$: 60%–80% of predicted
Severe persistent	Continual	Frequent	PEF or FEV$_1$: ≤60% of predicted

Abbreviations: FEV$_1$, forced expiratory volume in 1 second; PEF, peak expiratory flow.

Adapted from National Asthma Education and Prevention Program. Guidelines for the diagnosis and management of asthma: expert panel report 2. Bethesda (MD): US Department of Health and Human Service, National Institutes of Health, National Heart, Lung, and Blood Institute; 1997. NIH publication 97-4051:20.

challenge test can be used to quantify the bronchospastic response to a graded concentration of stimulus; however, this test is not routinely performed in clinical practice.

Some athletes who have no history of asthma may be found to have symptoms of bronchospasm during or after exercise. A distinction is sometimes made in the literature between exercise-induced asthma (EIA), a chronic inflammatory disease, and exercise-induced bronchospasm (EIB), a transient bronchospastic disorder that may not have an inflammatory cause but may be triggered by thermally or osmotically induced alterations in the airways [84]. In most studies, all types of commonly used asthma medications have been shown to be effective in either disorder.

In clinical practice, EIA and EIB are often difficult to distinguish. Up to 90% of asthmatic patients also have EIB, and EIB occurs in approximately 10% of the general population [85]. Symptoms are the same as with other forms of asthma but only occur during or after exercise of at least 5 minutes' duration. Spirometry testing demonstrates a normal FEV$_1$ at rest, with a significant decrease (usually of at least 10%) with exercise, peaking 5 to 10 minutes after onset of intense physical activity [86]. Environmental controls and alterations in exercise routines are often useful, as are standard asthma medications such as bronchodilators and inhaled corticosteroids. By warming up before vigorous exercise, for example, athletes can take advantage of a "refractory period" induced by short bouts of exercise [87,88].

Nonreversible changes can also occur with asthma over time, with chronic inflammation leading to structural changes and permanent remodeling of the airways. Over time, decrements seen on pulmonary function tests may not return to normal after bronchodilator administration. These changes can further compromise an athlete's physiologic reserve and lower his or her symptomatic threshold. Aggressive control of asthma should be sought to prevent this permanent remodeling.

Although the patient and the physician should be prepared to manage an acute asthma attack, asthma treatment should focus on preventing such acute attacks from occurring. An on-field medical bag should include an albuterol metered-dose inhaler and a spacer chamber. This combination has proved to be as effective as a nebulizer for delivering β-adrenergic agonist therapy during acute asthma exacerbations in emergency departments and should be an effective method of medication delivery in other settings like sports venues [89]. Following an exacerbation, baseline asthma control should be increased and then re-evaluated over the ensuing days and weeks.

Inhaled β-adrenergic agonists provide the fastest relief of bronchospasm and thus comprise the backbone of treatment, even in cases of status asthmaticus, which is a state of severe airway obstruction that is unresponsive to standard acute asthma treatment protocols. Additional medications used in severe asthma exacerbations may include systemic corticosteroids, anticholineric drugs such as ipratroprium, magnesium, leukotriene inhibitors, methylxanthines, and epinephrine. Oxygen should be provided to keep oxygen saturation at least 95%. Intubation should be avoided whenever possible because it may aggravate bronchospasm; however, exhaustion and deterioration of mental status are indications to protect the airway and initiate mechanical ventilation.

Six to 12 hours after an initial asthma exacerbation, many asthmatic patients suffer a late-phase reaction that is commonly more refractory to bronchodilators than the initial attack. Some degree of bronchospasm can also remain for weeks after an acute attack resolves. For this reason, other medications such as inhaled or oral steroids and long-acting β-adrenergic agonists should be considered even after an initial exacerbation appears controlled.

The long-term medical management of asthma is based on the classification system in Table 1. People who have mild intermittent asthma do not need daily medications, and short-acting β-adrenergic agonists should only be used when symptoms arise or before a triggering stimulus like exercise is encountered. Patients who have mild persistent asthma should be treated with a low-dose inhaled corticosteroid on a daily basis to minimize use of rescue medications. Moderate persistent asthmatics, however, are not sufficiently controlled with regular use of low-dose corticosteroids. Although an increase in the dose of corticosteroid will improve lung function, the addition of a long-acting β-adrenergic agonist to the inhaled corticosteroid will provide a superior response and better long-term control. Other recommended adjunctive second- and third-line agents include leukotriene modifiers, cromolyn, and theophylline. High-dose inhaled corticosteroids are usually reserved for use in conjunction with long-acting β-adrenergic agonists and other medications.

The safety of corticosteroids has been studied at length in growing children to determine effects of growth delay, osteoporosis, glaucoma, cataracts, and hypothalamic-pituitary-adrenal axis suppression. In all of these studies, adverse effects of corticosteroid use were negligible and were clearly outweighed by the reduction in hospitalizations and risk of death from asthma that were gained from regular inhaled corticosteroid use [90]. In particular, risks of growth reduction (commonly a concern in certain adolescent and pediatric athletes) are negligible because the small decrease in growth velocity seen in children in the first year of treatment was not sustained and no differences were present in target adult heights [91]. Risks of oral thrush and hoarseness can be minimized by using a spacer and rinsing with water after each dose.

In contrast to these reassuring studies on the safety of inhaled corticosteroids with or without long-acting β-adrenergic agonists, other studies have demonstrated adverse effects of long-acting β-adrenergic agonists being used in the absence of inhaled corticosteroids [92,93]. Although this risk of adverse effects may be more pronounced in black than in white patients [94], they should not be used as monotherapy for asthma, regardless of race.

When caring for an athlete who has asthma, the physician must also ensure that any treatment prescribed is allowed within that athlete's competitive arena and that appropriate permission for its use has been documented in all but emergent conditions. Rules for medications vary by sport, but up-to-date links to current therapeutic use exemption forms and medications that are permitted and prohibited can be found at the US Anti-Doping Agency Web site (β-adrenergic agonists) or at the World Anti-Doping Agency Web site (www.wada-ama.org/en). Because high school or college athletes may, in addition to interscholastic competition, participate at the international level, sports medicine providers and athletes should check for the most up-to-date rules for any relevant agencies (National Collegiate Athletic Association, International Olympic Committee) that may apply and ensure that permission has been granted for medication use, if applicable, before it is prescribed.

Given the tremendous variability in asthma severity in a given individual over time, the vast array of potential triggers for asthmatics in general, and the significant morbidity and mortality seen with the disease when it is inadequately controlled, it is imperative that each athlete is taught to effectively self-manage his or her asthma and maintain excellent communication with the treating physician. A myriad of resources are available to patients, including written action plans, peak flow meters, and other educational materials for patients and their families. Future updates, recommendations, and clinical guidelines developed by the National Asthma Education and Prevention Program (NAEPP) are available on-line at http://www.nhlbi. nih.gov/guidelines/asthma/asthgdln. htm.

Summary

Medical management of the athlete is a challenging endeavor. Many important conditions that are seen in the athletic population, such as sudden cardiac death, concussion, and MRSA infections, are areas of active research, and sports medicine physicians must stay current with new developments because treatment guidelines invariably evolve and change. Chronic conditions that can affect athletes such as HTN, the female athlete triad, diabetes mellitus, and asthma present their own difficulties because treatment plans often have to be tailored to the individual athlete and to the specific rigors and demands of their particular sport. Guiding the therapeutic program for an athlete and safely returning that athlete to competition following an illness or injury is an objective shared by all sports medicine physicians. Although the challenges that face physicians who care for athletes are many, so too are the rewards. Indeed, there is no greater reward for a sports medicine physician than witnessing an athlete who he or she has treated achieve success on the playing field.

Acknowledgments

The authors would like to acknowledge and thank Eva Perkins and Kathy Jeschke of the Northridge Hospital Medical Center library for their help in preparing this article.

References

[1] Maron BJ. Update: cardiovascular risks to young persons on the athletic field. Ann Intern Med 1998;129(5):379–86.
[2] Maron BJ, Gohman TE, Aeppli D. Prevalence of sudden cardiac death during competitive sports activities in Minnesota high school athletes. J Am Coll Cardiol 1998;32:1881–4.
[3] Maron BJ, Epstein SE, Roberts WC. Causes of sudden death in competitive athletes. J Am Coll Cardiol 1986;7:204–14.
[4] Maron BJ, Shirani J, Poliac LC, et al. Sudden death in young competitive athletes: clinical, demographic, and pathological profiles. JAMA 1996;276:199–204.
[5] Maron BJ. Hypertrophic cardiomyopathy: a systematic review. JAMA 2002;287:1308–20.
[6] Maron BJ, Gardin JM, Flack JM, et al. Prevalence of hypertrophic cardiomyopathy in a general population of young adults. Circulation 1995;92:785–9.
[7] Maron BJ. Medical progress: sudden death in young athletes. N Engl J Med 2003;349: 1064–75.
[8] Shirley KW, Adirim TA. Sudden cardiac death in young athletes. Clinical Pediatric Emergency Medicine 2005;6:194–9.
[9] Bader RS, Goldberg L, Sahn DJ. Risk of sudden cardiac death in young athletes: which screening strategies are appropriate? Pediatr Clin North Am 2004;51:1421–41.
[10] Maron BJ, Pelliccia A, Spirito P. Cardiac disease in young trained athletes: insights into methods for distinguishing athlete's heart from structural heart disease with particular emphasis on hypertrophic cardiomyopathy. Circulation 1995;91:1596–601.

[11] Maron BJ. Structural features of the athlete heart as defined by echocardiography. J Am Coll Cardiol 1986;7:190–203.

[12] Pelliccia A, Maron BJ, Spataro A, et al. The upper limit of physiologic cardiac hypertrophy in highly trained elite athletes. N Engl J Med 1991;324:295–301.

[13] Maron BJ, Zipes DP. 36th Bethesda Conference. Eligibility recommendations for competitive athletes with cardiovascular abnormalities: November 6, 2005. J Am Coll Cardiol 2005; 45(8):1313–75.

[14] Alexander RW, Griffith GC. Anomalies of the coronary arteries and their significance. Circulation 1956;14:800–5.

[15] Maron BJ. The athlete's heart and cardiovascular disease: risk profiles and cardiovascular preparticipation screening of competitive athletes. Cardiol Clin 1997;15:473–83.

[16] Roberts WC. Major anomalies of coronary arterial origin seen in adulthood. Am Heart J 1986;111(5):941–63.

[17] Roberts WC, Shirani J. The four subtypes of anomalous origin of the left coronary artery from the right aortic sinus (or from the right coronary artery). Am J Cardiol 1992;70(1): 119–21.

[18] Frommelt PC, Frommelt MA. Congenital coronary artery anomalies. Pediatr Clin North Am 2004;51:1273–88.

[19] Frommelt PC, Frommelt MA, Tweddell JS, et al. Prospective echo diagnosis and surgical repair of anomalous origin of a coronary artery from the opposite sinus with an interarterial course. J Am Coll Cardiol 2003;42:148–54.

[20] Zeppilli P, dello Russo A, Santini C, et al. In vivo detection of coronary artery anomalies in asymptomatic athletes by echocardiography screening. Chest 1998;114:89–93.

[21] Romp RL, Herlong JR, Landolfo CK, et al. Outcome of unroofing procedure for repair of anomalous aortic origin of left or right coronary artery. Ann Thorac Surg 2003;76:589–95.

[22] Chobanian AV, Bakris GL, Black HR, et al. The seventh report of the Joint National Committee on prevention, detection, evaluation, and treatment of high blood pressure: the JNC 7 report. JAMA 2003;289:2560–72.

[23] National High Blood Pressure Education Program Working Group on High Blood Pressure in Children and Adolescents. The fourth report on the diagnosis, evaluation, and treatment of high blood pressure in children and adolescents. Pediatrics 2004;114(Suppl):555–76.

[24] Pickering TG, Hall JE, Appel LJ, et al. Recommendations for blood pressure measurement in humans: an AHA scientific statement from the Council on High Blood Pressure Research, Professional, and Publications Subcommittee. Hypertension 2005;45:142–61.

[25] Vanhees L, Defoor JG, Schepers D, et al. Effect of bisoprolol and atenolol on endurance exercise capacity in healthy men. J Hypertens 2000;18:35–43.

[26] Centers for Disease Control and Prevention. Sports-related recurrent brain injuries: United States. MMWR Morb Mortal Wkly Rep 1997;46(10):224–7.

[27] McCrea M, Hammeke T, Olsen G, et al. Unreported concussion in high school football players: implications for prevention. Clin J Sport Med 2004;14(1):13–7.

[28] Congress of Neurological Surgeons. Report of Ad Hoc Committee to Study Head Injury Nomenclature: glossary of head injury including some definitions of injuries of the cervical spine. Clin Neurosurg 1966;12:386–94.

[29] American Academy of Neurology. Practice parameter: the management of concussion in sports (summary statement). Report of the Quality Standards Subcommittee of the American Academy of Neurology. Neurology 1997;48(3):581–5.

[30] Aubry M, Cantu R, Dvorak J, et al. Summary and agreement statement of the first International Conference on Concussion in Sport, Vienna 2001. Phys Sportsmed 2002;30(2):57–62 (also co-published in Br J Sport Med 2002;36:3–7 and Clin J Sport Med 2002;12:6-12).

[31] McCrory P, Johnston K, Meeuwisse W, et al. Summary and agreement statement of the 2nd International Conference on Concussion in Sport, Prague 2004. Clin J Sport Med 2005; 15(2):48–55.

[32] Erlanger D, Kaushik T, Cantu R, et al. Symptom-based assessment of the severity of concussion. J Neurosurg 2003;98(3):477–84.

[33] McCrea M, Kelly JP, Randolph C. Standardized Assessment of Concussion (SAC): on-site mental status evaluation of the athlete. J Head Trauma Rehabil 1998;13(2):27–35.

[34] McCrea M. Standardized mental status testing on the sideline after sport-related concussion. J Athl Train 2001;36(3):274–9.

[35] Johnston KM, Ptito A, Chankowsky J, et al. New frontiers in diagnostic imaging in concussive head injury. Clin J Sport Med 2001;11:166–76.

[36] Hovda DA, Lee SM, Smith ML, et al. The neurochemical and metabolic cascade following brain injury: moving from animal models to man. J Neurotrauma 1995;12:903–6.

[37] McIntosh TK, Smith DH, Meaney DF, et al. Neuropathological sequelae of traumatic brain injury: relationship to neurochemical and biomechanical mechanisms. Lab Invest 1996;74: 315–42.

[38] Lovell M, Collins M, Bradley J. Return to play following sports-related concussion. Clin Sports Med 2004;23:421–41.

[39] Cantu RC. Cerebral concussion in sport: management and prevention. Phys Sportsmed 1992;14:64–74.

[40] Cantu RC. Posttraumatic retrograde and anterograde amnesia: pathophysiology and implications in grading and safe return to play. J Athl Train 2001;36:244–8.

[41] Kelly JP, Nichols JS, Filley CM. Concussion in sports: guidelines for the prevention of catastrophic outcome. JAMA 1991;266:2867–9.

[42] Cantu RC. Second-impact syndrome. Clin Sports Med 1998;17(1):37–44.

[43] Lovell M, Iverson G, Collins M, et al. Does loss of consciousness predict neuropsychological decrements after concussion? Clin J Sport Med 1999;9:193–8.

[44] Collins MW, Iverson GL, Lovell MR, et al. On-field predictors of neuropsychological and symptom deficit following sports-related concussion. Clin J Sport Med 2003;13:222–9.

[45] Bleiberg J, Cernich A, Cameron K, et al. Duration of cognitive impairment after sports concussion. Neurosurgery 2004;54:1073–80.

[46] Guskiewicz KM, Bruce SL, Cantu RC, et al. National Athletic Trainers' Association position statement: management of sport-related concussion. J Athl Train 2004;39(3):280–97.

[47] Jevons MP. "Celbenin"-resistant staphylococci. Br Med J 1961;1:124–5.

[48] Zetola N, Francis JS, Nuermerger EL, et al. Community-acquired methicillin-resistant Staphylococcus aureus: an emerging threat. Lancet Infect Dis 2005;5:275–86.

[49] Centers for Disease Control and Prevention. Four pediatric deaths from community acquired methicillin-resistant Staphylococcus aureus—Minnesota and North Dakota, 1997–1999. MMWR Morb Mortal Wkly Rep 1999;48:707–10.

[50] Herold BC, Immergluck LC, Maranan MC, et al. Community-acquired methicillin-resistant Staphylococcus aureus in children with no identified predisposing risk. JAMA 1998;279: 593–8.

[51] Barrett TW, Moran GJ. Update on emerging infections: news from the Centers for Disease Control and Prevention. Ann Emerg Med 2004;43(1):43–7.

[52] Lowy FD. Staphylococcal aureus infections. N Engl J Med 1998;339:520–32.

[53] Charlebois ED, Perdreau-Remington F, Kreiswirth B, et al. Origins of community strains of methicillin-resistant Staphylococcus aureus. Clin Infect Dis 2004;39:47–54.

[54] Fey PD, Said-Salim B, Rupp ME, et al. Comparative molecular analysis of community or hospital-acquired methicillin-resistant Staphylococcus aureus. Antimicrob Agents Chemother 2003;47:196–203.

[55] Sattler CA, Mason EO, Kaplan SL. Prospective comparison of risk factors and demographic and clinical characteristics of community-acquired, methicillin-resistant versus methicillin-susceptible Staphylococcus aureus infection in children. Pediatr Infect Dis J 2002;21(10): 910–7.

[56] Fergie JE, Purcell K. Community-acquired methicillin-resistant Staphylococcus aureus in South Texas children. Pediatr Infect Dis J 2001;20:860–3.

[57] Metry D, Rajani K. New and emerging pediatric infections. Dermatol Clin 2003;21:269–76.

[58] Naimi TS, LeDell KH, Como-Sabetti K, et al. Comparison of community and health care-associated methicillin-resistant *Staphylococcus aureus* infection. JAMA 2003;290:2976–84.

[59] American Psychiatric Association. Diagnostic and statistical manual of mental disorders. 4th edition Text Revision. Washington, DC: American Psychiatric Association; 2000.

[60] Misra M, Aggarwal A, Miller KK, et al. Effects of anorexia nervosa on clinical, hematologic, biochemical, and bone density parameters in community-dwelling adolescent girls. Pediatrics 2004;114(6):1574–83.

[61] Mehler PS. Diagnosis and care of patients with anorexia nervosa in primary care settings. Ann Intern Med 2001;134:1048–59.

[62] Herzog DB, Nussbaum KM, Marmor AK. Comorbidity and outcome in eating disorders. Psychiatr Clin North Am 1996;19:843–59.

[63] Walsh JM, Wheat ME, Freund K. Detection, evaluation, and treatment of eating disorders: the role of the primary care physician. J Gen Intern Med 2000;15(8):577–90.

[64] De Souza MJ, Van Heest J, Demers LM, et al. Luteal phase deficiency in recreational runners: evidence for a hypometabolic state. J Clin Endocrinol Metab 2003;88(1):337–46.

[65] Rickenlund A, Eriksson MJ, Schenck-Gustafsson K, et al. Amenorrhea in female athletes is associated with endothelial dysfunction and unfavorable lipid profile. J Clin Endocrinol Metab 2005;90(3):1354–9.

[66] Rickenlund A, Eriksson MJ, Schenck-Gustafsson K, et al. Oral contraceptives improve endothelial function in amenorrheic athletes. J Clin Endocrinol Metab 2005;90(6):3162–7.

[67] American Academy of Pediatrics. Committee on Sports Medicine and Fitness. Medical concerns in the female athlete. Pediatrics 2000;106(3):610–3.

[68] NIH Consensus Statement. Osteoporosis prevention, diagnosis, and therapy. Statement online March 27–29, 2000;17(1):1–36.

[69] Birch K. Female athlete triad. BMJ 2005;330(7485):244–6.

[70] Snow-Harter CM. Bone health and prevention of osteoporosis in active and athletic women. Clin Sports Med 1994;13:389–404.

[71] Wulfers MC. Calcaneal ultrasonography for bone assessment. Am Fam Physician 2003; 67(3):462.

[72] Koenigsberg MR, Bartlett D, Cramer JS. Facilitating treatment adherence with lifestyle changes in diabetes. Am Fam Physician 2004;69(2):309–16.

[73] National Center for Chronic Disease Prevention & Health Promotion, Centers for Disease Control and Prevention. Behavioral risk factor surveillance system: trends data. Available at: http://apps.nccd.cdc.gov/brfss/Trends/TrendData.asp. Accessed October 7, 2006.

[74] Mokdad AH, Bowman BA, Ford ES, et al. The continuing epidemics of obesity and diabetes in the United States. JAMA 2001;286:1195–200.

[75] Pan XR, Li GW, Hu YH, et al. Effects of diet and exercise in preventing NIDDM in people with impaired glucose tolerance. The Da Qing IGT and Diabetes Study. Diabetes Care 1997; 20:537–44.

[76] Tuomilehto J, Lindstrom J, Eriksson JG, et al. Prevention of type II diabetes mellitus by changes in lifestyle among subjects with impaired glucose tolerance. N Engl J Med 2001; 344:1343–50.

[77] Knowler WC, Barrett-Connor E, Fowler SE, et al. Reduction in the incidence of type 2 diabetes with lifestyle intervention or metformin. N Engl J Med 2002;346:393–403.

[78] Hoffman RP. Eating disorders in adolescents with type 1 diabetes. A closer look at a complicated condition. Postgrad Med 2001;109(4):67–9, 73–74.

[79] Rodin GM, Johnson LE, Garfinkel PE, et al. Eating disorders in female adolescents with insulin-dependent diabetes mellitus. Int J Psychiatry Med 1986–1987;16(1):49–57.

[80] Zinman B, Ruderman N, Campaigne BN, et al. Physical activity/exercise and diabetes mellitus. Diabetes Care 2003;26(Suppl 1):S73–7.

[81] American Diabetes Association. Clinical practice guidelines. Diabetes Care 2006;29(Suppl 1):S1–85.

[82] McFadden ER Jr, Warren EL. Observations on asthma mortality. Ann Intern Med 1997;127: 142–7.

[83] Asthma in America. Asthma statistics. Accessed October 9, 2006, Available at: http://www. asthmainamerica.com.

[84] Hermansen CL. Exercise-induced bronchospasm vs. exercise-induced asthma. Am Fam Physician 2004;69(4):808.

[85] Parsons JP, Mastronarde JG. Exercise-induced bronchoconstriction in athletes. Chest 2005; 128(6):3966–74.

[86] Sinha T, David AK. Recognition and management of exercise-induced bronchospasm. Am Fam Physician 2003;67(4):769–74, 776.

[87] Reiff DB, Choudry NB, Pride NB, et al. The effect of prolonged submaximal warm-up exercise on exercise-induced asthma. Am Rev Respir Dis 1989;139:479–84.

[88] Schnall RP, Landau LI. Protective effects of repeated short sprints in exercise induced asthma. Thorax 1980;35:828–32.

[89] Cates CJ, Crilly JA, Rowe BH. Holding chambers (spacers) versus nebulisers for beta-agonist treatment of acute asthma. Cochrane Database Syst Rev 2006;2:CD000052.

[90] National Asthma Education and Prevention Program. Guidelines for the diagnosis and management of asthma: expert panel report 2. Bethesda (MD): U.S. Department of Health and Human Services, National Institutes of Health, National Heart, Lung, and Blood Institute; 1997. NIH publication 97–4051.

[91] Long-term effects of budesonide or nedocromil in children with asthma. The Childhood Asthma Management Program Research Group. N Engl J Med 2000;343:1054–63.

[92] Lemanske RF Jr, Sorkness CA, Mauger EA, et al. Inhaled corticosteroid reduction and elimination in patients with persistent asthma receiving salmeterol: a randomized controlled trial. JAMA 2001;285:2594–603.

[93] Mcivor RA, Pizzichini E, Turner MO, et al. Potential masking effects of salmeterol on airway inflammation in asthma. Am J Respir Crit Care Med 1998;158:924–30.

[94] Nelson HS, Weiss ST, Bleecker ER, et al. The Salmeterol Multicenter Asthma Research Trial: a comparison of usual pharmacotherapy for asthma or usual pharmacotherapy plus salmeterol. Chest 2006;129(1):15–26.

ELSEVIER
SAUNDERS

Clin Podiatr Med Surg
24 (2007) 159–189

CLINICS IN
PODIATRIC
MEDICINE AND
SURGERY

Diabetes: The Latest Trends in Glycemic Control

John M. Giurini, DPM, Emily A. Cook, DPM*,
Jeremy J. Cook, DPM

*Harvard Medical School, Division of Podiatric Surgery, Department of Surgery,
Beth Israel Deaconess Medical Center, Boston, MA 02215, USA*

A 1998 article published by Harris and colleagues [1] stated that the current prevalence of diabetes mellitus in the United States was approximately 7% of the population, with a notable increase across all age groups. It is projected that by 2025, more than 300 million people globally will have type 2 diabetes mellitus [2]. Studies have shown that for patients who have diabetes, the lifetime risk of developing a pedal ulceration is 15% and that 20% of all diabetic hospital admissions are related to a foot ulceration [3–5]. Approximately 2% of diabetics have a foot ulcer at any given time, with as many as 163,000 Americans hospitalized for these issues [5,6]. The Medicare costs associated with diabetic lower-extremity ulcerations were $1.5 billion in 1995 [7].

As these issues come to prominence, the role of the diabetic foot expert will become more sharply defined. Beyond the traditional roles of infection, wound, and deformity management, the modern diabetic foot expert will be charged with direct medical management while the patient is in the hospital. This article seeks to discuss the appropriate medical management of the diabetic patient in the hospitalized setting. The authors attempt to explain the most contemporary concepts and protocols for glycemic control and discuss future directions of diabetic care. Although this excerpt serves as a guide, the degree to which it is employed should be reflective of clinician training and comfort level with these topics. As dictated by the clinical situation, a medical or endocrinology consultation is reasonable whenever the clinician believes that the required care exceeds his or her level of expertise.

* Corresponding author.
E-mail address: ecook@bidmc.harvard.edu (E.A. Cook).

0891-8422/07/$ - see front matter © 2007 Elsevier Inc. All rights reserved.
doi:10.1016/j.cpm.2006.12.001   *podiatric.theclinics.com*

Glycemic goals

Determining glycemic control

Glycemic control can be determined by a variety of means including measures that evaluate immediate glucose levels and those that evaluate long-term control of up to 3 months. The fastest and most affordable method requires simply a lancet and a glucometer. These implements should be in every diabetic foot care professional's office because hypoglycemic emergencies have the potential to occur at any time. With a simple finger-stick, the current glycemic status of a patient can be quickly assessed.

Other measures include blood tests that require laboratory analysis. Two such measures are plasma glucose and hemoglobin A1c (HbA1c). The plasma glucose is a component of the chemistry seven or basic metabolic panel. Plasma glucose levels are considered more accurate than whole blood testing, which is used more commonly in glucometers. Typically, plasma glucose has a 10% to 15% higher concentration than whole blood testing [8].

The HbA1c illustrates the degree to which hemoglobin is glycosolated. Because the average life cycle of a blood cell is approximately 90 to 120 days, this value characterizes the average glycemic control maintained over an approximately 3-month period. This test has a high degree of variability depending on the assay used, and a normal (nondiabetic) value can be 4% to 6%. Therefore, this technique is not used for the diagnosis of diabetes mellitus but rather for monitoring. In response to the Diabetes Control and Complications Trial (DCCT) [9] and the United Kingdom Prospective Diabetes Study (UKPDS) [10], in 1996 the National Glycohemoglobin Standardization Program (NGSP) was initiated with the goal of standardizing HbA1c laboratory techniques nationwide to enable increased reliability and comparability to those glycemic goals detailed in the DCCT and UKPDS. As of 2000, 90% of surveyed laboratories provided evidence that their techniques produced accurate results, which was increased from 66% in 1996. Facilities which used NGSP-certified techniques were found to accurately determine the concentration of a nationally released test sample within 0.8% of the actual value [11].

Glycemic goals

Two medical–academic bodies have published glycemic goals to optimize care and minimize the complications associated with suboptimal glycemic control. The American Diabetes Association (ADA) in 2005 and the American College of Endocrinology and the American Association of Clinical Endocrinologists (AACE) in 2004 produced articles that summarized their respective goals of euglycemia. These goals are outlined in Table 1 [12–14].

There are some differences within the specific values set forth by each group. The ADA applies the same guidelines to inpatient and outpatient settings, whereas the AACE uses different standards for diabetics in the

Table 1
Summary of glycemic targets

	American diabetes association	American college of endocrinology and AACE
Outpatients		
HbA1c	<7.0%	<6.5%
Fasting/preprandial glucose	B: 80–120 mg/dL P: 90–130 mg/dL	P: <110 mg/dL
Postprandial glucose	P: <180 mg/dL[a]	P: <140 mg/dL[b]
Bedtime glucose	B: 100–140 mg/dL P: 110–150 mg/dL	—
Hospitalized patients		
Critical care	—	P: <110 mg/dL
Non–critical care patients		
Fasting/preprandial	—	P: <110 mg/dL
Maximum allowed	—	P: <180 mg/dL

Abbreviations: B, whole blood; P, plasma; —, data not available.
[a] At peak 1–2 hours after start of meal.
[b] At 2 hours.
Data from Refs. [12–14].

inpatient setting, with further delineation for intensive care and non–critical care patients. Overall, the AACE endorses a slightly more aggressive approach in glucose control. The AACE fasting or premeal plasma glucose target is less than 110 mg/dL compared with the ADA goal of between 90 and 130 mg/dL. Some mild disagreement also exists with regard to postmeal levels. The ADA endorses a postprandial peak level of no more 180 mg/dL compared with the AACE 2-hour postmeal target of less than 140 mg/dL in the outpatient setting. The AACE inpatient postprandial guidelines are slightly more lenient than their outpatient recommendations and state that an inpatient who never exceeds 180 mg/dL will be glycemically optimized for wound healing and elimination of infection [12,13].

Long-term glycemic control is evaluated as previously stated by way of the HbA1c test. A nondiabetic individual will have a value of less than 6%; these organizations state that a target value of less than 6.5% (AACE) or less than 7.0% (ADA) will minimize and delay the onset of diabetic complications such as neuropathy, retinopathy, and nephropathy [12,13]. In general, 1% on the HbA1c scale is reflective of approximately 30 to 35 mg/dL in the mean glucose level.

The benefits of glycemic control

The benefits of aggressive glycemic control are based on the widely held belief that euglycemia delays the onset and minimizes the severity of many diabetic complications. The DCCT was the first large type 1 diabetes mellitus study to demonstrate the potential benefits of glycemic control. In this trial, after 1400 type 1 diabetics were intensively treated, the rate of nephropathy and retinopathy decreased by 50% to 70%. Neuropathic occurrence was noted to decrease by 60% in the intensive-treatment arm; this group's mean HbA1c was noted to be 7.2%. Further analysis demonstrated that for every 10% decrease in HbA1c, the overall risk of complication decreased by 40% [9]. It was not until the 1998 UKPDS that tight glycemic controls were noted to be beneficial in patients who had type 2 diabetes mellitus. The UKPDS looked at 5000 recently diagnosed type 2 diabetes mellitus patients who were placed on an intensive regimen and evaluated for complications over a 10-year period. The study found a significant reduction in retinopathy and microalbuminuria. These results were achieved despite a mean difference in HbA1c of only 0.9% (7% versus 7.9%) between the control and intensive-therapy groups [10]. Although these goals are aggressive and carry hypoglycemic risks, their benefits are well detailed throughout the literature. The ADA and AACE goals require a concerted effort from the patient, especially given that the average HbA1c among American diabetics is near 9% [14]. It is important to realize that although these are guidelines, clinical judgment for the individual patient overrides them.

Infection

Beyond the long-term benefits of strict glycemic control, issues that impact the diabetic foot care provider include the effect on infection control and wound healing. For patients undergoing surgery, the increased risk of perioperative infection is thought to be partially linked to hyperglycemia. This topic is covered in greater detail in the Perioperative Glucose Management section. Some in vitro studies have shown that impaired neutrophilic chemotaxis is observed at glucose concentrations exceeding 240 mg/dL. Rassias and colleagues [15] noted that insulin infusion had a beneficial impact on neutrophil function. Many studies have found that patients who have elevated plasma glucose during the postoperative period were at increased risk for infection [16–18].

Wound healing

The direct impact of chronic hyperglycemia on wound healing is poorly understood. Diabetics demonstrate a diminished capacity toward wound healing; however, the significance of hyperglycemia compared with concomitant morbidities such as infection and micro- and macrovascular disease has not been isolated.

The literature shows that hyperglycemia has deleterious effects on essential wound healing events. The precise mechanism is still unknown, but some elements have been isolated, including a decrease in chemotaxis, polymorphonuclear leukocyte mobilization, and phagocytosis in the hyperglycemic state [19,20]. Skin fibroblasts from diabetics proliferate and function less effectively in a hyperglycemic milieu [21,22]. The role of decreased growth factor production in diabetics is another avenue of research being pursued. Mediators such as vascular endothelial growth factor, platelet-derived growth factor, and keratinocyte growth factor deficiencies are being investigated as possible contributors to poor wound healing [23–25].

It has also been postulated that hyperglycemia may impair endothelial-dependent vasodilation in micro- and macrocirculation. Insulin has a vasodilatory effect on skeletal muscle by way of its interaction with vascular endothelium, causing an increased production of nitric oxide. Therefore, if there is a transient decrease in the amount of perfusion to tissues during a state of hyperglycemia, then this further impedes wound healing [26–28].

To the authors' knowledge, only one clinical study to date has shown a direct link between hyperglycemia and a diminished capacity to heal a foot wound. Marston and colleagues' [29] study looked at 245 patients who had chronic diabetic foot ulcers (>6 weeks duration) and compared the rate of healing over a 12-week period between a bioengineered human dermal substitute and traditional normal saline dressing changes with frequent debridements. A determination was made as to the impact of glucose control on wound healing as measured by HbA1c. At the outset of the study, 32% of patients had a HbA1c of 7% or less, with the remaining 68% having a HbA1c greater than 7%. Of this latter group, 36% had a HbA1c of greater than 10%. At the conclusion of the study, 38% of patients who had a HbA1c of 7% or less healed their wounds ($P = .09$), whereas 68% of patients who had an elevated HbA1c ($>7\%$) failed to close their wounds by the study's end. A subset of 101 patients whose HbA1c worsened over the course of the study healed their wounds only 21% of the time, whereas patients able to improve or remain stable with glycemic control exhibited a healing rate of 36%.

Summary

Major organizations like the ADA are constantly re-evaluating and reissuing guidelines. The astute clinician must regularly review the literature to keep abreast of the changes that most significantly impact patient care.

Oral antihyperglycemic medication

Oral antihyperglycemic agents, insulin, and combination therapies

As previously mentioned, the goals of euglycemia are managed through a number of pharmacologic avenues. Patients who have type 2 diabetes mellitus and achieve suboptimal results with diet and exercise may require the addition of an oral antihyperglycemic medication. Most of these agents have a prolonged half-life and are poorly equipped for acute management; however, many patients taking these medications as an outpatient may wish to continue them while hospitalized. This practice is permissible, especially in the nonsurgical setting. This section attempts to delineate the wide array of oral medications that are available and to outline their relevance to the podiatric surgeon.

A pharmacologic ladder exists that logically leads the patient from oral monotherapy and terminates with insulin and select oral agents. The scope of this article does not include a review of the algorithm for initiation and modification of diabetic therapies but seeks to educate the practitioner about oral medications that may impact care. Only the medications available in the United States are reviewed. The four classes of medications covered in this discussion are biguanides, thiazolidinediones, alpha-glucosidase inhibitors, and insulin secretagogues. There are three basic mechanisms employed by the four classes of oral antihyperglycemic medication: stimulation of insulin secretion, improved insulin sensitivity, and inhibition of hepatic glucose production [30].

Bigaunides

This class of agents has been used in Europe for over 40 years, with the second generation arriving in the United States market in the 1990s. Although their specific mechanism of action is unclear, their impact on the liver, the gastrointestinal tract, and muscle is significant. These medications are thought to act by reducing glucose absorption from the gastrointestinal tract, by minimizing hepatic gluconeogenesis while enhancing glucose absorption in the liver, and by enhancing insulin-mediated glucose uptake in muscle. Because this class does not directly stimulate insulin secretion, hypoglycemia in monotherapy is rare.

Three preparations are available: classic metformin (Glucophage), extended release form, and liquid form. The most commonly occurring side effect appears to be dose-related diarrhea (20%–30%). A more notorious side effect plagued the first generation of this class, phenformin. Fatal lactic acidosis forced phenformin's withdrawal from the United States market in the late 1970s. The current iteration is less prone to this side effect. The likelihood of an adverse event increases in patients who have a creatinine clearance of less than 60 mL/min or hepatic insufficiency. Serum creatinine levels of 1.4 mg/dL or greater in women and 1.5 mg/dL or greater in men represent a contraindication to this medication. Patients who are at risk for induced renal failure secondary to radiocontrast dye use, fasting status, or general anesthesia should withhold metformin for 24 to 48 hours before and after the procedure to confirm a return to baseline renal function [10,30,31].

Thiazolidinediones

The second generation of these medications was introduced in 1999 and is thought to act primarily as an insulin sensitizer at the cellular level. These agents bind to a nuclear peroxisome proliferator–activated receptor (PPAR) that is believed to enhance insulin-mediated nuclear-based actions of insulin-like glucose absorption by adipose and muscle cells. They are also thought to inhibit gluconeogenesis in the liver. The peak onset of these medications is 4 to 6 weeks and has little utility in acute care [30].

The two agents used in the United States are pioglitazone (Actos) and rosiglitazone (Avandia). The first generation, troglitazone, was removed from the United States market for hepatic toxicity, and currently available agents (considered very safe) should be used with caution in patients who have possible hepatic insufficiency (alanine aminotransferase [ALT] >2.5 times high normal). Because fluid retention is another side effect associated with this class, these agents are relatively contraindicated in patients who have congestive heart failure (CHF). Recent literature by Tang [32] indicates that the fluid retention encountered is not associated with worsening cardiac function. This investigator advised that these agents are appropriate in mild CHF (class 2 or less) but recommended careful monitoring of fluid status [30,32].

Insulin secretagogues

Sulfonylureas

Considered first-line therapy when cost is of concern, these agents have been used for decades in the United States. They are classified as insulin secretagogues, meaning that their primary mechanism of action is to enhance insulin secretion from native pancreatic beta cells by way of cellular calcium channels, which in turn enhances glucose absorption in muscle and decreases gluconeogenesis in the liver.

Glyburide (Diabeta, Euglucon) and glipizide (Glucotrol) are considered second generation, whereas glimepiride (Amaryl) released in 1995 is sometimes referred to as a third generation. Their predecessors (chlorpropamide, tolazamide, tolbutamide) were associated with cardiovascular toxicity and antabuse-like–mediated abdominal cramping. These complications have not been frequently observed in the more recent agents. All medications in this class, however, still carry a significant risk of hypoglycemia if inadequate glucose is consumed. Hypoglycemia is the most significant of adverse reactions, and mild bouts occur in 2% to 4%, whereas severe hypoglycemic events that require hospitalization occur less than 1%. Geriatric patients, malnourished patients, and those who have renal or hepatic insufficiency are considered at high risk for hypoglycemic events [30].

Megalitinides

Megalitinides are also insulin secretagogues and share a mechanism similar to the action of sulfonylureas but bind to a different site on the beta cell membrane. They still stimulate insulin release but only in the presence of glucose. Therefore, the risk of hypoglycemia is minimized as they contribute primarily in the postprandial phase. Their shorter half-life (relative to sulfonylureas) makes them well tolerated in the hospital setting. This shorter half-life also makes it possible to give them premeal to prevent postprandial hyperglycemia. The first megalitinide was released in 1997, and currently available forms include nateglinide (Starlix) and repaglinide (GlucoNorm) [33].

Alpha-glycosidase inhibitors

This class of medication also exerts its primary effect in the postprandial phase but does so by delaying the absorption of dietary carbohydrates. Hypoglycemia does not typically occur as a result of this class (similar to the megalitinides) [34]. When a patient uses an alpha-glycosidase inhibitor in combination therapy and has a hypoglycemic episode, pure oral glucose or intravenous dextrose must be used because the absorption of dietary carbohydrates such as orange juice or candy is inhibited.

Acarbose (Prandase) and miglitol (Glyset) are examples of agents used in the United States. Due to its mechanism of action, this antihyperglycemic class is plagued by diarrhea, bloating, and abdominal discomfort in approximately 30% of patients. Acarbose is contraindicated in cirrhosis, whereas both agents should be avoided in patients who have inflammatory bowel disease or renal impairment [34–36].

Combinations

Fixed combinations exist and are warranted if additional agents are needed. At this time, five fixed combinations are available in the United States market. These agents carry the same benefits and risks associated with each individual medication.

Summary

With the recent flood of oral agents and classes, familiarity with their pharmacologic profiles is useful because many patients may be taking them on an outpatient basis. Given the relative duration and onset of these agents, however, their utility for glycemic control in the acute setting is somewhat limited. Immediate resolution can be achieved more effectively with a variety of currently available insulins, which are more appropriate in these settings.

Insulin

Insulin is a polypeptide hormone secreted by the beta cells within the islets of Langerhans in the pancreas. This regulatory peptide, which is required in all patients who have type 1 diabetes mellitus and in some who have type 2 diabetes mellitus, is secreted in response to increased glucose concentration within the bloodstream and facilitates a number of physiologic processes.

People who have type 1 diabetes mellitus lack the ability to produce insulin as a result of an autoimmune reaction resulting in the destruction of insulin-producing pancreatic beta cells, thus creating a requirement for exogenous insulin for survival [37]. Insulin therapy within type 1 diabetes mellitus patients is to reproduce physiologic insulin secretion as closely as possible. In this setting, insulin is typically used as monotherapy, without the need for adjunctive oral hypoglycemic medications, usually with multiple doses of insulin throughout the day [38]. In type 2 diabetics in whom more conservative measures fail to obtain adequate control, insulin may be employed as monotherapy or in combination with oral agents. Progression to more aggressive therapies may be linked to a number of causes including physiologic etiologies such as further loss of beta cell function, with diminishing insulin secretion and increased insulin resistance. Patient-mediated reasons like poor compliance with diet, exercise, and medication regimens are also likely contributors [39]. Because many of these patients have numerous comorbidities, other therapeutic agents may be the cause of a worsening diabetic state via inappropriate stimulated hepatic gluconeogenesis or even increased peripheral insulin resistance. Included within these potential antagonists are steroids, thiazide diuretics, oral contraceptives, tacrolimus, cyclosporine, β-blockers, and colchicines, to name a few [40].

Insulin side effects

It is fortunate that serious side effects of insulin are uncommon [41]. Local injection-site reactions occur in about 2.4% of people by way of an immunoglobulin E–mediated hypersensitivity reaction [42]. Since the advent of recombinant human insulin, systemic allergies have been rare, but some reported cases exist [43]. Lipohypertrophy and lipoatrophy as a result of multiple same-site injections have been well documented [44,45]. To avoid lipodystrophy, patients should rotate injection sites. Weight gain is also associated with insulin use, with approximately 4 kg or more documented in the literature. Lean muscle mass and trunk lipid mass account for this increased weight in type 1 and type 2 diabetes mellitus, respectively [46,47]. Hypoglycemia is one of the most emergent of the adverse reactions attributed to insulin therapy. To counter this threat, insulin users are advised to carry 15 g of carbohydrates or glucagon and glucose tablets with them at all times in addition to wearing medical identification.

Factors altering insulin action

Exogenous insulin pharmacokinetics are vulnerable to a variety of potential modulators. More than 50% intrapersonal variability in onset, peak, and duration has been demonstrated in some studies [48]. Insulin is typically injected subcutaneously; the location and the depth can have a significant impact on pharmacokinetics. Subcutaneous insulin is most rapidly absorbed into the abdomen, followed by the arms, the thighs, and the buttocks. The depth of the injection, which can be altered by different needle lengths, also matters. Deeper injections result in more rapid uptake, which is why intramuscular injections may be used during hyperglycemic emergencies. Any process that increases blood flow to injection areas, such as massage, exercise, hot water, and even sun bathing, speeds absorption. In contrast, tobacco use and other factors that decrease injection site perfusion, in turn, delay insulin absorption [49]. Xenogenic insulin derived from other species behaves differently than peptides derived from humans and carries alternative risks. The delivery system used to administer insulin also has an impact on pharmacokinetics and adverse reaction profiles; this topic is discussed in greater detail in the passages that follow. Variability of insulin action may result from a miscellany of factors such as stress, nutrition, gastroparesis, and patient errors. It is advisable to rotate sites within the same region for the same insulin and time of day, or further variability may ensue [50–52]. Due to the complex interactions that may contribute to day-to-day insulin variability, frequent self-monitoring of blood glucose is strongly advised.

Insulin types and pharmacokinetics

Subcutaneous insulin may be administered alone or mixed in a syringe with another insulin, with the exception of glargine (Lantus). Insulins are frequently categorized according to their onset and duration. These classifications include rapid-, short-, intermediate-, and long-acting insulins. Premixed insulin combinations are also available, which include an intermediate-acting insulin mixed with a set amount of rapid- or short-acting insulin. As previously mentioned, onsets, peaks, and durations vary; only reasonable estimations can be projected for each type of insulin.

Rapid-acting insulins start working within 5 to 30 minutes and peak anywhere from 30 minutes to 3 hours. Due to their rapid absorption, they are appropriate to administer immediately with meals to blunt the rise in serum glucose. Hypoglycemic complications may ensue if a meal is delayed, such as in a hospital setting. Their short duration (3–5 hours) may also predispose a patient to late postprandial hyperglycemia. The rapid acting insulins available in the United States are lispro (Humalog), aspart (NovoLog), and glulisine (Apidra) [53–55].

Subcutaneously injected regular insulin (Humulin R, Novolin R) is considered a short-acting form. Regular insulin must be timed so that it is taken 30 minutes before a meal. If the insulin is used immediately preceding the meal, as in a rapid-acting insulin, an early postprandial hyperglycemic peak occurs because its onset is approximately 30 minutes and its peak is predicted 1 to 5 hours later. This latent peak creates a tendency for some patients to become hypoglycemic if timed inappropriately.

The remaining insulins, intermediate- and long-acting, are not intended to be administered as a bolus like the previously described insulin subtypes but rather as a basal dose throughout the course of a day. Intermediate-acting insulin, such as neutral protamine Hagedorn (NPH) (Humulin N, Novolin N), is given once or twice a day to act as a basal insulin requirement. It works throughout the fasting and postabsorptive states, regulating hepatic glucose production and limiting lipolysis. Although used as a basal insulin, NPH has a peak, usually within 4 to 12 hours, and can last from 14 to 26 hours [56].

Peakless or long-acting insulins more closely mimic native basal insulin action. As before, their goal is to regulate fasting and basal serum glucose levels to ultimately achieve normoglycemic levels. The two peakless or nearly peakless insulins available commercially in the United States are glargine (Lantus) and detemir (Levemir). They can be given during any time of the day and last up to 24 hours, but due to variability, some patients benefit from twice-a-day regimens to maintain basal levels. When a change to a long-acting insulin is desired, it is recommended that the initial dose of long-acting insulin be 50% or less of the previous total daily insulin requirement. Great care should be taken when adjusting dosages of long-acting insulins due to their extended duration of action. Glargine has some distinguishing qualities. Its prolonged duration of action is due to its acidity. Glargine's pH is approximately 4 and, on entering the body, it slowly precipitates, allowing for a controlled release of insulin as it becomes neutralized. For this reason, glargine cannot be mixed with other insulins [57,58].

An intermediate-acting insulin may be mixed with a short- or rapid-acting insulin manually or purchased in a fixed premix form. The ADA [59] has specific guidelines to refer to for the proper mixing of insulin because the body may respond to mixed insulin differently than if each were given separately. This type of insulin is more preferable and convenient for some people who wish to have premeal and basal insulin included in one injection. This fixed mixed form may aid in compliance and can simplify dosing for the elderly; however, fixed mixed dosing is only recommended for patients who have type 2 diabetes mellitus [60]. Patients who have type 1 diabetes mellitus often require frequent adjustments, which are not possible with these combined insulin regimens. Fixed doses of mixed insulin are now widely available in many formulations [61]:

Humalog 75/25 = 75% lispro protamine suspension, 25% lispro
Humalog 50/50 = 50% lispro protamine suspension, 50% lispro
NovoLog 70/30 = 70% aspart protamine suspension, 30% aspart
Humalin 70/30 = 70% NPH, 30% regular
Humalin 50/50 = 50% NPH, 50% regular
Novolin 70/30 = 70% NPH, 30% regular

Insulin regimens

There are two major types of insulin regimens: conventional insulin therapy and intensive insulin therapy. Conventional insulin therapy consists of once- or twice-daily injections with a fixed mixed amount of short- and long-acting insulin. An example of this therapy would be a twice-daily split-mixed regimen. This regimen has been traditionally used to simplify treatment and increase compliance. Intensive insulin therapy achieves improved and personally designed insulin plans and usually consists of multiple daily injections [62]. One to two injections are given as a basal rate, with additional short- or rapid-acting insulin for each meal and snack. This therapy is known as basal-bolus therapy. In brief, the concept is that there is an intermediate- or long-acting insulin basal rate to suppress hepatic glucose production equal to the body's normal basal insulin requirement. Meals are then individually covered with a calculated amount of rapid- or short-acting insulin to cover additional carbohydrate intake [63–65]. An insulin pump is another delivery system that functions much the same way by providing an adjustable basal rate with mealtime bolus amounts. This approach is increasing in popularity and was once prescribed only for type 1 diabetes mellitus patients but has been extended to include certain type 2 diabetes mellitus patients who are willing to perform the requisite frequent self-monitoring of blood glucose.

Insulin sliding scales

Hospitalized patients who have diabetes are often placed on insulin sliding scales, especially during periods of fasting in preparation for a surgical procedure. Patients may be placed on a sliding scale for additional control regardless of whether they are simply diet-controlled or they are on oral hypoglycemic medications, insulin, or a combination of therapies [66].

Simply put, with sliding scales, glucose levels are checked by way of a glucometer before a meal and at bedtime. Based on a set range of glucose values, a predetermined amount of rapid- or short-acting insulin is administered.

The literature describes several types of sliding scales. Some are weight based, whereas others divide patients into type 1 or type 2 diabetes mellitus [67]. Other scales focus on dosing insulin by calculating the total daily insulin requirement for a patient in order to take into account the level of insulin resistance [68]. Hospitals may give the physician a choice between an approved standard sliding scale or a customized sliding scale [69]. A feature common to all scales is that the bedtime insulin sliding scale should be less than the daytime insulin sliding scale. At the authors' institution, the bedtime sliding scale is also used for periods of fasting, such as in preparation for surgery when additional insulin coverage may be needed. Sliding scales can be further individualized based on the response the patient had to the ordered amount of insulin given for the premeal glucose reading. For example, to correct a consistently elevated noontime blood glucose level, the amount of insulin ordered prebreakfast may be increased. By identifying the insulin that is responsible for each glucose reading, the insulin can be adjusted appropriately.

The type of insulin used in the scale, rapid or fast acting, should also be taken into consideration. Proponents for rapid-acting insulin argue that its onset most closely matches the rise in glucose levels, as long as it is given immediately before a meal. If regular insulin is given in the same manner, however, the patient will undergo a period of hyperglycemia and potential postprandial hypoglycemia as previously detailed. Other practitioners believe that regular insulin is safer to administer than rapid-acting insulin in a hospital setting because patients must rely on others to bring them food and a delay may result in hypoglycemia [70].

In recent years, sliding scales have fallen under criticism. Wide glucose fluctuations are possible due to the fact that the patient is receiving insulin based on a prior glucose reading. These fluctuations may be further exacerbated if concomitant basal insulin is not used. If a regular insulin sliding scale dose is given at every meal alone based on the premeal glucose reading, then one is essentially chasing a previous high or low reading and not actually controlling current glucose levels. Many endocrinologists' goal for the bolus portion of insulin is to adjust it so that it maintains a near normal glucose value during the peak. Critics argue that it is not known how high the glucose level peaks postprandially when it is only tested before a meal [71].

Furthermore, glucometer readings provide only estimates of blood glucose and can vary in accuracy, but despite this, changes in sliding scales may be based on a small change in blood glucose from a glucometer reading [72]. Other causes of suboptimal control of patients managed with insulin sliding scales include the previously outlined factors that alter subcutaneous insulin pharmacokinetics. It is widely reported that patients are frequently poorly controlled on insulin sliding scales, and a greater understanding and diligence is needed among physicians [73].

When a more precise and consistent level of glucose control is required, such as in the critically ill, intravenous insulin may be a more effective option and is discussed in a later section. Despite the enhanced control, insulin infusions require frequent monitoring, which is not possible in most hospital settings unless a patient is in an ICU.

Insulin pumps

The use of continuous subcutaneous insulin infusion (CSII), also known as the insulin pump, has increased in recent years, with more than 50,000 participants worldwide. The CSII is a battery-operated device that delivers an operator-determined quantity of insulin through a nonmetallic cannula. The insulin is administered in two ways: basal and bolus. The patient programs into the CSII a constant basal rate, which varies from day to day based on activity and stressors. The additional bolus delivery form of a rapid-acting insulin is typically used during meals and periods when glucose levels surpass the coverage anticipated by the basal rate. Traditionally reserved for type 1 diabetics, these devices require dedication and intensive monitoring on the patient's part.

On admission to the hospital, it is important to decide whether an insulin pump should be continued. This decision must be made with the primary team and the patient, if able. A recent article by Cook and colleagues [74] outlined general factors that may be considered contraindications to continued CSII use in the hospitalized patient. Primarily, these factors include altered mental status or patients in critically ill states such as sepsis or trauma. Cook and colleagues [74] included a patient–doctor contract that clearly delineates the patient's role while maintaining the physician's clinical authority. Other times to temporarily discontinue the use of an insulin pump are during and immediately following a surgery. There are also certain radiologic studies and procedures that may interfere with pump function and result in complications. In this setting, the pump should be deactivated and kept separate from hazardous devices.

When the patient is unable or unwilling to manage the device in the acute setting, a temporary calculated basal-bolus regimen, an insulin sliding scale, or a continuous intravenous insulin course is considered an acceptable alternative. If possible, therapy should be initiated 1 hour before discontinuing the insulin pump. Insulin sliding scales are generally reserved for temporary glucose coverage. When it is anticipated that the patient will not be able to resume the use of his or her insulin pump for an extended period, the safest method of glycemic control is continuous intravenous insulin therapy. Regardless, an endocrinology consultation is wise in any of these circumstances because the risk of poor glucose control and ketoacidosis increases and should be closely monitored.

A noncompromised patient who has an insulin pump is generally well educated with the device and can maintain tight control of blood glucose levels. If possible, patients are allowed to continue insulin pump administration while hospitalized.

After the decision has been made to continue use of an insulin pump, several specific parameters should be determined and documented. The name of the manufacturer of the specific device should be obtained. Nursing staff should be alerted to the necessary amount of frequent finger-stick levels, and concurrent endocrinology consultation is strongly recommended. The patient's basal rate, typically recorded as units per hour, is the first set of parameters to determine. There may be several rates reported based on the time of day. For instance, the rate between midnight and 6 AM will likely be different than the rate between noon and 6 PM. Next, the bolus rate is based on an insulin-to-carbohydrate ratio as determined by the patient's carbohydrate counting. An example would be a 1:5 ratio. This method is used to determine how many units of insulin are required to cover a particular number of grams of carbohydrates in a meal. Patients typically report four such ratios that correspond to all three meals and snacks; some of these ratios may be identical. Occasionally, a higher-than-desired glucose level is recorded; therefore, a temporary high bolus is required. In this situation, a correction factor must be determined, which is similar to the carbohydrate ratio but is used only until the patient returns to the desired plasma glucose level. Afterward, the patient may resume his or her normal routine [74].

Perioperative glucose management

As the role of the podiatric service becomes more integral to a multidisciplinary approach at an increasing number of institutions nationwide, perioperative assessment and preparation have become essential elements, especially for successful limb salvage. This section serves as a primer in glucose management for podiatric surgeons working in this capacity and in no way supersedes the utility of a medical consultation when indicated. Evaluation and assessment of other common comorbidities such as impaired cardiovascular and renal function are also equally important in the preoperative examination and the determination of overall optimization of the patient.

Metabolic response to surgery and anesthesia

With regard to glycemic control, there are no standardized perioperative protocols in existence [75,76]. This lack of standardized protocols is largely due to the variety of available treatment regimens and requires a degree of customization and flexibility to optimize the patient. Many confounding factors such as the type of diabetes, level of insulin resistance, overall metabolism, and stresses placed on the body cause the patient to respond differently to insulin and other hypoglycemic medications. A complex metabolic process ensues in response to surgery and anesthesia, which is beyond the intended emphasis of this article. Although most physicians and patients fear hypoglycemia while fasting, the more frequent physiologic state is that of hyperglycemia. Briefly, the effects of general anesthesia and overall increased sympathetic response cause less insulin to be secreted. Furthermore, insulin resistance becomes more prevalent due to the increased secretion of varying amounts of the counter-regulatory hormones produced during times of stress. This increased insulin resistance causes the body produce more glucose through the liver and decrease overall peripheral glucose use [77–79]. This catabolic fasting state of gluconeogenesis, glycogenolysis, ketosis, proteolysis, and lipolysis places diabetic patients at risk for developing severe hyperglycemia and even potentially ketoacidosis if they have type 1 diabetes mellitus [80]. In addition, studies have shown that the type of anesthesia and the extent and duration of surgical intervention creates large variations of the counter-regulatory hormones glucagon, epinephrine, norepinephrine, cortisol, and growth hormone, making glucose homeostasis difficult to predict and highly variable [78–80].

Importance of perioperative glycemic control

Even though the importance of glycemic control seems obvious, hyperglycemia is still a frequent finding in the perioperative setting. The reasons to maintain an inpatient's blood glucose levels somewhat higher than normal in preparation for surgery are often multifactorial; however, recent literature has been ripe with data advocating tighter control of glucose in the perioperative setting.

Primarily, tighter glucose control minimizes overall perioperative morbidity and mortality. The classic prospective randomized study Diabetes Mellitus Glucose Infusion in Acute Myocardial Infarction (DI-GAMI) showed that long-term benefit and reduction in mortality from myocardial infarction were due to tight glucose control with the use of initial intravenous insulin infusion [81]. There have been several studies since then looking at the positive impact that insulin may have on improving operative outcomes, particularly with regard to cardiothoracic surgery [82]. The reason for improved survival is likely multifaceted and includes improved glucose homeostasis and possible improved oxygenation of the tissues through insulin's vasodilatory effects to skeletal muscle by way of increased production of nitric oxide in vascular endothelium [27,28].

It is also well documented that perioperative hyperglycemia increases the risk of developing a postoperative infection [17,83,84]. Most of this research was performed in the 1990s, and the exact mechanism is still unknown [18,85]. Furthermore, the higher the level of blood glucose, the greater the chance of experiencing an infection postoperatively, especially if the blood glucose is greater than 200 mg/dL [17,83]. In a recent study by Hruska and colleagues [86], it was clearly shown that before initiating tighter blood glucose control, there was a statistically significant increase in postoperative infections in the diabetic population compared with the nondiabetic population ($P = .0014$). After initiating an insulin drip protocol to maintain blood glucose levels between 120 and 160 mg/dL, the postoperative infection rate decreased significantly in the diabetic patients ($P = .0092$). Although these studies assessed infection rates in cardiac surgery, the improvement in postoperative infections by tightly controlling glucose levels in the immediate postoperative period still warrants further investigation in patients undergoing noncardiac surgery. It is not practical or necessary to place every diabetic patient undergoing surgery on an insulin drip with intensive care monitoring postoperatively; however, future studies may set higher standards of tighter glucose management.

Hyperglycemia has been shown to have deleterious effects on essential wound healing events. As mentioned before, multiple studies at the cellular level have demonstrated that there is overall impaired cell migration and a deficiency of proangiogenic growth factors such as platelet-derived growth factor and vascular endothelial growth factor [23–25]. Complex physiologic processes contribute to the prolonged inflammatory state and to delayed wound healing and contraction in the diabetic wound [22]. For these and previously discussed reasons, postoperative surgical wound healing may be further optimized in a well-controlled diabetic patient.

Hyperglycemic avoidance is desirable for a multitude of reasons, even when glucose is elevated for short intervals. Therefore, it is probably not ideal to aim for higher glucose levels than outpatient goals to avoid perioperative hypoglycemia. Future prospective, controlled, randomized studies are needed to further evaluate safe modalities to improve glycemic control in the perioperative period.

Goals of perioperative glycemic control

Regardless of the aforementioned factors, four primary glycemic goals remain paramount: prevention of hypoglycemia, hyperglycemia, and ketosis, and the reduction of morbidity and mortality. The risks associated with hypoglycemia are easily understood because this state carries a significant risk of mortality. Events such as cardiac arrhythmias or altered mental status may be triggered by this state and can be difficult to detect in the immediate postoperative period. Diabetic ketoacidotic and hyperosmolar nonketotic states may be induced by severe hyperglycemia, as is the potential for volume depletion secondary to osmotic diuresis. Although patients who have type 2 diabetes mellitus are less likely to develop ketosis, without insulin, type 1 diabetics may progress to ketoacidosis. Understanding the differences between each type of diabetes becomes imperative when managing elevated glucose levels as each type of diabetes carries different consequences if treated incorrectly. Although a patient who has type 2 diabetes mellitus can tolerate some mildly elevated plasma glucose values and still withhold insulin dosing, this may prove catastrophic for type 1 diabetics who may become ketotic as a result. Patients who have type 2 diabetes mellitus are more prone to nonketotic states but may develop ketoacidosis at the extremely high range [68].

Beyond these prime directives, the necessary stringency of glycemic control is unclear. The long-term benefits of tight glucose control are well documented in both diabetic types, as evidenced by the DCCT [9] and the UKPDS [10]; however, fewer reports address the perioperative period. The studies that consider this sensitive period generally are in reference to major surgical interventions and those in critical care units. Although these studies have shown promise (with decreases in morbidity and mortality), the applicability to less critically ill patients is poorly understood.

Optimally, surgery is scheduled in the early morning. Most physicians aim to maintain a blood glucose concentration between 150 and 200 mg/dL. Patients actively receiving an insulin infusion can obtain tighter control, with a blood glucose goal between 101 and 150 mg/dL [68,87].

The Beth Israel Deaconess Medical Center (BIDMC) enjoys a close relationship with the staff and services of the Joslin Diabetes Center. This partnership allows for regular consultation and education. Many of the perioperative glycemic control protocols presented here are a result of those interactions and are based on unpublished data from the Joslin Diabetes

Center clinical guidelines. A variety of strategies exists and practitioners must use their own clinical judgment to select the best regimen for their patients.

A systematic approach with logical considerations of all significant variables can assist in the decision-making process. The initial variable to consider is the extent of the procedure, which can be divided into major and nonmajor surgery. Examples of major lower-extremity surgery include lower-extremity bypass surgery, severe polytrauma, and only the most severe limb-threatening infections often seen with septicemia. In general, most foot and ankle procedures are considered nonmajor surgery and may include but are not limited to all elective foot procedures regardless of the anatomic location. In addition, procedures that seek to eliminate mild to moderate infections such as osteomyelitis and abscesses are also included. Even more complex procedures such as mild to moderate trauma, joint replacements, and extensive lower-extremity deformity reconstructions are considered nonmajor surgery.

Other important considerations are the type of diabetes and the degree of patient insulin resistance. These considerations are addressed by separating patients into two primary groups. The first group comprises all patients who have type 1 diabetes mellitus and type 2 diabetics who require multiple daily insulin injections. The second group includes the remainder of diabetics not included within group 1: type 2 diabetics who are diet controlled, are taking oral hypoglycemics, and are taking subcutaneous insulin once or twice daily. Regardless of which group a patient is in, surgery at the earliest time is recommended to avoid prolonging the fasting state.

Major surgery

Preparation for major surgery of the lower extremity is less likely to fall within the range of the typical podiatric patient, but as previously mentioned, major surgery includes lower-extremity bypass surgery, severe polytrauma, and severe limb-threatening infections. Patients in these circumstances are more appropriate candidates for intravenous insulin infusion regardless of the type of diabetes.

Initiation of an insulin drip requires careful deliberation, but certain circumstances can impact the decision to start an insulin infusion. These circumstances include prolonged surgical procedures, some emergent surgeries, anticipated ICU transfers, unstable type 1 diabetes mellitus with ketoacidosis, and unstable glucose concentrations such as is seen with septicemia [68]. The insulin infusion allows for the tightest level of glucose control with very close monitoring. Insulin has also been shown to independently improve operative outcomes in the previously described DIGAMI study, possibly decreasing acute myocardial infarctions. More recent studies have further supported the use of insulin infusion with cardiothoracic surgery and critically ill patients [82]. Insulin has well-described vasodilatory effects on skeletal muscle by inducing vascular endothelium to increase production of nitric oxide

[27,28]. Insulin itself may contribute to lowering infection rates by normalizing defense mechanisms and inflammatory mediators [17,84]. Further research is warranted to help with patient selection to determine which patients would benefit from continuous intravenous insulin therapy.

Nevertheless, the authors' approach has been to place patients on closely monitored insulin infusions when major surgery is to be performed. Endocrinologist or primary care physician consultation is highly recommended during this time because the decision to initiate insulin infusion should not be taken lightly and should be closely and cautiously monitored. In some instances, patients may require transfer to an ICU or a step-down unit for closer monitoring.

Patients who are septic with limb-threatening infections must also be aggressively managed surgically. Undrained abscesses in the lower extremity are not well tolerated in the diabetic patient, and attempts to control blood glucose levels will fail until incision and drainage with debridement has occurred. Many of these situations are considered surgical emergencies requiring immediate surgical intervention.

Although a variety of methods have been reported that determine insulin infusion rates and many protocols have been studied, no consensus on a universal approach exists. One may give an intermittent small bolus of regular insulin every 2 hours, a combined glucose-potassium-insulin solution, or varying amounts of separate continuous glucose and insulin infusions. The authors' approach varies somewhat and is based on unpublished data from the Joslin Diabetes Center, 2006.

After the decision for insulin infusion has been made, all hypoglycemic oral medications and standing insulin orders are discontinued. If the patient's blood glucose level is currently less than 200 mg/dL, then 5% dextrose, 0.45% normal saline ($D_5\frac{1}{2}NS$) at 60 to 100 mL/h is started concurrently to avoid rapid hypoglycemia. Most patients will have a blood glucose level of greater than 300 mg/dL because uncontrolled hyperglycemia is often the reason for starting an insulin drip. If this is the case, a stat dose of rapid-acting intravenous insulin is given based on body weight (0.1 U/kg). The initial insulin rate is determined by whether the patient is insulin naive. If the patient was already on an insulin regimen, then the total current 24-hour insulin requirement is determined and divided by 24 to obtain an initial hourly rate. If the patient does not routinely use insulin, then a conservative starting dose at 0.02 U/kg body weight per hour is initiated.

Blood glucose levels are checked in 1 hour, and the infusion rate is adjusted as necessary to maintain a blood glucose level between 101 and 150 mg/dL. If the glucose level is at this goal, then no change in the insulin infusion is needed, unless the patient experiences a large fluctuation in glucose levels. If fluctuations greater than 200 mg/dL are reported within 1 hour of adjustment, then the insulin infusion rate is lowered 25% or by 1 U/h, whichever is greater. When the blood glucose levels are between 101 and 150 mg/dL without fluctuations, glucose checks can be reduced from hourly to every 2 hours.

If the glucose level is less than 100 mg/dL, then the insulin infusion must be lowered based on how low the glucose level has become and whether there were large fluctuations within the blood glucose level. If it is very low (<60 mg/dL), then the insulin drip is immediately held, 1 ampule of 50% glucose is given, and the glucose level is checked every 30 minutes until the level is greater than 100 mg/dL.

If the glucose level is above the goal of 101 to 150 mg/dL, then the insulin drip must be adjusted based on the severity of glucose elevation and the amount of fluctuation that is occurring. Regardless of the amount of fluctuation, if the glucose level is between 301 and 400 mg/dL, then the insulin drip is increased by 40% or 3 U/h, whichever is greater. If the glucose level is very high (>400 mg/dL), then the insulin drip is doubled or increased by 4 U/h, whichever is greater.

The last consideration that should be given to a patient placed on an insulin infusion is how to appropriately discontinue it. Abrupt discontinuation is not recommended. The patient's home regimen of insulin or oral medication should be given 1 to 2 hours before discontinuing insulin infusion. If the patient was diet controlled, then a rapid- or short-acting subcutaneous insulin equal to or twice the amount of the hourly insulin infusion rate requirement is administered. A tapering effect of the intravenous insulin occurs to the point that the insulin infusion can then be safely discontinued as opposed to an abrupt halt. This tapering should help to avoid a large fluctuation in glucose levels. A backup subcutaneous insulin sliding scale should also be ordered if additional insulin coverage is needed. If the patient cannot tolerate foods and liquids, then discontinuation of the intravenous insulin is not yet recommended.

Nonmajor surgery

Nonmajor surgery encompasses most podiatric procedures. These procedures include everything from elective cases to extensive reconstructions. As noted before, patients are divided into two major groups for managing glucose. Group 1 includes all patients who have type 1 diabetes mellitus and type 2 diabetic patients who require multiple insulin injections. Group 2 includes all other diabetic patients: type 2 diabetics on once- or twice-daily insulin regimens, patients taking oral hypoglycemic medication with or without insulin, and diet-controlled patients.

Day before surgery

Both groups require little intervention on the day before surgery. Outpatient insulin regimens and diets may be continued without alterations. If the patient is on a basal-bolus regimen of insulin, this is continued. For those taking oral hypoglycemics, no change is required until the day of surgery. Finger-stick glucose levels should be checked before every meal and at bedtime. When the glucose is poorly controlled (a common occurrence in the face of infection), a sliding scale of fast-acting insulin can be used to supplement control. The BIDMC podiatry service uses a weight-based sliding scale developed by the Joslin Diabetes Center. Sliding scales may need to be adjusted and individualized for each patient to optimize glucose control.

Group 1: day of surgery

On the day of surgery, the patient begins fasting at midnight and 5% dextrose in water (D_5W) or ($D_5\frac{1}{2}NS$) is initiated unless the blood glucose level is greater than 200 mg/dL (normal saline is usually an acceptable alternative during hyperglycemic situations). Exceptions to this regimen exist and medical judgment should override these recommendations as needed. All scheduled rapid- or short-acting insulin is held. Intermediate-acting insulin is reduced by one half to two thirds. Peakless or relatively peakless insulins such as glargine or detemir are typically reduced to one half to two thirds of the usual dose, although if the glucose levels have been very high, then the entire dose may still be given. If a patient receives an insulin mixture, then the rapid-acting portion of the mixture should be held and the intermediate-acting portion should be cut in half to two thirds. Glucose levels are monitored every 2 hours before and during surgery. An insulin sliding scale with rapid-acting insulin supplements glucose control using the reduced bedtime portion of the sliding scale. If glucose levels cannot be controlled and are greater than 400 mg/dL, then an insulin infusion may be initiated. If the glucose falls below 80 mg/dL, then one ampule of 10% dextrose in water ($D_{10}W$) is given intravenously and the glucose is rechecked in 30 minutes. The most important distinguishing characteristic of patients in group 1 is that all type 1 diabetes mellitus patients require basal insulin at all times for survival, even when fasting.

Group 1: postoperatively

Postoperatively, the glucose levels are checked when the patient reaches the postoperative unit. The bedtime insulin sliding scale and the previously noted protocol is continued until the patient can tolerate at least 50% of his or her prescribed diet.

Group 2: day of surgery

On the day of surgery, the patient begins fasting at midnight and D_5W or $D_5\frac{1}{2}NS$ is initiated unless the blood glucose level is greater than 200 mg/dL. Medical judgment should again determine the type, amount, and rate of intravenous fluid administered, if any. All oral hypoglycemic medications are held, as is all scheduled rapid- or short-acting insulin. Intermediate- or long-acting insulin is cut in half. If a patient receives an insulin mixture, then the fast-acting portion of the mixture should be held and the intermediate-acting portion should be reduced in half. Glucose levels are monitored every 2 hours before and during surgery. An insulin sliding scale supplements glucose control using the bedtime portion of the sliding scale. A continuous intravenous insulin infusion may be initiated if glucose cannot be controlled and is greater than 400 mg/dL. If the glucose level is below 80 mg/dL, then one ampule of D10W is given intravenously and the glucose is rechecked in 30 minutes.

Group 2: postoperatively

Glucose levels are checked when the patient reaches the postoperative unit. The bedtime insulin sliding scale is continued until the patient can tolerate at least 50% of the prescribed diet. Serum creatinine levels should also be checked if the patient receives metformin as an outpatient. If the serum creatinine levels are greater than or equal to 1.4 mg/dL in women or 1.5 mg/dL in men, then metformin should be held and glucose control should be achieved with an insulin sliding scale until creatinine levels normalize.

Additional considerations

As previously mentioned, the insulin pump is managed differently than other forms of insulin delivery systems. Briefly, patients are usually maintained on their insulin pumps (if not contraindicated) while hospitalized and allowed to make adjustments as needed. Special attention is required during or immediately following a surgery. A temporary calculated basal-bolus regimen, insulin sliding scale, or continuous intravenous insulin course is needed based on the duration of surgery. This regimen is continued until the patient can again manage the pump.

Deep venous thrombosis prophylaxis in diabetics

Although still controversial, diabetes may also accentuate risk of thrombotic complications such as venous thromboembolism (VTE) or pulmonary embolism [88]. It is not known whether diabetes or hyperglycemia independently increases the risk for VTE in patients who have diabetes or whether associated comorbidities and the tendency for increased cardiovascular events increase the risk. The literature is scarce and limited with regard to diabetes and VTE risk. The Framingham Study from 1979 demonstrated that there was no increased risk of VTE in diabetics and that the level of hyperglycemia also did not impact risk [89]. Other antiquated studies agree [90–92]. In more current literature, diabetes as a risk factor has been re-evaluated. Despite controversies, it is agreed that diabetic patients often have other comorbidities that have well-established, independent VTE risk factors such as obesity, venous stasis associated with prolonged immobilization, and CHF [93]. Many studies further state that diabetes independently increases the risk of a thromboembolic event [88,94,95]. Regardless, additional studies are needed, and recommended VTE prophylaxis in diabetic lower-extremity surgery is unknown. The overall incidence of VTE or pulmonary embolism in foot and ankle surgery is extremely low, with most cases related to traumatic events [96–98]. Little is known about the incidence in high-risk diabetic patients. Because of this, the authors' institution anecdotally advocates for deep venous thrombosis prophylaxis in all hospitalized diabetic patients for foot and ankle surgery unless otherwise contraindicated. Multiple concomitant comorbidities frequently exist, and this precaution will likely remain the authors' mainstay of treatment until further studies suggest a modification.

Summary

This section gives only a brief presentation on the perioperative glycemic controls used at the authors' institution. A well-considered protocol is important in delivering consistent, quality care, but each patient has unique metabolic needs and requires careful scrutiny. When the complexity of a patient's medical status exceeds a clinician's comfort level for management, the authors strongly advise medical or endocrinology consultation.

Future directions in diabetic glycemic control

Beyond transplant and the hard-sought-after cure, the medical-research community remains resolute in its determination to enhance glycemic control to stave off diabetic complications. With the advent of new technologies and research, many innovations are on the horizon that may offer greater control and fewer adverse effects. New oral medications and noninjectable insulins are just a few of the agents that show promise.

Glucagon-like peptide-1 agonists

As of April 2005, the US Food and Drug Administration (FDA) approved the first drug in this class (exenatide) as an adjunct to sulfonylurea or metformin. Secreted by intestinal L cells, glucagon-like peptide-1 (GLP-1) normally enhances insulin secretion in the presence of glucose, inhibits glucagon secretion, and may up-regulate insulin gene expression. GLP-1 agonists have been found to increase insulin secretion by stimulating beta cells and enhance satiation by delaying gastric emptying. Therefore, its greatest effect is in the postprandial phase. Some data suggest that this class may also protect beta cells.

Because the naturally occurring peptide has a half-life of only minutes, analogs such as exenatide and liraglutide that have longer half-lives and prolonged duration of action were developed. Liraglutide is currently in phase 3 testing and is being evaluated for stand-alone therapy. These drugs are for use in type 2 diabetics only and are administered subcutaneously.

The most commonly associated side effect is nausea (31%). Patients who have gastroparesis treated with metoclopramide (Reglan) should avoid this class [99,100].

Dipeptidyl peptidase-IV inhibitors

This class of medication prolongs the action of endogenous GLP-1 by inhibiting the enzyme that breaks it down. Therefore, it has the same benefits as GLP-1.

Vildagliptin (Galvus), currently under FDA review, and the recently approved sitagliptin (Januvia) are once-daily oral agents for type 2 diabetes mellitus. These medications work through the incretin system by inhibiting the enzyme dipeptidyl peptidase-4 in order to enhance glucose control by addressing both beta-cell and alpha-cell production [101]. Adverse reactions include hypoglycemia, nasopharyngitis, and pruritus [102].

Amylin analogs

Amylin is a hormone secreted by pancreatic beta cells with insulin. It reduces glucagon secretion and, like the GLP-1 agonists, slows gastric emptying. Patients who produce inadequate insulin have a concomitant shortage of amylin release.

In March 2005, pramlintide (Symlin), an amylin analog, was approved by the FDA for patients who have type 1 and type 2 diabetes mellitus. Pramlintide is given as a separate subcutaneously administered adjunct to insulin therapy with or without other oral anti-hyperglycemics [103]. It is renally cleared; therefore, dose adjustments need to be made in the renally impaired. Approximately 10% of patients experience nausea and headache, and hypoglycemic events are equivalent to placebo after the first 4 weeks of therapy [104].

Glitazars

Also known as the dual-action PPARs, these agents represent a class of drugs that have combined PPAR-α and PPAR-Γ receptor agonism. Thiazolidinediones are PPAR-Γ agonists that reduce insulin resistance in peripheral tissues. PPAR-α agonists are well-documented lipid-controlling agents. Because dyslipidemia is typically concomitant in type 2 diabetes mellitus, medications that treat hyperglycemia and dyslipidemia are of obvious benefit. To date, however, many agents within this class have failed to pass phase 3 testing as a result of a variety of safety concerns [105].

Endocannabinoid receptor antagonist

This class of medication was developed to inhibit endocannabinoid receptors and thus designed to exploit a group of physiologic pathways that affect appetite and satiety. Current research supports the belief that with inhibition of this system, satiation will occur more rapidly and patients will subsequently lose weight. Other hypothesized actions include regulation of blood pressure and lipid modulation. Scheen [106] presented data from the Rimonabant in Obesity–Diabetes Study at the 2005 ADA Scientific Sessions meeting. This study looked at over 1000 diabetics who had a mean body mass index of 34 and an HbA1c of 7.5% who were treated with rimonabant for a year. Substantial improvements were noted in weight, HbA1c, and lipid profiles.

Rimonabant was released in July 2006 in the European Union. At this time, the FDA is still reviewing the application in the United States. The most significant adverse reactions were nausea (11.2%), anxiety, and depression [107].

Oral insulin

A highly anticipated product with little previous success but recent advances includes oral insulin. An orally administered insulin has been researched for quite some time. Bioavailability is largely limited by its size and the deactivation that occurs within the gastric and intestinal environments [108]. At the 2006 ADA Scientific Sessions meeting, data were presented regarding an oral form of regular insulin in early clinical trials. This oral agent was compared with a subcutaneous injection of aspart insulin. Serum glucose was compared serially between groups. Onset occurred within 15 minutes and it had 60% to 70% of the biopotency of subcutaneous regular insulin. Per report, no adverse reactions such as hypoglycemia or gastrointestinal symptoms were recorded [109,110].

Inhaled insulin

Less invasive insulin is highly desirable. Exubera (insulin human [rDNA origin]) was FDA approved in January 2006 and is the first commercially available noninjectable insulin that has onset and duration comparable to regular insulin while maintaining comparable glucose control. Its bioavailability relative to regular subcutaneous insulin has been reported to be anywhere from 10% to 20%.

At this time, only those type 1 and type 2 diabetics who have normal pulmonary function can use this insulin. A mild cough, usually occurring within minutes of use, was reported in approximately 30% of subjects. Hypoglycemic events were reported less frequently than with the regular insulin control [111–113]. Patients still require long-acting insulins if they have type 1 diabetes mellitus but may use Exubera as monotherapy or with another oral antihyperglycemic medication or long-acting insulin if they have type 2 diabetes mellitus. Cost appears to be a significant concern, and further long-term studies of pulmonary function are being continued [114,115].

Summary

The projected impact of diabetes on future generations is cause for concern, especially in industrialized nations. Improved understanding of the significance of serum glycemic variability may provide clinicians with a more universal goal for their patients. Constant innovation in this rapidly evolving field of study offers the potential to develop medications and treatments that treat diabetes and commonly associated conditions.

References

[1] Harris MI, Flegal KM, Cowie CC, et al. Prevalence of diabetes, impaired fasting glucose, and impaired glucose tolerance in U.S. adults: the third National Health and Nutrition Examination Survey, 1988–1994. Diabetes Care 1998;21:518–24.

[2] King H, Aubert RE, Herman WH. Global burden of diabetes, 1995–2025: prevalence, numerical estimates, and projections. Diabetes Care 1998;21:1414–31.

[3] Basu S, Hadley J, Tan RM, et al. Is there enough information about foot care among patients with diabetes? Int J Low Extrem Wounds 2004;3(2):64–8.

[4] Reiber GE, Lipsky BA, Gibbons GW. The burden of diabetic foot ulcers. Am J Surg 1998; 176(2A Suppl):5S–10S.

[5] Ramsey SD, Newton K, Blough D, et al. Incidence, outcomes, and cost of foot ulcers in patients with diabetes. Diabetes Care 1999;22(3):382–7.

[6] Jeffcoate WJ, Harding KG. Diabetic foot ulcers. Lancet 2003;361(9368):1545–51.

[7] Harrington C, Zagari MJ, Corea J, et al. A cost analysis of diabetic lower-extremity ulcers. Diabetes Care 2000;23:1333–8.

[8] D'Orazio P, Burnett RW, Fogh-Andersen N, et al. The International Federation of Clinical Chemistry Scientific Division Working Group on selective electrodes and point of care testing. Approved IFCC recommendation on reporting results for blood glucose. Clin Chem 2005;51:1573–6.

[9] The Diabetes Control and Complications Trial Research Group. The effect of intensive therapy of diabetes on the development and progression of long-term complications in insulin-dependent diabetes mellitus. N Engl J Med 1993;329:977–86.

[10] United Kingdom Prospective Diabetes Study Group (UKPDS). Intensive blood-glucose control with sulphonylureas or insulin compared with conventional treatment and risk of complications in patients with type 2 diabetes. Lancet 1998;352:853–7.

[11] Little R, Rohlfing CL, Wiedmeyer H, et al. NGSP Steering Committee. The national glycohemoglobin standardization program: a five-year progress report. Clin Chem 2001; 47:1985–92.

[12] American Diabetes Association Consensus Statement: standards of medical care in diabetes. Diabetes Care 2006;29:S4–42.

[13] Garber AJ, Moghissi ES, Bransome ED Jr, et al. American College of Endocrinology position statement on inpatient diabetes and metabolic control. Endocr Pract 2004;10:77–82.

[14] Deeg MA. Basic approach to managing hyperglycemia for the nonendocrinologist. Am J Cardiol 2005;96(Suppl):38E–40E.

[15] Rassias AJ, Marrin CA, Arruda J, et al. Insulin infusion improves neutrophil function in diabetic cardiac surgery patients. Anesth Analg 1999;88(5):1011–6.

[16] Golden SH, Peart-Vigilance C, Kao WH, et al. Perioperative glycemic control and the risk of infectious complications in a cohort of adults with diabetes. Diabetes Care 1999;22(9): 1408–14.

[17] Furnary AP, Zerr KJ, Grunkemeier GL, et al. Continuous intravenous insulin infusion reduces the incidence of deep sternal wound infection in diabetic patients after cardiac surgical procedures. Ann Thorac Surg 1999;67:352–62.

[18] Pomposelli JJ, Baxter JK III, Babineau TJ, et al. Early postoperative glucose control predicts nosocomial infection rate in diabetic patients. JPEN J Parenter Enteral Nutr 1998;22:77–81.
[19] Shaw JE, Boulton AJ. The pathogenesis of diabetic foot problems: an overview. Diabetes 1997;46(Suppl 2):S58–61.
[20] Bagdade JD, Stewart M, Walters E. Impaired granulocyte adherence: a reversible defect in host defense in patients with poorly controlled diabetes. Diabetes 1978;27:677–81.
[21] Takehara K. Growth regulation of skin fibroblasts. J Dermatol Sci 2000;24(Suppl 1):S70–7.
[22] Mansbridge JN, Liu K, Pinney RE, et al. Growth factors secreted by fibroblasts: role in healing diabetic foot ulcers. Diabetes Obes Metab 1999;1:265–79.
[23] Werner S, Breeden M, Hubner G, et al. Induction of keratinocyte growth factor expression is reduced and delayed during wound healing in the genetically diabetic mouse. J Invest Dermatol 1994;103:469–73.
[24] Doxey DL, Ng MC, Dill RE, et al. Platelet-derived growth factor levels in wounds of diabetic rats. Life Sci 1995;57:1111–23.
[25] Lerman OZ, Galiano RD, Armour M, et al. Cellular dysfunction in the diabetic fibroblast: impairment in migration, vascular endothelial growth factor production, and response to hypoxia. Am J Pathol 2003;162(1):303–12.
[26] Akbari CM, Saouaf R, Barnhill DF, et al. Endothelium-dependent vasodilatation is impaired in both microcirculation and macrocirculation during acute hyperglycemia. J Vasc Surg 1998;28(4):687–94.
[27] Vincent MA, Montagnani M, Quon MJ. Molecular and physiologic actions of insulin related to production of nitric oxide in vascular endothelium. Curr Diab Rep 2003;3(4):279–88.
[28] Steinberg HO, Brechtel G, Johnson A, et al. Insulin-mediated skeletal muscle vasodilation is nitric oxide dependent. A novel action of insulin to increase nitric oxide release. J Clin Invest 1994;94(3):1172–9.
[29] Marston WA. Dermagraft Diabetic Foot Ulcer Study Group. Risk factors associated with healing chronic diabetic foot ulcers: the importance of hyperglycemia. Ostomy Wound Manage 2006;52(3):26–8.
[30] DeFronzo RA. Pharmacologic therapy for type 2 diabetes mellitus. Ann Intern Med 1999;131(4):281–303.
[31] Garber AJ, Duncan TG, Goodman AM, et al. Efficacy of metformin in type II diabetes: results of a double-blind, placebo-controlled, dose-response trial. Am J Med 1997;103:491–7.
[32] Tang WH. Do thiazolidinediones cause heart failure? A critical review. Cleve Clin J Med 2006;73(4):390–7.
[33] Horton ES, Clinkingbeard C, Gatlin M, et al. Nateglinide alone and in combination with metformin improves glycemic control by reducing mealtime glucose levels in type 2 diabetes. Diabetes Care 2000;23:1660–5.
[34] Chiasson J-L, Josse RG, Hunt JA, et al. The efficacy of acarbose in the treatment of patients with non-insulin-dependent diabetes mellitus. A multicenter controlled clinical trial. Ann Intern Med 1994;121:928–35.
[35] Hoffmann J, Spengler M. Efficacy of 24-week monotherapy with acarbose, glibenclamide, or placebo in NIDDM patients. The Essen Study. Diabetes Care 1994;17:561–6.
[36] Holman RR, Cull CA, Turner RC. A randomized double-blind trial of acarbose in type 2 diabetes shows improved glycemic control over 3 years (U.K. Prospective Diabetes Study 44). Diabetes Care 1999;22:960–4.
[37] Atkinson MA, Maclaren NK. The pathogenesis of insulin-dependent diabetes mellitus. N Engl J Med 1994;331:1428–36.
[38] Clement S. Guidelines for glycemic control. Clin Cornerstone 2004;6(2):31–9.
[39] Stumvoll M, Goldstein BJ, van Haeften TW. Type 2 diabetes: principles of pathogenesis and therapy. Lancet 2005;365:1333–46.

[40] Doyle ME, Egan JM. Pharmacological agents that directly modulate insulin secretion. Pharmacol Rev 2003;55(1):105–31.

[41] Brunton SA, Davis SN, Renda SM. Overcoming psychological barriers to insulin use in type 2 diabetes. Clin Cornerstone 2006;8(Suppl 2):S19–26.

[42] Wonders J, Eekhoff EM, Heine R, et al. [Insulin allergy: background, diagnosis and treatment.]. Ned Tijdschr Geneeskd 2005;149(50):2783–8.

[43] Wittrup M, Pildal J, Rasmussen AK, et al. [Systemic and local allergy to human insulin.] Ugeskr Laeger 2003;165(21):2207–8.

[44] De Villiers FP. Lipohypertrophy—a complication of insulin injections. S Afr Med J 2005; 95(11):858–9.

[45] Beltrand J, Guilmin-Crepon S, Castanet M, et al. Insulin allergy and extensive lipoatrophy in a child with type 1 diabetes. Horm Res 2006;65(5):253–60.

[46] Sinha A, Formica C, Tsalamandris C, et al. Effects of insulin on body composition in patients with insulin-dependent and non-insulin-dependent diabetes. Diabet Med 1996; 13(1):40–6.

[47] Jacob AN, Salinas K, Adams-Huet B, et al. Potential causes of weight gain in type 1 diabetes mellitus. Diabetes Obes Metab 2006;8(4):404–11.

[48] Gin H, Hanaire-Broutin H. Reproducibility and variability in the action of injected insulin. Diabetes Metab 2005;31(1):7–13.

[49] Hildebrandt P. Skinfold thickness, local subcutaneous blood flow and insulin absorption in diabetic patients. Acta Physiol Scand Suppl 1991;603:41–5.

[50] Hildebrandt P. Subcutaneous absorption of insulin in insulin-dependent diabetic patients. Influence of species, physico-chemical properties of insulin and physiological factors. Dan Med Bull 1991;38(4):337–46.

[51] Heinemann L. Variability of insulin absorption and insulin action. Diabetes Technol Ther 2002;4(5):673–82.

[52] Guerci B, Sauvanet JP. Subcutaneous insulin: pharmacokinetic variability and glycemic variability. Diabetes Metab 2005;31(4 Pt 2):4S7–24.

[53] NovoLog [package insert]. Princeton, NJ: Novo Nordisk Pharmaceuticals; 2001.

[54] Apidra [package insert]. Kansas City, Mo: Aventis Pharmaceuticals, Inc; 2004.

[55] Humalog [package insert]. Indianapolis, IN: Eli Lilly and Company; 2000.

[56] Humulin/Humalog [package insert]. Indianapolis, IN: Eli Lilly and Company; 2004.

[57] Lantus [package insert]. Kansas City, MO: Aventis Pharmaceutical Inc; 2001.

[58] Levemir [package insert]. Princeton, NJ: Novo Nordisk Inc; 2005.

[59] American Diabetes Association. Continuous subcutaneous insulin infusion. Diabetes Care 2004;27(Suppl 1):S110.

[60] Rolla AR, Rakel RE. Practical approaches to insulin therapy for type 2 diabetes mellitus with premixed insulin analogues. Clin Ther 2005;27(8):1113–25.

[61] Garber AJ. Premixed insulin analogues for the treatment of diabetes mellitus. Drugs 2006; 66(1):31–49.

[62] Hanaire-Broutin H, Melki V, Bessieres-Lacombe S, et al. Comparison of continuous subcutaneous insulin infusion and multiple daily injection regimens using insulin lispro in type 1 diabetic patients on intensified treatment. A randomized study. Diabetes Care 2000;23:1232–5.

[63] Rašlová K, Bogoev M, Raz I, et al. Insulin detemir and insulin aspart: a promising basal-bolus regimen for type 2 diabetes. Diabetes Res Clin Pract 2004;66:193–201.

[64] Raskin P, Guthrie RA, Leiter L, et al. Use of insulin aspart, a fast-acting insulin analog, as the mealtime insulin in the management of patients with type 1 diabetes. Diabetes Care 2000;23(5):583–8.

[65] Rosenstock J, Park G, Zimmerman J, for the U.S. Insulin Glargine (HOE 901) Type 1 Diabetes Investigator Group. Basal insulin glargine (HOE 901) versus NPH insulin in patients with type 1 diabetes on multiple daily insulin regimens. Diabetes Care 2000;23(8): 1137–42.

[66] Dickerson LM, Ye X, Sack JL, et al. Glycemic control in medical inpatients with type 2 diabetes mellitus receiving sliding scale insulin regimens versus routine diabetes medications: a multicenter randomized controlled trial. Ann Fam Med 2003;1(1):29–35.

[67] Rosenthal A, Skarbinski J, Masharani U. Endocrine. Available at: http://medicine.ucsf.edu/housestaff/handbook/HospH2002_C9.htm#_INSULIN_SLIDING_SCALE. Accessed August, 2006.

[68] Jacober SJ, Sowers JR. An update on perioperative management of diabetes. Arch Intern Med 1999;159(20):2405–11.

[69] Rafoth RJ. Standardizing sliding scale insulin orders. Am J Med Qual 2002;17(5):175–8.

[70] Alfonso A, Koops MK, Mong DP, et al. Glycemic control with regular versus lispro insulin sliding scales in hospitalized type 2 diabetics. J Diabetes Complications 2006; 20(3):153–7.

[71] Queale WS, Seidler AJ, Brancati FL. Glycemic control and sliding scale insulin use in medical inpatients with diabetes mellitus. Arch Intern Med 1997;157(5):545–52.

[72] Djakoure-Platonoff C, Radermercker R, Reach G, et al. Accuracy of the continuous glucose monitoring system in inpatient and outpatient conditions. Diabetes Metab 2003; 29(2 Pt 1):159–62.

[73] Golightly LK, Jones MA, Hamamura DH, et al. Management of diabetes mellitus in hospitalized patients: efficiency and effectiveness of sliding-scale insulin therapy. Pharmacotherapy 2006;26(10):1421–32.

[74] Cook CB, Boyle ME, Cisar NS, et al. Use of continuous subcutaneous insulin infusion (insulin pump) therapy in the hospital setting: proposed guidelines and outcome measures. Diabetes Educ 2005;31(6):849–57.

[75] Hoogwerf BJ. Perioperative management of diabetes mellitus: how should we act on the limited evidence? Cleve Clin J Med 2006;73(Suppl 1):S95–9.

[76] Clark JDA, Currie J, Hartog M. Management of diabetes in surgery: a survey of current practice by anaesthetists. Diabet Med 1992;9:271–4.

[77] Hirsch IB, McGill JB, Cryer PE, et al. Peri-operative management of surgical patients with diabetes mellitus. Anesthesiology 1991;74:346–59.

[78] Zaloya GP. Catecholamines in anesthetic and surgical stress. Int Anesthesiol Clin 1988;26: 187–98.

[79] Werb MR, Zinman B, Teasdale SJ, et al. Hormone and metabolic responses during coronary artery bypass surgery: role of infused glucose. J Clin Endocrinol Metab 1989; 69:1010–8.

[80] Monk TG, Mueller M, White PF. Treatment of stress response during balanced anesthesia. Anesthesiology 1992;76:39–45.

[81] Malmberg K. Prospective randomised study of intensive insulin treatment on long term survival after acute myocardial infarction in patients with diabetes mellitus. DIGAMI (Diabetes Mellitus, Insulin Glucose Infusion in Acute Myocardial Infarction) Study Group. BMJ 1997;314(7093):1512–5.

[82] Furnary AP, Gao G, Grunkemeier GL, et al. Continuous insulin infusion reduces mortality in patients with diabetes undergoing coronary artery bypass grafting. J Thorac Cardiovasc Surg 2003;125(5):1007–21.

[83] Zerr KJ, Furnary AP, Grunkemeier GL, et al. Glucose control lowers the risk of wound infection in diabetics after open heart operations. Ann Thorac Surg 1997;63: 356–61.

[84] Butler SO, Btaiche IF, Alaniz C. Relationship between hyperglycemia and infection in critically ill patients. Pharmacotherapy 2005;25(7):963–76.

[85] Black CT, Hennessey PJ, Andrassy RJ. Short-term hyperglycemia depresses immunity through nonenzymatic glycosylation of circulating immunoglobulin. J Trauma 1990;30: 830–3.

[86] Hruska LA, Smith JM, Hendy MP, et al. Continuous insulin infusion reduces infectious complications in diabetics following coronary surgery. J Card Surg 2005;20:403–7.

[87] Rehman H, Mohammed K. Perioperative management of diabetic patients. Curr Surg 2003;60(6):607–11.
[88] Petrauskiene V, Falk M, Waernbaum I, et al. The risk of venous thromboembolism is markedly elevated in patients with diabetes. Diabetologia 2005;48:1017–21.
[89] Kannel WB, McGee DL. Diabetes and glucose tolerance as risk factors for cardiovascular diseases: the Framingham study. Diabetes Care 1979;2:120–6.
[90] Partamian JO, Bradley RF. Acute myocardial infarction in 258 cases of diabetes: immediate mortality and five year survival. N Engl J Med 1965;273:455–61.
[91] Asplund K, Hagg E, Helmers C, et al. The natural history of stroke in diabetic patients. Acta Med Scand 1980;207:417–24.
[92] Jones EW, Mitchell JRA. Venous thrombosis in diabetes mellitus. Diabetologia 1983;25:502–5.
[93] Tsai AW, Cushman M, Rosamond WD, et al. Cardiovascular risk factors and venous thromboembolism incidence: the longitudinal investigation of thromboembolism etiology. Arch Intern Med 2002;162:1182–9.
[94] Humar A, Johnson EM, Gillingham KJ, et al. Venous thromboembolic complications after kidney and kidney–pancreas transplantation. Transplantation 1998;65:229–34.
[95] Kikura M, Takada T, Sato S. Preexisting morbidity as an independent risk factor for perioperative acute thromboembolism syndrome. Arch Surg 2005;140:1210–7.
[96] Mizel MS, Temple HT, Michelson JD, et al. Thromboembolism after foot and ankle surgery. A multicenter study. Clin Orthop Relat Res 1998;348:180–5.
[97] Solis G, Saxby T. Incidence of DVT following surgery of the foot and ankle. Foot Ankle Int 2002;23(5):411–4.
[98] Slaybaugh RS, Beasley BD, Massa EG. Deep venous thrombosis risk assessment, incidence, and prophylaxis in foot and ankle surgery. Clin Podiatr Med Surg 2003;20(2):269–89.
[99] Parkes DG, Pittner R, Jodka C, et al. Insulinotropic actions of exendin-4 and glucagon-like peptide-1 in vivo and in vitro. Metabolism 2001;50:583–9.
[100] Nauck MA, Wollschlager D, Werner J, et al. Effects of subcutaneous glucagon-like peptide 1 (GLP-1 [7-36 amide]) in patients with NIDDM. Diabetologia 1996;39:1546–53.
[101] Caremark: RxPipeline Insider. Available at: www.rxpipelineinsider.com. Accessed August 9, 2006.
[102] Ahren B, Simonsson E, Larsson H, et al. Inhibition of dipeptidyl peptidase IV improves metabolic control over a 4-week study period in type II diabetes. Diabetes Care 2002;25:869–75.
[103] Kruger DF, Gloster MA. Pramlintide for the treatment of insulin-requiring diabetes mellitus. Drugs 2004;64:1419–32.
[104] Hollander PA, Levy P, Fineman MS, et al. Pramlintide as an adjunct to insulin therapy improves long-term glycemic and weight control in patients with type 2 diabetes. Diabetes Care 2003;26:784–90.
[105] Uwaifo GI, Ratner RE. Novel pharmacologic agents for type 2 diabetes. Endocrinol Metab Clin North Am 2005;34:155–97.
[106] Scheen A. Late breaking clinical trials. Presented at the 65th Scientific Sessions of the ADA. San Diego, June 10–14, 2005.
[107] Pi-Sunyer FX, Aronne LJ, Heshmati HM, et al. RIO-North America Study Group. Effect of rimonabant, a cannabinoid-1 receptor blocker, on weight and cardiometabolic risk factors in overweight or obese patients: RIO-North America: a randomized controlled trial. JAMA 2006;295(7):761–75.
[108] Crane CW, Luntz GR. Absorption of insulin from the human small intestine. Diabetes 1968;17:625–7.
[109] Walter A. Drug Topics. Available at: http://www.drugtopics.com/drugtopics/article/articleDetail.jsp?id=367627. Accessed September 5, 2006.

[110] Davis SS. Overcoming barriers to the oral administration of peptide drugs. Trends Pharmacol Sci 1990;11:353–5.

[111] Exubera [package insert]. New York, NY: Pfizer; 2006.

[112] Barclay L. Exubera approved despite initial lung function concerns. Available at: http://www.medscape.com/viewarticle/523294?rss. Medscape Medical News Accessed May 1, 2006.

[113] Freed S. Exubera update: lungs, bioavailability and hypoglycemia. Available at: http://www.diabetesincontrol.com/modules.php?name=News&file=article&sid=3481. Accessed August 14, 2006.

[114] Norwood P, Dumas R, England RD, et al. Exubera Phase 3 Study Group. Inhaled insulin (Exubera) achieves tight glycemic control and is well tolerated in patients with type 1 diabetes. Program and abstracts of the European Association for the Study of Diabetes 41st Annual Meeting. Athens, Greece, September 12–15, 2005. Abstract 73.

[115] DeFronzo RA, Bergenstal RM, Cefalu WT, et al. Exubera Phase III Study Group. Efficacy of inhaled insulin in patients with type 2 diabetes not controlled with diet and exercise: a 12-week, randomized, comparative trial. Diabetes Care 2005;28(8):1922–8.

ELSEVIER
SAUNDERS

Clin Podiatr Med Surg
24 (2007) 191–222

CLINICS IN
PODIATRIC
MEDICINE AND
SURGERY

Obesity and Considerations in the Bariatric Surgery Patient

Aileen M. Takahashi, MD

*Association of South Bay Surgeons, 23451 Madison Street, Suite 340, Torrance,
CA 90505, USA*

Nearly 130 million adults in the United States are overweight or obese, accounting for 64% of the population [1]. Since 1980, the prevalence of obesity has increased by more than 75% [2]. Adults are not the only individuals affected by this disease. In children and adolescents, obesity has nearly doubled over the last 30 years to total nearly one fourth of this population [3]. There is a clear association between obesity and medical problems including diabetes, hypertension, cardiovascular disease, and shortened longevity. Significant weight loss, however, can reduce these risks and improve the morbidity and mortality associated with obesity. In response to the rising trend in the American population's weight, the number of surgical weight loss or bariatric procedures increased from 13,365 in 1998 to 72,177 in 2002 and to an estimated 140,000 procedures in 2005 [4]. This explosion is in part supported by the advent of minimally invasive surgery, with the annual rate of laparoscopic bariatric surgery during this same period increasing 44-fold [5].

Most physicians have encountered someone in their practice who is morbidly obese or who has had bariatric surgery. These patients are multifaceted, with comorbidities that may be undertreated or not yet identified, further complicating their operative risk. The purpose of this article is to provide a clinical definition of morbid obesity and to discuss its associated medical and economic impact. Surgical options currently available for the treatment of morbid obesity are reviewed, including expected success rates and potential risks and side effects. The preoperative workup of the morbidly obese patient is described in relation to undergoing major surgery, and the long-term implications of bariatric surgery and massive weight loss are reviewed. By the end of this article, clinicians should not only be

E-mail address: asbs@southbaysurgeons.com

podiatric.theclinics.com

Table 1
"Ideal" weights for women

Height			Ideal weight		Multiplier (lb)		
Feet	Inches	Centimeters	Pounds	Kilograms	2X	2.5X	3X
4	10	147.3	115	52.2	230	287.5	345
4	11	149.9	117	53.1	234	292.5	351
5	0	152.4	119.5	54.2	239	298.7	358.5
5	1	154.9	122	55.3	244	305	366
5	2	157.5	125	56.7	250	312.5	375
5	3	160.0	128	58.1	256	320	384
5	4	162.6	131	59.4	262	327.5	393
5	5	165.1	134	60.8	268	335	402
5	6	167.6	137	62.1	274	342.5	411
5	7	170.2	140	63.5	280	350	420
5	8	172.7	143	64.9	286	357.5	429
5	9	175.3	146	66.2	292	365	438
5	10	177.8	149	67.6	298	372.5	447
5	11	180.3	152	68.9	304	380	456
6	0	182.9	155	70.3	310	387.5	465

Weights are middle values for medium frame.

aware of the challenges of morbidly obese patients but also feel comfortable caring for them in their podiatric practice.

Definition of morbid obesity

Morbid obesity is no longer considered a simple problem related to poor self-control. It is a chronic, lifelong, multifactorial disease of excessive fat

Table 2
"Ideal" weights for men

Height			Ideal weight		Multiplier (lb)		
Feet	Inches	Centimeters	Pounds	Kilograms	2X	2.5X	3X
5	2	157.5	136	61.7	272	340	408
5	3	160.0	138	62.6	276	345	414
5	4	162.6	140	63.5	280	350	420
5	5	165.1	142.5	64.6	290	362.5	435
5	6	167.6	145	65.8	274	342.5	411
5	7	170.2	149	67.6	298	372.5	447
5	8	172.7	151	68.5	302	377.5	453
5	9	175.3	154	69.8	308	385	462
5	10	177.8	157	71.2	314	392.5	471
5	11	180.3	160	72.6	320	400	480
6	0	182.9	163.5	74.2	327	408.7	490.5
6	1	185.4	167	75.7	334	417.5	501
6	2	188.0	171	77.6	342	427.5	513
6	3	190.5	174.5	79.2	349	436.2	523.5
6	4	193.0	179	81.2	358	447.5	537

Weights are middle values for medium frame.

storage. More objectively, the National Institutes of Health (NIH) defines it as being 100 lb over ideal body weight (based on the 1999 Metropolitan Life Table) (Tables 1 and 2) or having a body mass index (BMI) greater than 40 kg/m^2. A BMI as low as 35 kg/m^2 also meets the "morbid" criteria for morbid

Body Mass Index (BMI)

	4'8"	4'9"	4'10"	4'11"	5'0"	5'1"	5'2"	5'3"	5'4"	5'5"	5'6"	5'7"	5'8"	5'9"	5'10"	5'11"	6'0"	6'1"	6'2"	6'3"	6'4"	6'5"	6'6"
200	45	43	42	41	39	38	37	36	34	33	32	31	30	30	29	28	27	26	26	25	24	24	23
205	46	44	43	42	40	39	38	36	35	34	33	32	31	30	29	29	28	27	26	26	25	24	24
210	47	46	44	43	41	40	39	37	36	35	34	33	32	31	30	29	29	28	27	26	26	25	24
215	48	47	45	44	42	41	39	38	37	36	35	34	33	32	31	30	29	28	28	27	26	26	25
220	49	48	46	45	43	42	40	39	38	37	36	35	34	33	32	31	30	29	28	28	27	26	25
225	51	49	47	46	44	43	41	40	39	38	36	35	34	33	32	31	31	30	29	28	27	27	26
230	52	50	48	47	45	44	42	41	40	38	37	36	35	34	33	32	31	30	30	29	28	27	27
235	53	51	49	48	46	45	43	42	40	39	38	37	36	35	34	33	32	31	30	29	28	28	27
240	54	52	50	49	47	45	44	43	41	40	39	38	37	36	35	34	33	32	31	30	29	29	28
245	55	53	51	50	48	46	45	44	42	41	40	38	37	36	35	34	33	32	32	31	30	29	28
250	56	54	52	51	49	47	46	44	43	42	40	39	38	37	36	35	34	33	32	31	31	30	29
255	57	55	53	52	50	48	47	45	44	43	41	40	39	38	37	36	35	34	33	32	31	30	30
260	58	56	54	53	51	49	48	46	45	43	42	41	40	39	37	36	35	34	33	33	32	31	30
265	60	58	56	54	52	50	49	47	46	44	43	42	41	40	38	37	36	35	34	33	32	32	31
270	61	59	57	55	53	51	50	48	46	45	44	42	41	40	39	38	37	36	35	34	33	33	31
275	62	60	58	56	54	52	50	49	47	46	45	43	42	41	40	38	37	36	35	34	34	33	32
280	63	61	59	57	55	53	51	50	48	47	45	44	43	41	40	39	38	37	36	35	34	33	32
285	64	62	60	58	56	54	52	51	49	48	46	45	43	42	41	40	39	38	37	36	35	34	33
290	65	63	61	59	57	55	53	52	50	48	47	46	44	43	42	41	40	39	38	37	36	35	34
295	66	64	62	60	58	56	54	52	51	49	48	46	45	44	42	41	40	39	38	37	36	35	34
300	67	65	63	61	59	57	55	53	52	50	49	47	46	44	43	42	41	39	39	38	37	36	35
305	69	66	64	62	60	58	56	54	52	51	49	48	47	45	44	43	41	40	39	38	37	36	35
310	70	67	65	63	61	59	57	55	53	52	50	49	47	46	45	43	42	41	40	39	38	37	36
315	71	68	66	64	62	60	58	56	54	53	51	49	48	47	45	44	43	42	41	39	38	37	37
320	72	69	67	65	63	61	59	57	55	53	52	50	49	47	46	45	44	42	41	40	39	38	37
325	73	71	68	66	64	62	60	58	56	54	53	51	50	48	47	45	44	43	42	41	40	39	38
330	74	72	69	67	65	63	61	59	57	55	53	52	50	49	47	46	45	44	42	41	40	39	38
335	75	73	70	68	66	63	61	60	58	56	54	53	51	50	48	47	46	44	43	42	41	40	39
340	76	74	71	69	67	64	62	60	59	57	55	53	52	50	49	48	46	45	44	43	41	40	39
345	78	75	72	70	68	65	63	61	59	58	56	54	53	51	50	48	47	46	44	43	42	41	40
350	79	76	73	71	69	66	64	62	60	58	57	55	53	52	50	49	48	46	45	44	43	42	41
355	80	77	74	72	70	67	65	63	61	59	57	56	54	53	51	50	48	47	46	44	43	42	41
360	81	78	75	73	71	68	66	64	62	60	58	57	55	53	52	50	49	48	46	45	44	43	42
365	82	79	76	74	71	69	67	65	63	61	59	57	56	54	53	51	50	48	47	46	45	43	42
370	83	80	78	75	72	70	68	66	64	62	60	58	56	55	53	52	50	49	48	46	45	44	43
375	84	81	79	76	73	71	69	67	65	63	61	59	57	55	54	52	51	50	48	47	46	45	43
380	85	82	80	77	74	72	70	67	65	63	62	60	58	56	55	53	52	50	49	48	46	45	44
385	87	84	81	78	75	73	71	68	66	64	62	60	59	57	55	54	52	51	50	49	47	46	45
390	88	85	82	79	76	74	72	69	67	65	64	62	60	58	57	55	53	52	50	49	48	46	45
395	89	86	83	80	77	75	72	70	68	66	64	62	60	58	57	55	54	52	51	50	48	47	46
400	90	87	84	81	78	76	73	71	69	67	65	63	61	59	58	56	54	53	51	50	49	48	46
405	91	88	85	82	79	77	74	72	70	68	66	64	62	61	59	57	55	54	53	51	50	48	47
410	92	89	86	83	80	78	75	73	71	68	66	64	63	61	59	57	56	54	53	51	50	49	48
415	93	90	87	84	81	79	76	74	71	69	67	65	63	61	60	58	56	55	53	52	51	49	48
420	94	91	88	85	82	80	77	75	72	70	68	66	64	62	60	59	57	56	54	53	51	50	49
425	96	92	89	86	83	81	78	75	73	71	69	67	65	63	61	59	58	56	55	53	52	51	49
430	97	93	90	87	84	81	79	76	74	72	70	68	66	64	62	60	58	57	55	54	52	51	50
435	98	94	91	88	85	82	80	77	75	73	70	68	66	64	63	61	59	58	56	55	53	52	50
440	99	95	92	89	86	83	81	78	76	73	71	69	67	65	63	62	60	58	57	55	54	52	51
445	100	97	93	90	87	84	82	79	77	74	72	70	68	66	64	62	61	59	57	56	54	53	52
450	101	98	94	91	88	85	83	80	77	75	73	71	69	67	65	63	61	60	58	56	55	54	52
455	102	99	95	92	89	86	83	81	78	76	74	71	69	67	65	64	62	60	59	57	56	54	53
460	103	100	96	93	90	87	84	82	79	77	74	72	70	68	66	64	63	61	59	58	56	55	53
465	105	101	97	94	91	88	85	83	80	78	75	73	71	69	67	65	63	62	60	58	57	55	54
470	106	102	98	95	92	89	86	83	81	78	76	74	72	70	68	66	64	62	61	59	57	56	54
475	107	103	100	96	93	90	87	84	82	79	77	75	73	70	68	66	65	63	61	60	58	56	55
480	108	104	101	97	94	91	88	85	83	80	78	75	73	71	69	67	65	64	62	60	59	57	56
485	109	105	102	98	95	92	89	86	83	81	78	76	74	72	70	68	66	64	63	61	59	58	56
490	110	106	103	99	96	93	90	87	84	82	79	77	75	73	71	69	67	65	63	61	61	59	57
495	111	107	104	100	97	94	91	88	85	83	80	78	75	73	71	69	67	65	64	62	60	59	59

Fig. 1. Body mass index chart. (*Courtesy of* Ethicon Endo-Surgery, Inc. All rights reserved; with permission.)

obesity when severe obesity-related comorbidities such as hypertension or dyslipidemia are present. BMI is calculated as weight in kilograms divided by height in meters squared (Fig. 1). As BMI increases, so do the incidences of medical and surgical illnesses. The percentage of obese persons in the United States increased from 14.5% during 1976 to 1980 to 22.5% during 1988 to 1994 [2] and is continuing to increase. Part of this explosion is due to ready access to high-fat, high-calorie processed foods; a trend toward larger portions; and lack of exercise. Fast-food industries taking over food service operations at schools and the abundance of vending machines on campus promote excessive calorie intake among children and adolescents. The convenience of drive-through businesses and access to escalators and moving walkways contribute to a lack of physical activity. Sedentary pastimes such as computer-based activities, video games, and watching television expend little energy. The number of hours watching television directly correlates with BMI scores, further illustrating the effect of inactivity [6].

Other factors contributing to morbid obesity include mental and psychologic disorders, medications, mobility issues, and other environmental and hereditary influences. Hormonal imbalances such as hypothyroidism or Cushing's disease, or genetic defects like Prader-Willi syndrome contribute to only a minority of obesity cases.

The medical impact of morbid obesity

Morbidity and mortality rise sharply with increasing weight, beginning at a BMI of 30 [7,8], with the risk of death doubling in individuals who have a BMI greater than 35 (Table 3) [9,10]. Early death results from complications of diabetes, cardiovascular and cerebrovascular disorders, pulmonary disease, and various cancers, and these risks are proportional to the duration of obesity (Box 1). The location of excess fat distribution has also been found to be an important predictor of morbidity in the obese. Central or abdominal obesity, defined as a high waist-to-hip circumference ratio, is associated with higher risks of death and serious illness [7,8,11–13]. Ischemic cardiac disease is especially prevalent in the presence of central obesity. It has been hypothesized that central adipose tissue is more metabolically active than peripheral fat and that these breakdown products directly enter the portal circulation. Fat metabolism leads to metabolic imbalance and an increased incidence of dyslipidemias, glucose intolerance, diabetes, and increased mortality from ischemic cardiac disease [7,8,14]. In addition, adipose tissue can produce cortisol and angiotensin II, further contributing to cardiovascular risks related to obesity [15].

Cardiovascular disease

The NIH reported in 1996 that nearly 70% of diagnosed cardiovascular disease is obesity related [16], and in 1997, the American Heart Association

Table 3
Body mass index and mortality risk

BMI	Classification	Mortality risk
20	Normal	—
27 (20% overweight)	Overweight	Mortality increases sharply
		10% increase in death from stroke
35 (40% overweight)	Obese	55% increase in mortality from all causes
		70% increase in coronary artery disease
		75% increase in stroke
		400% increase in mortality from diabetes
40 (60% overweight)	Morbidly obese	2 to 12 fold increase in total mortality depending on age and severity of obesity
		Greater than twofold increase in mortality due to cerebrovascular disease
		cardiovascular disease
		diabetes

Data from Refs. [8,10,25].

announced that obesity is an independent modifiable cardiovascular risk factor. Hypertension is six times more likely to occur in obese individuals [8]. Cardiac output and blood volume rises with increasing weight to perfuse the additional body tissue, contributing to cardiac hypertrophy, which is characteristic of obesity-induced hypertension. Hyperinsulinemia and insulin resistance, also prevalent in the obese, may contribute to sodium retention through activation of the sympathetic nervous system and vasopressor activity of norepineprine and angiotensin II [17]. As cardiac hypertrophy progresses, the left ventricle is less compliant. With the additional blood volume, this decrease in compliance may lead to cardiac failure.

Not only is obesity an independent risk factor for ischemic disease but diabetes, dyslipidemia, and hypertension also contribute to the problem. Cardiac arrhythmias may develop from hypoxemic or hypercarbic episodes during apneic events inherent to the increased incidence of sleep apnea in the obese and from electrolyte disturbances from diuretic therapy, cardiac hypertrophy, and fatty infiltration of the conduction system.

The extent of cardiovascular impairment in morbidly obese individuals may not be apparent on the surface because overall, these individuals are less mobile and may not be active enough to experience symptoms of cardiac insufficiency. Aggressive preoperative evaluation in any morbidly obese patient to look for evidence of hypertension, dyslipidemias, ischemic cardiac disease, or cardiomyopathy is necessary to prevent anesthetic catastrophes.

Diabetes

The prevalence of type 2 diabetes mellitus, or non–insulin-dependent diabetes mellitus, has paralleled the rise in obesity in the United States. Nearly

Box 1. Medical conditions associated with morbid obesity

Cardiovascular
Hypertension
Dyslipidemia
Congestive heart failure
Ischemic heart disease
Sudden cardiac death
Obesity cardiomyopathy

Pulmonary
Restrictive disease
Dyspnea on exertion
Obstructive sleep apnea
Obesity hypoventilation syndrome
Pulmonary hypertension

Endocrine
Insulin resistance
Diabetes
Hypothyroidism
Hypogonadism and impotence
Menstrual irregularities and infertility
Polycystic ovarian syndrome
Hirsuitism
Gynecomastia

Gastrointestinal
Gallstones
Reflux and hiatal hernias
Pancreatitis
Fatty liver
Nonalcoholic steatohepatitis and cirrhosis

Genitourinary
End-stage renal disease
Urinary stress incontinence

Immunologic
Impaired wound healing
Impaired immune response

Musculoskeletal
Osteoarthritis
Low back pain and disc herniation
Gout

Integumentary
Venous stasis
Deep venous thrombosis and pulmonary embolism
Cellulitis
Panniculitis
Postoperative wound infections

Neurologic
Pseudotumor cerebri
Cerebrovascular event

Malignancy
Colon and rectal cancer
Renal cell cancer
Prostate cancer
Breast, ovarian, and endometrial cancer

Psychologic
Depression
Migraine headaches
Social isolation
Lack of professional advancement

80% of patients who have type 2 diabetes mellitus are obese [18]. In one study, a gain in abdominal fat was positively associated with an increased risk of type 2 diabetes mellitus, independent of weight change [15]. Insulin normally drives blood glucose into cells and stimulates the liver to convert calories into their storable form. When a nondiabetic individual consumes excess calories and gains weight, the body becomes increasingly resistant to insulin and elevated blood glucose levels. Higher levels of insulin production are required to maintain normal glucose levels; however, eventually the pancreas is unable to keep up with the demand, resulting in lower levels of blood insulin despite high glucose levels and, thus, non–insulin-dependent diabetes mellitus [19]. Pediatric and adolescent diabetes have traditionally been attributed to type 1 diabetes mellitus, or juvenile-onset diabetes mellitus, which is the result of a lack of insulin production from pancreatic islet cells. As the prevalence of obesity has increased in this population, so has the number of new cases of type 2 diabetes mellitus. In 1990, less than 4% of newly diagnosed pediatric cases of diabetes was type 2; however, in 2000, that proportion has increased by 500% [20]. These individuals are invariably obese.

In the pediatric and adult populations, modest sustained weight loss can increase insulin sensitivity and lower blood glucose and insulin levels [21]. An estimated 10-kg weight loss can eliminate the 35% reduction in life expectancy seen in type 2 diabetes mellitus [19].

Metabolic syndrome describes a cluster of metabolic disorders that predisposes individuals to atherosclerotic disease and diabetes. Components of the syndrome include abdominal obesity (waist circumference greater than 40 inches for men and 35 inches for women), hypertension, abnormal cholesterol levels such as elevated triglycerides or low high-density lipoprotein cholesterol, and insulin resistance [22]. Having at least three of these conditions meets criteria for the syndrome. A prothrombotic state with elevated fibrinogen or plasminogen activator inhibitor-1 and a proinflammatory state defined as an elevated C-reactive protein have also been described. Having at least three of the primary criteria indicates metabolic syndrome, putting these individuals at increased risk of coronary heart disease, cerebrovascular accidents, peripheral vascular disease, and diabetes. One study found that total and cardiovascular mortality risk was increased by 40% to 60% in the presence of metabolic syndrome [23].

Pulmonary disease and obstructive sleep apnea

Approximately 76% of morbidly obese patients have obstructive sleep apnea (OSA). Complications related to prolonged disease can be deadly, especially when challenged with such stresses as general anesthesia. OSA is caused by the collapse of the pharyngeal airway as muscle tone is lost during sleep. With the airway narrowed, snoring results and can at times be completely obstructive, resulting in brief episodes of oxygen desaturation. Hypercapnia and acidosis stimulate an increase in inspiratory drive, which typically awakens the individual and restores pharyngeal muscle tone. This cycle is repeated multiple times throughout the night. Alcohol and drugs that decrease the respiratory drive further exacerbate the problem. Initially, inspiration is driven by hypercarbia, but eventually, with desensitization, hypoxia becomes the primary drive. Over time, polycythemia develops in response to chronic hypoxia, increasing the risk of ischemic heart and cerebrovascular disease. Hypoxic episodes may also contribute to cardiac arrhythmias. Morning headaches are common and are due to nocturnal carbon dioxide retention and cerebral vasodilation. More significantly, chronic episodes of hypoxia cause pulmonary vasoconstriction and contribute to right heart failure [14]. Polysomnography, or sleep studies, can diagnose OSA, and if present, respiratory support by way of continuous positive airway pressure (CPAP) can be prescribed and titrated to effect. Most individuals on CPAP report that their sleep is more restful and that they are able to be more productive during waking hours.

Cancer risk

Cancer risk is higher in obese individuals. Compared with their nonobese counterparts, obese males have a higher mortality from cancer of the colon [24] and rectum. Men who are greater than 130% of their ideal weight are

twice more likely to die from prostate cancer [8]. In addition, postmenopausal obese women demonstrate a higher mortality from cancer of the gallbladder, biliary tract, uterus, ovaries, and breast [9,25].

Other medical conditions

Other medical problems related to or exacerbated by obesity include gallstones, liver disease, hiatal hernias and reflux, osteoarthritis, gout, recurrent
skin infections, urinary stress incontinence, female infertility, chronic venous
stasis, and deep venous thrombosis (DVT) [3,26]. Idiopathic intracranial
hypertension, or pseudotumor cerebri, is another disease associated with
obesity and increased intra-abdominal pressure and can lead to blindness.
Nonalcoholic fatty liver disease is widely prevalent among the obese. It is
typically a benign condition; however, nonalcoholic steatohepatitis (NASH)
represents inflammatory disease with risk of development of fibrosis of the
liver parenchyma and eventually cirrhosis and liver failure. Obesity is seen in
greater than 70% of NASH patients, and up to 75% have diabetes. The
progression of liver disease is often asymptomatic until advanced disease
has developed. Which patients progress from the benign disease to NASH
is unknown; however, diabetes, like obesity, is closely linked [27].

There is a significant relationship between obesity and depression [28].
Depression can be related to body image, isolation, dissatisfaction with re-
lationships, and discrimination in social and professional environments. The
inability to sit in booths at restaurants or fit into airline seats or being over-
looked for job promotions may contribute to an already low self-esteem. It
is ironic and unfortunate that food is often used as a comfort measure in
these situations, further exacerbating the original problem.

Effects on longevity

Lastly, obesity shortens life expectancy by 10 to 15 years. Even modest
elevations in weight increase the risk of death. When a person is overweight
and 50 years old, there is a 20% to 40% increase in the risk of death compared with individuals of the same age at normal weight. The correlation of
mortality and weight is steeper in men and women under age 50 years compared with older individuals [11], which emphasizes the need to intervene in
these younger individuals because there is the greatest potential to make
a significant impact.

The socioeconomic impact of morbid obesity

In 1999, the total health care costs of treating obese United States adults
reached $238 billion, and similar health care costs have been reported in
Canada, Australia, and France [3]. Morbidly obese patients cost more to
treat compared with nonobese patients. In Northern California, Kaiser-

Permanente looked at the health care costs of all members over a 1-year period and found that the annual costs of treating morbidly obese versus nonobese patients was 44% more per year [29]. Studies indicate that most direct
health care costs of obesity are from hypertension, cardiovascular disease,
and diabetes.

Modifications required to treat morbidly obese patients within the health
care system are also significant. Hospitals require larger gowns, blood pressure cuffs, beds, reinforced chairs, and wheelchairs. Structural changes include larger doorways, wider halls, and floor-mounted toilets. Nurses and
hospital staff require specialized training to move these patients. Within
the health care system, almost 85% of back injuries result from lifting heavy
patients [30]. This socioeconomic burden includes loss of productivity not
only of the obese patient but also of the injured health care provider (and
thus pay-out from workman's compensation insurance). One group-
purchasing survey found that 51% of hospitals have seen a decrease in
workplace injuries since making equipment modifications and providing
specialized training to care for bariatric patients [30]. "Sensitivity" training
is also needed for all health care providers within the hospital system to promote polite, respectful, and sensitive care.

Currently, most radiology departments have significant limitations in imaging the obese patient and will ultimately need to make appropriate and
expensive modifications. Most fluoroscopy tables are unable to accommo-
date weights greater than 300 lb. Often CT scanners and MRI tables do
not have heavy-duty motors to move the patients into the imaging machines. When weight is not an issue, girth may prevent entrance into the
imaging equipment. Open MRI imaging, although more expensive, may
provide one answer to imaging difficulties.

The impact of bariatric surgery

Sustained weight loss significantly reduces morbidity and mortality associated with obesity. Even as little as 10% weight loss can significantly lower
blood pressure and improve lipid profiles and insulin sensitivity. Individuals
greater than 100 pounds over the ideal body weight are a unique population,
and dietary changes and exercise alone are usually not enough. In most cases,
any weight lost is not maintained and these individuals rebound and gain even
more weight than originally lost. Most morbidly obese patients presenting for
weight loss surgery report they have lost hundreds of pounds over the years
but were unable to keep it off. The 1992 to 1996 NIH Consensus compared dieting alone against surgical intervention for weight loss and found that both
groups lost weight initially, but that after 2 years, the diet-alone group had re-
gained the weight lost, whereas the surgical-treatment group maintained medically significant weight loss. The NIH concluded that surgery is the only tool
available for sustained and effective long-term weight loss [16].

Effective bariatric surgery is defined as sustained excess weight loss of greater than 50% and resolution of comorbid conditions. Improvement or resolution of obesity-related comorbidities in association with weight loss after bariatric surgery has been significant. Resolution of diabetes has been reported in as high as 77% to 83% [31–34]. Pories and colleagues reported that 99% of patients who had glucose impairment were able to maintain normal levels of plasma glucose, glycosylated hemoglobin, and insulin for an average of 7.6 years. Normalization of glucose metabolism occurred within days of surgery, before significant weight loss, and was durable even if patients remained above their ideal body weight after surgery [33]. Resolution of hypertension has been reported in 60% to 74% [32,35]. In addition to diabetes and hypertension, surgically induced weight loss has corrected or alleviated hyperlipidemia (>70%) [34], OSA (86%) [34], arthritis, and infertility [31]. Improvements are not limited to medical conditions; quality-of-life questionnaires have reported that 58% of respondents believe their quality of life is "greatly improved" and 37% report quality of life as "improved" [31]. Improvements in comfort, mobility, social involvement, sexual functioning, self-confidence, and self-esteem are added benefits of massive weight loss after bariatric surgery. Productivity also has the potential to improve, with reports of unemployment rates decreasing from 80% to 53% in postoperative patients [36]. Increased life expectancy is another potential benefit. Christou and colleagues [37] studied gastric bypass patients over 5 years and reported a mean percentage excess weight loss of 67% and significant reductions in risk for cardiovascular disease, cancer, type 2 diabetes mellitus, respiratory conditions, and psychiatric disorders. Mortality in the bariatric surgery cohort was 0.68% over 5 years compared with 6.17% in controls; the reduction in relative risk of death was 89% ($P < .001$).

An historical overview of bariatric surgery

Surgical intervention for sustained weight loss arose in the 1950s. Even at that time, it was obvious that morbidly obese individuals were refractory to diet and available drug therapies. Initial operations were based on clinical experience gained with management of short-gut syndrome patients. In these patients, the total absorptive surface area is massively reduced, resulting in malabsorption of nutrients and significant amounts of weight loss. Pioneers in bariatric surgery took this experience and applied it to morbidly obese patients. One of the first procedures was the jejunoileal bypass, which consisted of transecting the small bowel at the proximal jejunum and anastomosing it to the terminal ileum. The bypassed bowel was not removed but was separately anastomosed to the cecum to prevent a closed loop segment. With most of the small bowel diverted, weight loss ensued but so did significant degrees of diarrhea, malnutrition, and electrolyte disturbances.

Multiple complications developed from the defunctionalized small bowel. Bacterial overgrowth and translocation through the atrophic small bowel into the portal venous system resulted in acute hepatic failure and, at times, cirrhosis and death. As serious complications with the jejunoileal bypass became apparent, the second generation of bypass procedures was developed. The biliopancreatic diversion (BPD) was introduced by Dr. Nicola Scopinaro in 1979 and eliminated the risk of defunctionalized bowel by keeping this limb intact with the biliopancreatic outflow. Multiple modifications have been made since its initial introduction; however, it remains the most accepted malabsorptive procedure.

In 1966, Dr. Edward Mason at the University of Iowa presented the gastric bypass in an attempt to rely less on malabsorption for sustained weight loss. By limiting the size of the resected stomach or gastric "pouch," food would pass slower, providing prolonged satiety. In addition, a significant length of small bowel was bypassed to provide a limited component of malabsorption. Since then, the size of the pouch, the outlet of the pouch, the length of the roux limb, and antecolic versus retrocolic passage of the roux limb are some of the modifications that have been fine-tuned to provide optimal weight loss while limiting complication risks. The gastric bypass, performed laparoscopically, remains the most common bariatric procedure performed in the United States today.

The advent of surgical stapling devices led to "gastric stapling" procedures in the 1970s. These procedures were attempts to reduce the long-term effects of malabsorption and to create a safer, more physiologic procedure. Gastric stapling procedures were purely restrictive and based on limiting the gastric pouch and outlet. The vertical banded gastroplasty (VBG) was an example of these procedures.

In the 1990s, stapling devices were further modified for use in laparoscopic surgery, thus expanding the bariatric surgery frontier. Traditionally, the only option to perform these procedures was with a supraumbilical laparotomy incision. Wound infections, incisional hernias, adhesions, and cosmesis were difficult. Since the advent of laparoscopy, these issues have significantly changed. Performing the surgery by video guidance using long instruments accessed through multiple small incisions allows faster recuperation times, fewer problems with wound healing and hernias, and overall, the body perceives the procedure as less stress [38]. Hospital stays are 2 to 3 days instead of 5 to 6 days. Comparing laparoscopic versus open gastric bypass, the wound infection rate is 1% versus 10% and the hernia rate is 0% versus 8% [39]. Overall, weight loss outcomes and resolution of obesity-related comorbidities are comparable between laparoscopic and open procedures. These outcomes have made these surgical procedures more attractive, and in some cases, they may be performed in an outpatient setting.

In June 2001, the Lap-Band system (Inamed Health, Santa Barbara, California) was released for use in the United States by the Food and Drug

Administration (FDA). Placed laparoscopically, it is purely restrictive and provides a reversible, adjustable means to significant weight loss. Although more common in European countries, its popularity in the United States is on the rise and will soon likely be placed more frequently than performing the gastric bypass.

Even with the various surgical options available, less than 10% of those eligible undergo surgical therapy. The reasons for this are multiple. Family physicians are not aware of or do not believe the reported benefits of bariatric surgery. Patients' fear of surgery and possible complications, family and societal disapproval, the previous "bad" reputation of bariatric surgery, and ignorance are also likely contributors. Some of these fears are not unfounded. The American Society of Bariatric Surgery (ASBS) and the American College of Surgeons (ACS) have tried to improve the delivery of bariatric surgery and have developed the concept of Centers of Excellence (COE) to direct patients to quality, competent, and safe programs. The ASBS founded the Surgical Review Corporation (www.surgicalreview.org) and the ACS founded the Bariatric Surgery Center Network Accreditation Program (www.facs.org) to which hospitals and surgeons voluntarily apply. The review includes evaluation of the surgeons' laparoscopic and bariatric experience and confirmation that a multidisciplinary approach is used involving psychologic, nutritional, pharmacologic, and nursing support. Preoperative classes and support group meetings are held to facilitate education about the lifestyle commitment and to promote realistic expectations. Hospitals must be properly equipped to care for the morbidly obese patient. Outcomes must be documented using a patient database. All of these issues are reviewed and when all criteria are met, the bariatric program and its surgeons receive accreditation. Currently, Medicare will not pay for patients to go to non-COE bariatric programs for their surgery, and many other insurance companies may soon follow.

Surgical options for weight loss

There are many surgical procedures available today to treat morbid obesity. The various options are typically described as malabsorptive, restrictive, or a combination of the two types of procedures. Malabsorptive procedures rely on bypassing significant amounts of bowel so that calories are not absorbed. Restrictive procedures are based on limiting calories taken in.

Malabsorptive procedures

The BPD and its variant with the duodenal switch (BPD+DS) is the primary malabsorptive procedure performed today (Fig. 2). In the BPD, approximately two thirds of the stomach is removed and a large amount of the small intestine is bypassed, creating a common channel of 50 to 75 cm in length. A long Roux-en-Y reconstruction results in delayed mixing of food in the "enteric limb" with digestive juices in the "biliopancreatic limb" until the common channel is reached. In one modification—maintaining the duodenum—the "duodenal switch" preserves the pylorus with the stomach and decreases the occurrence of dumping, which is a syndrome composed of nausea, vomiting, diarrhea, and tachycardia related to a large load of undigested food entering the small intestine. The BPD and the BPD+DS work primarily by malabsorption rather than by restriction. By minimizing the length of the common channel, digestion and absorption are delayed and weight loss ensues. This weight loss is based on malabsorption of calories not only from fat but also from protein. Stools are frequent and unusually malodorous. Malnutrition, vitamin deficiencies, and dehydration are common postoperative complications. Usually this operation is reserved for patients needing to lose several hundred pounds (ie, BMI >60). Reports of 80% excess weight loss at 2 years [40,41] and 91% at 5 years [40] have been reported, with a 9% morbidity rate and a 0.5% mortality rate [41]. Complications from malabsorption include anemia, bone demineralization, and protein malabsorption. Iron, calcium, vitamin D, vitamin B_{12}, and protein supplementation are required. Close follow-up with frequent laboratory checks is mandatory to prevent severe malnutrition. In some cases, a revision to lengthen the common channel may be necessary if there is significant

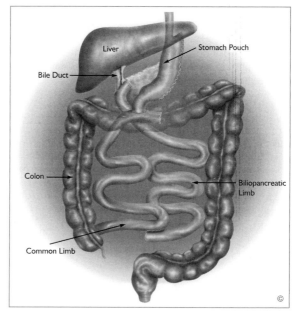

Fig. 2. Biliopancreatic diversion with duodenal switch. (*Courtesy of* Ethicon Endo-Surgery, Inc. All rights reserved; with permission.)

hypoproteinemia and protein/calorie malnutrition. Although typically performed through an "open" approach, some centers are able to perform the surgery laparoscopically. This is a much more complex and invasive procedure, requiring a longer period of recovery.

Restrictive procedures

Restrictive procedures are based on limiting the size of the stomach and its outlet. Previously, the vertical banded gastroplasty was the primary restrictive procedure (Fig. 3). The VBG involved stapling across the top portion of the stomach, making it smaller and limiting the outlet of the "new" stomach with mesh reinforcement. This procedure soon fell out of favor because it was not able to consistently induce or maintain weight loss due to the "pouch" or "stoma" enlarging in response to the restriction. Other causes of failure included mesh erosion and disruption of the staple line with the development of a gastrogastric fistula, both resulting in loss of the restrictive effect and regaining weight.

The laparoscopic adjustable gastric band (LAGB) has replaced the VBG as the restrictive procedure of choice (Fig. 4). Although only used in the United States for the last 5 years, it has been the most commonly performed

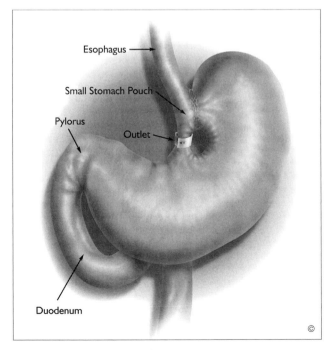

Fig. 3. Vertical banded gastroplasty. (*Courtesy of* Ethicon Endo-Surgery, Inc. All rights reserved; with permission.)

bariatric procedure in Australia and Sweden. Early United States reports with the LAGB were not as favorable, with more complications and reoperative rates as high as 41% [42]. A different surgical approach, along with modifications of the band itself, has led to a new era of the LAGB with comparable weight loss and complication rates. Placed laparoscopically, a silastic band with an inflatable inner balloon is placed around the top portion of the stomach. The balloon is connected to a port, which is placed subcutaneously on the abdominal wall and can be percutaneously accessed to size the outlet of the pouch. By adding saline to the port, the balloon is inflated and the pouch outlet is constricted. Over several adjustments, the band is inflated to provide restriction without dysphagia. Although the band can be adjusted to limit oral intake, there is also a true feeling of satiety that limits the patient's "food seeking" behavior. Success depends on the adjustability of the band and good communication between the patient and the bariatric surgeon. Weight loss with the band is gradual, with an expected loss of 1 to 2 pounds per week during the first 2 years. A plateau is usually seen by the third year. Excess weight loss of 40%, 53%, and 64% at 12, 24, and 48 months, respectively, has been reported [43]. The band is attractive to many patients who want surgical intervention but are afraid of their anatomy being changed forever. It is completely reversible and because no intestine is bypassed, there is no risk of vitamin malabsorption, protein deficiency, or dumping. Supplemental vitamins are typically recommended

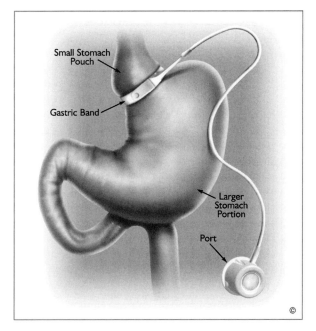

Fig. 4. Laparoscopic adjustable gastric band. (*Courtesy of* Ethicon Endo-Surgery, Inc. All rights reserved; with permission.)

in these patients because of their limited oral intake. Proceeding laparos-copically, the procedure can be performed with an overnight stay. Risks in-clude slippage (1%–3%), erosion (0.2%–0.6%), and port malfunction (1.2%–4.5%) [43,44]. Esophageal dilation seen during early trials with the LAGB was more a function of improper band adjustment and was com-pletely reversible with removal of saline from the band. Not all patients are candidates for the band. Because the band is a foreign body, those who have inflammatory bowel disease and connective tissue disorders may be at higher risk of erosion of the band.

Combined restrictive and malabsorptive procedures

The laparoscopic Roux-en-Y gastric bypass (LRYGB) uses restriction and malabsorption to achieve significant sustained weight loss. Currently, it is the most frequently performed bariatric procedure in the United States (Fig. 5). The top portion of the stomach is cut away to create a "pouch" 15 to 30 milliliters in size. The remnant stomach is left in its anatomic position, and approximately 100 cm of small bowel is bypassed. The alimentary limb consists of the gastrojejunostomy (pouch to small bowel) and approximately 100 cm of small bowel, whereas the biliopancreatic limb consists of the by-passed stomach, duodenum, and approximately 30 to 50 cm of small bowel. The enteroenterostomy (small bowel to small bowel anastomosis) rejoins

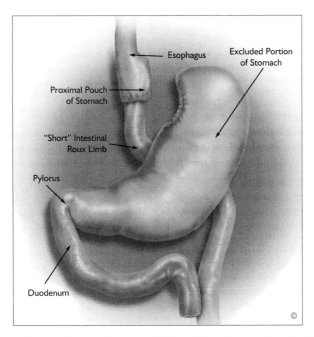

Fig. 5. Roux-en-Y gastric bypass. (*Courtesy of* Ethicon Endo-Surgery, Inc. All rights reserved; with permission.)

both limbs. Patients benefit from the restrictive component by feeling full earlier, and what they eat is not completely absorbed, thus reducing their calorie absorption. Over time, the pouch stretches out, but not usually to more than the size of a small orange. Success rates of 77% excess weight loss at 1 year have been reported, with most patients maintaining 60% excess weight loss after 10 to 14 years [45]. Mortality rates of 0.58% have been reported [46]. Similar to the BPD, risks include anastomotic leaks, dumping, bowel obstruction, and internal hernias. Vitamin and protein deficiencies may occur, but not to the same degree as in the more complex BPD. Unique to the LRYGB, the remnant stomach is left in its anatomic position; however, it is no longer accessible endoscopically, which may become significant in ulcer disease or cancer. A fistula may develop between the gastric pouch and the remnant stomach, resulting in failure to lose weight. In addition, obstruction of the biliopancreatic limb can cause distension of the remnant stomach as outflow becomes backed up. The patient may present with abdominal pain, but not the usual nausea and vomiting associated with pouch problems. If undiagnosed, severe gastric distension and even bowel and stomach necrosis can develop.

Because there are multiple surgical options for morbidly obese patients, their treatment must be individualized based on the extent of comorbidities, how much excess weight is to be lost, tolerance of anesthesia, surgical risks versus benefits, and personal preference. A multidisciplinary team can help morbidly obese individuals seeking surgical treatment choose the right operation. Despite which procedure they undergo, sensible dietary habits and exercise are still important components of success.

Preoperative preparation

The major motivating factor in this population is a concern over worsening health as related to rising weight. Previously healthy, a patient may now have developed weight-related comorbidities such as diabetes, hypertension, and weight-bearing joint pain. Morbidly obese patients often find that they no longer can keep up with their children and, at some point, have encountered an embarrassing social event such as not fitting into a theater seat or a booth in a public restaurant. Patients tend to fear early death and not being around for their loved ones. By the time patients present to a physician for bariatric surgery, they have usually committed to a lifestyle change that will finally allow them to have control over their bodies. They are looking for a "new lease on life." Bariatric surgery is an elective procedure and its success is based on proper patient education and commitment and the use of the surgery as a "tool" rather than a "quick fix."

Patients who may not be appropriate candidates for bariatric surgery include those who have portal hypertension; untreated mental illness such as schizophrenia, bipolar disease, and eating disorders; malignant hyperphagia as in Prader-Willi syndrome; and untreated addictions to alcohol, illicit drugs, or nicotine. Failure to follow instructions such as an inability to lose weight with physician-supervised programs, an inability to understand the lifestyle changes needed to take place to be successful after surgery, and hostility toward office staff are other characteristics of an unfavorable candidate. Patients at high risk for complications include those who have had previous gastric surgery or intestinal resection. Patients who have a history of lower abdominal procedures such as colon surgery may be more appropriate candidates for laparoscopic gastric banding because the upper abdomen should have minimal adhesions.

The process begins with a thorough interview to elicit the patient's medical history, previous weight loss attempts, current eating habits, and family and support structure. Documented weight loss with a medically supervised program, even if short-lived, is important in demonstrating that the individual is capable of following instructions. After a thorough physical is completed, a psychologist familiar with eating disorders performs an evaluation to identify any unresolved conflicts that may result in maladaptive eating behavior or self-sabotage after surgery. The psychologic evaluation is also used to determine the patient's appropriateness for surgery, whether the patient has realistic expectations, and to ensure that the individual is well informed, motivated, and has an intact support system. Some individuals may not be ideal candidates at initial presentation, but may become more appropriate after psychotherapy. Tobacco cessation is mandatory. Nutritional education and counseling is provided to help patients make better food choices and to encourage behavioral change, and instruction in an individualized exercise program is initiated. Laboratory serologies are obtained to look for endocrinologic reasons for obesity such as hypothyroidism and to document the baseline lipid profile, C-reactive protein level, and vitamin levels such as vitamins A and D. These levels can be further monitored as a means of assessing improvement. All patients are tested for *Helicobacter pylori* and, if found, treated because there is an increased ulcerogenic risk after surgery in untreated seropositive patients. An upper gastrointestinal study is performed, looking for hiatal hernias and documenting reflux, if present. Endoscopic evaluation is reserved for those who have a high suspicion of Barrett's esophagus, a precancerous condition, in the presence of a long history of gastroesophageal reflux. When patients report a history of symptoms suspicious for biliary lithiasis, an abdominal ultrasound is performed to confirm the presence of gallstones, in which case the gallbladder may be removed during the same operation. (Gallbladders and appendices are no longer routinely removed.)

Cardiac workup is based on the patient's suspicion for cardiac disease. All patients previously on phentermine-fenfluramine undergo echocardiography to look for valvular disease. An echocardiogram also provides information about wall motion (indicating a possible prior myocardial infarction if motion is poor), evaluation of right and left ventricular function, and pulmonary hypertension. Functional stress testing may be indicated in patients who have a prior history of myocardial infarction, congestive heart failure, angina, diabetes, and chronic renal insufficiency. Other risk factors to consider include advanced age, hypertension, tobacco use, and family history of heart disease. Many obese patients cannot tolerate a treadmill test. Dobutamine simulates the oxygen demands of exercise by increasing heart rate and contractility. Utilized as a stress echocardiogram, it can give information on potential ischemic areas and damaged cardiac muscle. Adenosine or persantine thallium stress tests are nuclear studies to simulate exercise and cause heterogeneity between segments of the heart with normal versus abnormal blood flow. Cardiac catheterization is performed in patients who have high-risk symptoms or significant degrees of ischemia on stress testing, and further interventions are based on the cardiologist's recommendations.

Pulmonary function tests are used when appropriate, and a baseline arterial blood gas is obtained to guide postoperative management. A carboxyhemoglobin level can also be obtained from the arterial blood gas to check patient compliance with smoking cessation. Patients are diligently screened for OSA and hypopnea syndromes and, if indicated, placed on CPAP.

In addition to the medical workup, patients attend support group meetings and education programs focusing on the new lifestyle changes they are to adopt to be successful in their weight loss. Appropriate social support is key to success. In addition, patients are often required to lose 10% to 20% of their weight preoperatively. Preoperative weight loss reflects an active exercise program and appropriate dietary changes. The weight loss promotes loss of intra-abdominal fat and shrinkage of the liver, especially the left lobe, which facilitates intraoperative exposure of the gastroesophageal junction.

Perioperative management

The perioperative management of the morbidly obese patient undergoing any major procedure should include these same guidelines. Surgical preparation for morbidly obese patients must include DVT and pulmonary embolism (PE) prophylaxis. Currently, there is no consensus or FDA-approved protocol, and prophylaxis is based on clinical experience. The author's program recommends withholding exogenous hormones (such as birth control pills) 6 weeks before and after surgery. A dose of 5000 units of heparin is injected subcutaneously on call to the operating room and continued three times a day postoperatively. Alternatively, 30 mg or 40 mg of enoxaparin (Lovenox) is used twice a day. Tedhose and thigh-high lower-extremity intermittent pneumatic compression stockings are placed before anesthesia induction and are continued in the postoperative period. Prophylaxis with

Lovenox is continued for 2 weeks postoperatively. If a patient already has a history of PE, then a temporary inferior vena cava filter should be placed preoperatively. Other high-risk patients include those who have a history of DVT, severe leg edema, or severe chronic venous stasis disease or those who are wheelchair bound.

Anesthetic management

Preoperative anesthesia consultation is recommended. A short neck, limited range of motion, redundant pharyngeal tissue, and a small mouth may limit airway management in the obese. OSA must be aggressively identified preoperatively because there is an approximate 13% incidence of difficult intubation in this population [14]. An experienced anesthesiologist is mandatory because fiberoptic awake intubation may be required in select cases.

After induction, obese patients typically desaturate quickly despite preoxygenation because they have increased oxygen consumption, restrictive pulmonary disease, and reduced functional residual capacity [14]. The supine position alone increases oxygen consumption, cardiac output, and pulmonary artery pressure. Chest wall compliance is restricted from the weight of the chest, and there is limited diaphragmatic motion from increased intra-abdominal pressure. Higher peak inspiratory pressures are needed to maintain ventilation. Trendelenberg positioning, if necessary, further restricts lung capacity.

In the morbidly obese, increases in blood volume, distribution, and cardiac output demand larger dosages of intravenous induction agents; however, intramuscular and subcutaneous injections of opioids and sedatives should be avoided because absorption is unreliable.

With the higher incidence of hiatal hernia and subsequent reflux seen in morbidly obese patients, precautions must be taken for aspiration. A combination of ketorolac (Toradol), ondansetron (Zofran), H_2 blockers, and metoclopramide (Reglan) is often used. Electrolyte disturbances from diuretic use should be suspected and ruled out preoperatively to prevent cardiac arrhythmias during induction. Most preoperative home medications should be continued except for oral hypoglycemic medications, insulin, and anticoagulants. Caution should be used with diuretics because they typically predispose the patient to overall fluid deficits, and angiotensin-converting enzyme inhibitors should be stopped the day before surgery secondary to the risk of profound hypotension during anesthesia [14].

Positioning, proper padding of the operating table, and minimizing anesthesia time is important in prevention of pressure sores, peripheral nerve injuries, and rhabdomyolysis due to pressure ischemia. Rhabdomyolysis is rare but can occur in the gluteal and lumbar areas. Risk factors include BMI greater than 50, long surgical duration, hypovolemia, and inadequate padding [47]. Aggressive hydration along with proper padding and reduction of anesthetic time minimize this risk. Increased intra-abdominal pressure compressing the inferior vena cava in the supine position can lead to hypotension from limited venous return. Consideration for a slight lateral decubitus position in nonabdominal surgery should be considered to shift the abdominal pannus and reduce intra-abdominal pressure.

Laparoscopic procedures, which increase already elevated intra-abdominal pressures and limit functional residual capacity, are actually well tolerated in the obese. Hypercapnia is present due to the carbon dioxide insufflation; however, further desaturation is not common. Increased minute ventilation is the primary means of correcting the hypercapnia; otherwise, there is an increased risk of acidosis and subsequent cardiac arrhythmias. After the insufflation is released, pulmonary compliance returns to baseline.

Pain management

Epidural anesthesia is an important consideration in "open" laparotomy incisions to facilitate pulmonary toilet, early mobilization, and minimal systemic narcotic usage. The combined use of opioids and local anesthetic is most effective in providing pain control safely with less drowsiness, nausea, and respiratory depression. Intramuscular injections are not recommended because inadvertently administered drugs to fatty tissue have variable uptake and distribution. When an epidural is unwarranted, such as in laparoscopic surgery in which there is less pain, a safe alternative is patient-controlled analgesia. Intravenous administration of opioids is effective in pain control; however, caution must be exercised to avoid respiratory depression. Doses should be based on ideal body weight rather than on actual obese weight.

Early ambulation is key to minimizing mortality following abdominal surgery. DVT is twice as common in obese patients undergoing surgery than in nonobese patients (48% versus 23%) [14] and is likely attributed to the greater blood volume and relative polycythemia seen in obese patients. Prolonged immobilization; increased intra-abdominal pressure, which limits venous return; and decreased fibrinolytic activity [14] also contribute to DVT.

Tight glucose control in diabetics must be maintained postoperatively. In hyperglycemic states, neutrophil function is decreased, resulting in a higher incidence of wound infections. There is also an increased risk of myocardial infarction during periods of myocardial ischemia in the presence of hyperglycemia.

Postoperative lifestyle changes

Patients are initially placed on liquids for 1 to 2 weeks, progressing thereafter to puree and then to soft foods, and are eventually able to eat most food consistencies by 4 to 6 weeks but in a greatly reduced quantity. Strict dietary modifications must be followed to prevent stretching of the new stomach. Red meats may be more difficult to digest, especially if overcooked or reheated. Breads, pasta, and rice intake should be limited because in some patients, they may be "trigger foods" (ie, foods that are associated with or initiate overeating). Liquids are separated from solids during mealtimes not only to maximize the restrictive benefit but also to prevent expansion of food in the small pouch, which may lead to a gastric outlet obstruction.

Because the volume taken in is significantly less, consumed meals must be of high quality and nutrient dense; that is, high in protein and low in fat and carbohydrates. High-quality meals are especially needed after the BPD and LRYGB because of the malabsorptive component. It is recommended that all patients take a multivitamin. Other recommendations for the BPD and LRYGB patient include 40 to 65 mg of iron, 350 μg of vitamin B_{12}, 800 to 1000 mg of folate, and 1200 to 1500 mg of calcium with 400 to 1600 IU of vitamin D per day. Calcium citrate is preferred over calcium carbonate (as in antacids) because there are less parietal cells after gastric resection and decreased acid production, resulting in less calcium absorption. When a patient is unable to maintain iron levels with standard supplementation, 300 mg of iron sulfate is recommended three times a day along with ascorbic acid for better absorption. Rarely, intravenous iron supplementation is needed. Iron and calcium replacements should not be taken at the same time because of impaired absorption when taken together. Time-release medications are changed over to regular-release so as to offset altered absorption. Pills are crushed or converted to elixirs initially. As the anastamosis heals, patients need to keep pill size smaller than 8 mm to prevent obstruction and pill erosion. Aspirin, nonsteroidal anti-inflammatory drugs (NSAIDs), cyclo-oxygenase inhibitors, macrolides, and tetracycline antibiotics are avoided postoperatively and long-term in gastric bypass patients to limit ulcer and bleeding risk, which can be substantial (Box 2). Because drug absorption and distribution can vary after bypass surgery, serum drug levels may need to be monitored such as with antipsychotics, antiepileptics, and thyroid supplementation. Patients are referred back to the internists for adjustments in their antihypertensive and hypoglycemic medications. Patients are followed closely for their weight loss progress and nutritional status. Laboratory samples are taken at increasing intervals to monitor prealbumen, uric acid, lipid, and iron profiles and to rule out anemia and vitamin deficiencies.

Potential postoperative complications

Although bariatric surgery is usually a safe, effective means of sustained weight loss, complications can occur (Table 4). Close follow-up with

Box 2. Drugs to be avoided after malabsortive procedures[a]

Salicylates
Aspirin
Anacin (aspirin)
Ascriptin (buffered aspirin)
Bufferin Ecotrin (aspirin)
Uracel (sodium salsalate)

NSAIDs
Advil (ibuprofen)
Alleve (naproxen)
Anaprox (naproxen)
Butazolidin (phenylbutazone)
Feldene (piroxicam)
Excedrin (ibuprofen)
Toradol (ketorolac)
Ibuprin (ibuprofen)
Motrin (ibuprofen)
Naprosyn (naproxen)
Nuprin (ibuprofen)
Voltaren (diclofenac)

Cyclo-oxidase-2 inhibitors
Bextra (valdecoxib)
Celebex (celecoxib)

Analgesics
Darvon (propoxyphene/aspirin)
Equagesic (meprobamate/aspirin)
Percodan (oxycodone/aspirin)

Macrolide antibiotics
Biaxin (clarithromycin)
E-mycin (erythromycin)
Erythrocin (erythromycin)
Robimycin (erythromycin)
Zithromax (azithromycin)

Tetracycline antibiotics
Brodspec (tetracycline)
Panmycin (tetracycline)
Sumycin (tetracycline)
Tetracap (tetracycline)

---

[a] This table is not all-inclusive.

a bariatric program and seeking medical attention immediately can often prevent a lethal consequence. What may seem to be minor complaints may be sentinels of a much more serious condition. Often (but not always), precise questioning, physical examination, and imaging studies can help differentiate a serious problem from a minor one; however, if indicated, surgical exploration may be needed.

Early postoperative period

Nausea and vomiting

Nausea and vomiting are common complaints and may be seen in most patients at some point postoperatively. Is the patient eating too fast, swallowing too large a piece of food, or developing a particular food intolerance? Is it medication related? Dehydration is common and must be aggressively treated. Prolonged vomiting can contribute to thiamine deficiency, which by itself can stimulate nausea and vomiting. Most often, patients may need to return to a liquid diet for a short time; however, if unresponsive to 24 hours of treatment or if abdominal pain is also present, then a proactive approach must be taken and may include imaging studies, endoscopy, and if suspicion is high, diagnostic laparoscopy.

Bleeding

Bleeding along the anastomotic staple lines can be intra-abdominal or intraluminal. If a drain was placed near the pouch at the time of surgery as in the LRYGB, then output will likely indicate an intra-abdominal bleed. When the drain has clotted or has slipped out of position, it will not be a reliable indicator. Intraluminal bleeds may present with bleeding per rectum,

Table 4
Surgical risks following bariatric surgery

Surgical risk	BPD	LRYBP	LAGB
Wound infection	√[a]	√[a]	√[b]
Incisional hernia	√[a]	√[a]	√[b]
Internal hernia	√	√	
Gallstones	√	√	√
Marginal ulcer	√	√	
Stricture		√	
Pouch dilation		√	√
Erosion or slippage of band			√
Port complications			√
Gastric remnant distension		√	
Anastomotic leak	√	√	
DVT or PE	√	√	√
Nutrient deficiency	√	√	
Dumping	√	√	

[a] If done with the open technique.
[b] At the port site.

hematemesis, or bowel obstruction from clot formation. Most bleeding stops with supportive care, although if it presents in the recovery room as hematemesis or bowel obstruction in the acute period, then surgical re-exploration is warranted.

Anastomotic leak

Breakdown and leakage of gastric or enteric contents may occur with BPD and LRYGB. Ischemia or tension at the staple lines, inadequate closure of the enterotomy, and inadvertent bowel injury are possible etiologies. Anastomotic leak is a potentially life-threatening complication and should always be considered true until proven false in any postoperative patient who is not progressing as expected. Patients who have unexplained tachycardia, tachypnea, fever, shoulder and back pain, and abdominal pain out of proportion to what is expected are subtle signs of a more serious problem. If a drain was placed at the time of surgery, drainage might turn bilious or resemble motor oil. Leaks usually present in the acute postoperative period but may present 7 to 10 days after surgery. The risk of a leak has been reported to be between less than 1% and 3%. Management varies depending on the patient's condition and includes drainage, bowel rest, and total parenteral nutrition or emergent surgical exploration, repair, drainage, and placement of a gastrostomy tube into the remnant stomach (for the LRYGB patient).

Pulmonary embolism

All morbidly obese patients undergoing major surgery are at risk for DVT and PE. For bariatric patients, the most common cause of death after surgery is not from a leak but from a PE. Despite multiple interventions, the incidence of a symptomatic PE ranges from 0.7% to 2.4% [48]. The prevalence of asymptomatic thromboembolism is unknown and likely even higher than reported. General anesthesia and obesity are two important predisposing factors for venous thromboembolism. Obesity-related comorbidities such as diabetes, hypertension, OSA, and lymphedema are also significant. In addition, morbidly obese individuals have a high plasma concentration of fibrinogen, von Willebrand's factor, and factor VII and tend to be deficient in antithrombin III. They also have enhanced platelet aggregation and elevated plasminogen activator inhibitor-1 relative to nonobese patients [49]. With weight loss, this thrombophilic diathesis corrects [50]. Full prophylaxis is warranted. In individuals at high risk, such as a prior history of DVT or PE, a prophylactic temporary Greenfield filter should be considered, along with the usual precautions.

Late postoperative period

Nutritional deficiencies

Because patients have a limited portion size, calories consumed must be nutrient dense. With the malabsorptive procedures, excess amounts of protein and certain vitamins must be consumed to absorb enough to meet daily requirements. Hair loss occurs in most patients within the first 6 months and usually recovers as weight stabilizes and more protein is taken in. Protein deficiency can also present with anemia, edema, muscle wasting, and weakness. Parathyroid hormone levels should be checked periodically. Because calcium is mostly absorbed in the duodenum, deficiencies can occur if not regularly supplemented. If not enough calcium is absorbed, then parathyroid hormone levels increase and stimulate the release of calcium from bones to stabilize blood calcium levels, leading to loss of bone mass. Annual bone scans are recommended to look for occult bone density loss.

Peripheral neuropathies may occur in patients who lose weight too rapidly; have prolonged nausea and vomiting postoperatively; do not take prescribed supplements such as vitamin B_{12}, multivitamins, calcium, and so forth; and fail to comply with follow-up appointments and laboratory draws.

Wernicke's encephalopathy has been described following gastric bypass. Usually seen in alcoholic patients who have chronic malnutrition and frequent vomiting, it frequently presents with confusion and ataxia and is due to thiamine deficiency. Because thiamine is absorbed in the stomach and proximal small bowel, deficiencies can also be significant in the gastric bypass patient who does not take appropriate supplementation [51].

Cholelithiasis

Cholelithiasis may develop in response to rapid weight loss. The solubility of bile salts is reduced when gaining or losing weight and may precipitate into sludge and eventually result in stone formation. Gallbladders are no longer being routinely removed at the time of surgery and should still be in the differential diagnosis of right upper-quadrant abdominal pain. The incidence of developing gallstones after rapid weight loss is approximately 30% [52], and some institutions recommend screening for biliary disease preoperatively and removal of the gallbladder at the time of the bariatric surgery, if indicated. Prophylaxis with ursodeoxycholic acid (Actigall, Ursodiol), which decreases cholesterol production and decreases its content in bile to prevent stone formation, is usually poorly tolerated. Side effects include abdominal pain, constipation, diarrhea, dizziness, vomiting, and cough.

Gout

Gout is typically an inherited disease of abnormal excretion or production of uric acid. Morbid obesity and rapid weight loss disrupt uric acid metabolism and may lead to the development of gout. Weight loss can induce attacks because of increased uric acid production from the breakdown of endogenous muscle and production of ketones from fat metabolism. Diuretics, which are commonly used in the obese to assist with water retention, prevent the excretion of uric acid and may trigger an attack. Often in the initial post-operative period, uric acid levels are elevated and a short course of allopurinol (Zyloprim) is used to limit uric acid production. Minimizing loss of muscle during rapid weight loss should be attempted with mild exercise.

Dumping syndrome

Dumping syndrome is a phenomenon that occurs in response to a large load of undigested food introduced to the small intestine. Dumping usually occurs when there is rapid entry of foods high in carbohydrates and sugars directly into the small bowel, resulting in a high osmolar load. "Early" dumping syndrome occurs during or right after the meal and presents with nausea, vomiting, severe diarrhea, abdominal cramping, sweating, and tachycardia. "Late" dumping syndrome occurs 1 to 3 hours later as a large load of insulin is released to combat the high carbohydrate load. The blood sugar then drops, resulting in symptoms of hypoglycemia such as weakness, diaphoresis, anxiety, palpitations, and dizziness. The symptoms vary among individuals, with some experiencing both syndromes. The unpleasantness of symptoms can result in a sort of "forced behavior modification."

Bowel obstruction

Adhesions and internal hernias are the most common cause of bowel obstruction after bariatric surgery, with the latter being more dangerous. Internal hernias can occur after BPD and LRYGB because bowel and sometimes mesentery have been cut and the bowel rerouted. Closure of mesenteric defects should be performed to minimize this risk, which has been reported to be 3% to 4% [53]. Antecolic passage of the roux limb may also minimize the occurrence of internal hernias [54]. When an obstruction occurs along the biliopancreatic limb, the patient does not necessarily present with nausea or vomiting because there is no connection with the pouch. Enteric contents may back up into the gastric remnant and cause severe dilatation and even stomach necrosis. Nasogastric tube decompression does nothing for this type of obstruction. Diagnosis is difficult; however, subtle findings include elevated amylase and bilirubin, along with fluid distension of the biliopancreatic limb on CT scan. Patients often present late or the diagnosis may be delayed, and removal of small bowel or stomach may be necessary due to necrosis.

Marginal ulcers

Marginal ulcers and stomal stenosis may occur after LRYGB as a result of technique or chronic use of aspirin or NSAIDs. All postoperative patients are recommended to find alternatives to aspirin and NSAIDs, but if absolutely necessary, prophylaxis with proton pump inhibitors should be prescribed. The same is true for short courses of steroids.

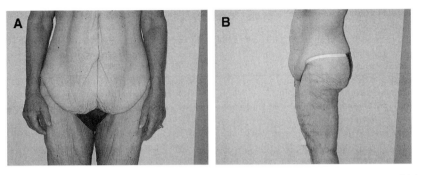

Fig. 6. (*A, B*) After massive weight loss. (*Courtesy of* Charles W. Spenler, MD, Torrance, CA.)

Excess skin

After patients lose massive amounts of weight, they may encounter yet another problem. With the fat lost, collagen-damaged excess skin now hangs on the new body frame, much like oversized clothes on a small person (Fig. 6A, B). Multiple areas are affected, including the chin, upper arms, breasts, abdomen, trunk, and thighs. This excessive skin can limit mobility and make hygiene difficult. Aside from cosmetic reasons, in some cases, it may become a medical necessity to remove the excess skin and tissue (eg, in the patient who burns her upper arms while trying to cook over a hot stove). A distorted body image is common in bariatric patients and some may still perceive themselves as obese even though they have lost massive amounts of weight. Body contouring procedures performed by plastic surgeons remove the excess skin, recreate support to the anterior abdominal wall, and can improve cosmesis and self-esteem (Fig. 7A, B). In most cases, multiple surgeries are required to address various parts of the body, and often, insurance companies do not reimburse for these procedures.

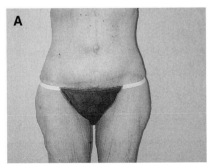
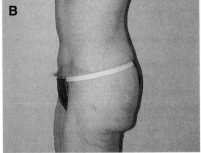

Fig. 7. (*A, B*) After belt lipectomy. (*Courtesy of* Cnarles W. Spenler, MD, Torrance, CA.)

Summary

Morbidly obese patients are a unique population that presents special considerations and risks for surgical intervention. Obesity-related comorbidities include but are not limited to hypertension, cardiac disease, diabetes, OSA, cancer of the gastrointestinal and reproductive systems, gallstones, and depression. Multiple bariatric procedures are now available to obese individuals willing to make a lifelong commitment to their health. As patients lose significant amounts of weight, resolution of many of the comorbidities improves or resolves; however, even with massive weight loss, some of the health risks remain, especially if the damage while being obese is already done. At some point in the future, a medical treatment for obesity will be discovered, but until that time comes, surgical intervention provides a safe, reliable, and sustained alternative.

Acknowledgments

The author would like to acknowledge Eric P. Dutson, MD, for his assistance and guidance in preparation of this article.

References

[1] Hedley AA, Ogden CL, Johnson CL, et al. Prevalence of overweight and obesity among US children, adolescents, and adults, 1999-2002. JAMA 2004;291(23):2847–50.
[2] Flegal KM, Carrol MD, Kuczmarski RJ, et al. Overweight and obesity in the United States: prevalence and trends, 1960-1994. Int J Obes Relat Metab Disord 1998;22:39–47.
[3] Rubin R. Obesity: the public health crisis. Presented at the American Obesity Association Conference. Washington, DC, September, 1999.
[4] Santry HP, Gillen DL, Lauderdale DS. Trends in bariatric surgery procedures. JAMA 2005; 294:1909–17.
[5] Nguyen NT, Root J, Zainabadi K, et al. Accelerated growth of bariatric surgery with the introduction of minimally invasive surgery. Arch Surg 2005;140:1198–202.
[6] Viner RM, Cole TJ. Television viewing in early childhood predicts adult body mass index. J Pediatr 2005;147(4):429–35.
[7] Peeters A, Barendregt J, Willekens F, et al. Obesity in adulthood and its consequences for life expectancy: a life-table analysis. Ann Intern Med 2003;138:24–32.
[8] Blumenkrantz M. Obesity: the world's oldest metabolic disorder, obesity & health—an overview. Available at: www.quantum.hcp.com/obesity.htm. Accessed February 2, 1999.
[9] Garrison RJ, Castelli WP. Weight and thirty-year mortality of men in the Framingham study. Ann Intern Med 1985;103:1006–9.
[10] Drenick EJ, Ament ME, Finegold SM, et al. Excessive causes of death in morbidly obese men. JAMA 1980;243(5):443–5.
[11] Health implications of obesity. NIH consensus statement. Available at: http://www.lapsurgery.com/BARIATRIC%20SURGERY/nih.htm. 1985;5(9):1–7.
[12] Scaglione R, Argano C, Di Chiara T, et al. Obesity and cardiovascular risk: the new public health problem of worldwide proportions. Expert Rev Cardiovasc Ther 2004; 2(2):203–12.
[13] Cikim AS, Ozbey N, Orhan Y. Relationship between cardiovascular risk indicators and types of obesity in overweight and obese women. J Int Med Res 2004;32(3):268–73.

[14] Adams JP, Murphy PG. Obesity in anaesthesia and intensive care. Br J Anaesth 2000;85: 91–108.

[15] Pantanetti P, Garrapa GG, Mantero F, et al. Adipose tissue as an endocrine organ? A review of recent data related to cardiovascular complications of endocrine dysfunctions. Clin Exp Hypertens 2004;26(4):387–98.

[16] The National Institutes of Health. NIH Publication No. 96-1468, Bethesda, MD: Weight Control Info Network. July, 1996.

[17] Mikhail N, Golub MS, Tuck ML. Obesity and hypertension. Prog Cardiovasc Dis 1999;42: 39–58.

[18] Diabetes in America. 2nd Edition. The National Institutes of Diabetes and Digestive and Kidney Diseases; NIH Publication No. 95-1468, Bethesda, MD: Weight Control Info Network. 1995.

[19] Bray GA. Medical consequences of obesity. J Clin Endocrinol Metab 2004;89(6):2583–9.

[20] American Diabetes Association. Type 2 diabetes in children and adolescents. Diabetes Care 2000;23(3):381–98.

[21] Goldstein DJ. Beneficial health effects of modest weight loss. Int J Obes Relat Metab Disord 1992;16(6):397–415.

[22] Lakka HM, Laaksonen DE, Lakka TA, et al. The metabolic syndrome and total and cardiovascular disease mortality in middle-aged men. JAMA 2002;288(21):2709–16.

[23] Sundstrom J, Riserus U, Byberg L, et al. Clinical value of the metabolic syndrome for long term prediction of total and cardiovascular mortality: prospective, population based cohort study. BMJ 2006;332:878–81.

[24] Lee IM, Paffenbarger RS. Quetelet's index and risk of colon cancer in college alumni. J Natl Cancer Inst 1992;84:1326–31.

[25] Huang Z, Hankinson SE, Colditz GA, et al. Dual effects of weight and weight gain on breast cancer risk. JAMA 1997;278:1407–11.

[26] The National Institutes of Health. NIH Publication No. 94-3680, Bethesda, MD: Weight Control Info Network. November, 1993.

[27] Beymer C, Kowdley KV, Larson A, et al. Prevalence and predictors of asymptomatic liver disease in patients undergoing gastric bypass surgery. Arch Surg 2003;138:1240–4.

[28] Simon GE, Von Korff M, Saunders K, et al. Association between obesity and psychiatric disorders in the US adult population. Arch Gen Psychiatry 2006;63(7):824–30.

[29] Quesenberry CP Jr, Caan B, Jacobson A. Obesity, health services use, and healthcare costs among members of a healthcare maintenance organization. Arch Intern Med 1998;158:466–72.

[30] Diconsiglio J. Hospitals equip to meet the bariatric challenge. Rising number of obese patients necessitates specific supplies. Mater Manag Health Care 2006;15(4):36–9.

[31] Schauer PR, Burguera B, Ikramuddin S, et al. Effect of laparoscopic Roux-en-Y gastric bypass on type 2 diabetes mellitus. Ann Surg 2003;238:467–83.

[32] Ponce J, Haynes B, Paynter S, et al. Effect of lap-band-induced weight loss on type 2 diabetes and hypertension. Obes Surg 2004;14(10):1335–42.

[33] Pories WJ, Swanson MS, MacDonald KG, et al. Who would have thought it? An operation proves to be the most effective therapy for adult-onset diabetes mellitus. Ann Surg 1995;222: 339–50.

[34] Buchwald H, Avidor Y, Braunwald E, et al. Bariatric surgery: a systematic review and meta-analysis. JAMA 2004;292:1724–37.

[35] Schauer PR, Ikramuddin S, Gourash W, et al. Outcomes after laparoscopic Roux-en-Y gastric bypass for morbid obesity. Ann Surg 2000;232:515–29.

[36] van Germert WG, Adang EM, Greve JW, et al. Quality of life assessment of morbidly obese patients: effect of weight-reducing surgery. Am J Clin Nutr 1998;67:197–201.

[37] Christou NV, Sampalis JS, Liberman M, et al. Surgery decreases long-term mortality, morbidity, and health care use in morbidly obese patients. Ann Surg 2004;240:416–23.

[38] Nguyen NT, Goldman CD, Ho HS, et al. Systemic stress response after laparoscopic and open gastric bypass. J Am Coll Surg 2002;194(5):555–66.

[39] Nguyen NT, Goldman C, Rosenquist CJ, et al. Laparoscopic versus open gastric bypass: a randomized study of outcomes, quality of life, and costs. Ann Surg 2001;234(3):279–91.

[40] Baltasar A, Bou R. Duodenal switch: an effective therapy for morbid obesity-intermediate results. Obes Surg 2001;11(1):54–8.

[41] Hess DS, Hess DW. Biliopancreatic diversion with a duodenal switch. Obes Surg 1998;8: 267–82.

[42] DeMaria EJ, Sugerman HJ, Meador JG, et al. High failure rate after laparoscopic adjustable silicone gastric banding for treatment of morbid obesity. Ann Surg 2001;233(6):809–18.

[43] Ponce J, Paynter S, Fromm R. Laparoscopic adjustable gastric banding: 1014 consecutive cases. J Am Coll Surg 2005;201(4):529–35.

[44] Sarker S, Herold K, Creech S, et al. Early and late complications following laparoscopic adjustable gastric banding. Am Surg 2004;70(2):146–9.

[45] Wittgrove AC, Clark GW. Laparoscopic gastric bypass, Roux-en-Y 500 patients: technique and results, with 30-60 months follow up. Obes Surg 2000;10(3):233–9.

[46] O'Connell TL. An overview of obesity and weight loss surgery. Clin Diab 2004;22(3):115–20.

[47] De Freitas, Carvalho DA, Valezi AC, et al. Rhabdomyolysis after bariatric surgery. Obes Surg 2006;16:740–4.

[48] Sapala JA, Wood MH, Schunknecht MP, et al. Fatal pulmonary embolism after bariatric operations for morbid obesity: a 24-year retrospective analysis. Obes Surg 2003;13:819–25.

[49] De Pergola G, Pannacciulli N. Coagulation and fibrinolysis abnormalities in obesity. J Endocrinol Invest 2002;25(10):899–905.

[50] Primrose JN, Davies JA, Prentice CR, et al. Reduction in factor VII, fibrinogen, and plasminogen activator inhibitor-1 activity after surgical treatment of morbid obesity. Thromb Haemost 1992;68(4):396–9.

[51] Parsons JP, Marsh CB, Mastronarde JG. Wernicke's encephalopathy in a patient after gastric bypass surgery. Chest 2005;128(4):453S–4S.

[52] Sugarman HJ, Brewer WH, Shiffman ML, et al. A multicenter, placebo-controlled, randomized, double-blind, prospective trial of prophylactic ursodiol for the prevention of gallstone formation, following gastric-bypass-induced rapid weight loss. Am J Surg 1995;169(1):91–6.

[53] Higa KD, Ho T, Boone KD. Internal hernias after laparoscopic Roux-en-Y gastric bypass: incidence, treatment and prevention. Obes Surg 2003;13:350–4.

[54] Champion JK, Williams M. Small bowel obstruction and internal hernias after laparoscopic Roux-en-Y gastric banding. Obes Surg 2003;13(4):596–600.

ELSEVIER
SAUNDERS

Clin Podiatr Med Surg
24 (2007) 223–244

CLINICS IN
PODIATRIC
MEDICINE AND
SURGERY

Perioperative Management of the Podiatric Surgical Patient

Bruce I. Kaczander, DPM, FACFAS[a,b,*],
Jeffrey G. Cramblett, DPM, FACFAS[b],
Gurbir S. Mann, DPM[b]

[a]William Beaumont Hospital, 3601 W. Thirteen Mile Road, Royal Oak,
Michigan 48073, USA
[b]Botsford General Hospital, Botsford Podiatry Clinic, 28100 Grand River Avenue,
Suite 200, Farmington Hills, MI 48336, USA

The effects of podiatric surgery and anesthesia on the health of patients with or without coexisting disease can be dramatic. For this reason, optimal care and planning in the perioperative period, defined as that period of time just before, during, and after a surgical procedure, is crucial. More often than not, this term is equated with consultation by internists or other non-surgical physicians who attempt to evaluate a patient's health status before surgery, define medical issues, and anticipate the effects of anesthesia and surgery [1]. Surgeons, anesthesiologists, and other health care providers who bring their own expertise and the perspectives of their discipline to the management of patients undergoing surgery also provide perioperative medical care. Optimal perioperative medication management requires an understanding of the disease-specific pharmacologic therapies. As the number of pharmacologic agents continues to grow and each agent has some special action or effect, it becomes difficult for physicians to maintain a working familiarity with all of these agents [2]. In this article, the authors describe the impact of these drugs on the care of patients and current information on drug management in the perioperative period.

Diabetes

The worldwide prevalence of diabetes is steadily rising, with an estimated 16 million people with diabetes mellitus in the United States [3]. Patients

* Corresponding author. Michigan Foot and Ankle Center, 24725 W Twelve Mile Road #270, Southfield, MI 48034.
E-mail address: drkaczdpm@aol.com (B.I. Kaczander).

0891-8422/07/$ - see front matter © 2007 Elsevier Inc. All rights reserved.
doi:10.1016/j.cpm.2006.12.006

with diabetes are at increased risk for perioperative complications, namely, infectious, metabolic, electrolyte, renal, and cardiac complications during and after surgery [4–9]. The primary goal of perioperative management in the diabetic patient is a safe and effective outcome without complications, which requires communication and coordination of care between the internist or endocrinologist and the surgical team [4]. During any surgical procedure, numerous metabolic changes occur that have an effect on diabetes mellitus. Secretion of insulin antagonists, including epinephrine, norepinephrine, cortisol, and growth hormone, occurs. These hormones cause insulin resistance at the tissue level as well; epinephrine causes a decrease in insulin secretion, which effectively contributes to hyperglycemia during and after surgery. In addition, there is an increase in gluconeogenesis, net protein catabolism, and an increase in metabolic rate, which can result in poor control of blood glucose, ketosis, and acidosis [4,5,10].

Patients with diabetes mellitus are also at risk of hypoglycemia in the perioperative period owing to prolonged fasting, hypoglycemic medications, inadequate nutritional therapy, sedation, and postoperative gastrointestinal problems (ie, ileus, vomiting) [4]. Factors that affect the extent of the endocrine and metabolic changes during and after surgery include the type of diabetes, preoperative diabetic control, the magnitude of the surgery, and perioperative complications [4]. Impaired wound healing is one of the most important consequences of perioperative hyperglycemia. It has been shown in patients with type I/II diabetes that granulocyte chemotaxis and phagocytic function are adversely affected by hyperglycemia, particularly when blood glucose levels are greater than 250 mg/dL [4,11]. Collagen synthesis is suppressed by hyperglycemia when glucose levels are higher than 200 mg/dL [4]. These physiologic changes lead to impaired wound healing, which contributes to the increased rate of postoperative infections, septicemia, and mortality observed in patients with diabetes mellitus [12,13].

How a patient's diabetes mellitus will be managed during surgery is dependant on several patient-specific issues and surgical factors [4]. When evaluating a diabetic patient with respect to medication management in the perioperative period, one should ascertain the type and duration of diabetes mellitus, the patient's current therapy for diabetes, and his or her status of glycemic control. One must also identify other comorbidities and consider the type of surgery planned to assess the surgical risk. For patients undergoing minor or major surgery whose diabetes is well controlled with oral medications, it is recommended that the oral medications be discontinued the morning of surgery or 24 to 48 hours preoperatively if they are on metformin or chlorpropamide [4]. If the diabetes is poorly controlled with oral medications and the patient is scheduled for major surgery, insulin and glucose infusion is advised. For patients undergoing minor surgery and taking insulin to control their diabetes, it is recommended that one half to two thirds of their usual morning insulin can be given, and less if it is anticipated that they will be given nothing by mouth past their noon meal. Their intravenous fluids during surgery should be D-5-W/0.45 NS to prevent hypoglycemia [4].

For patients taking insulin and undergoing major surgery, it is recommended that a continuous intravenous insulin and glucose infusion be administered [10]. The continuous intravenous glucose infusion is given to prevent hypoglycemia and to provide a source of carbohydrates to minimize the risk for ketosis and acidosis during fasting and the stress of surgery. In addition, potassium chloride should be included in the insulin and glucose infusion unless the patient has hyperkalemia or chronic renal failure [4]. It is deemed inappropriate to use only intravenous push insulin to manage diabetes perioperatively, because intravenous push insulin has a half-life of only 5 to 10 minutes [10]. The metabolic and hormonal stresses of surgery persist during the early postoperative period, especially the day of surgery and the first postoperative day, and can last for up to 4 days [14,15]. For patients receiving insulin and glucose infusion, this regimen can be discontinued once the patient begins eating. Subcutaneous regular insulin can be given every 6 hours until the patient begins tolerating regular meals, and, at this point, the patient can resume a regular preoperative insulin regimen. For patients on oral medications, the medications can be restarted when the patient resumes a usual diet.

Oral contraceptives

Oral contraceptives are the most important cause of thrombosis in young women. For this reason, the decision to continue or stop oral contraceptives before surgery must balance the risk of unwanted pregnancy against the risk of thromboembolism. Although a clear picture of the exact mechanism is not yet established, certain aspects are known. The medications do not consistently alter bleeding or clotting times; however, there is an increase in factors VII, VIII, IX, and X, and a decrease in antithrombin III [16]. The risk of thrombosis increases threefold [16] when compared with the risk in women not talking contraceptives within 4 months of the initiation of therapy and is unaffected by the duration of use; the risk decreases to previous levels within 1 to 3 months of stopping treatment [16,17]. Two types of preparations are used for oral contraception: (1) combinations of estrogens and progestins and (2) continuous progestin therapy without concomitant administration of estrogens (Table 1) [16]. Oral contraceptives with greater estrogen content (> 50 mg) have a higher risk of thromboembolism when compared with formulations with lower estrogen content (30 mg); however, even the lower dose estrogen content pills carry a risk of thrombosis [17]. In surgical patients who are at low risk for venous thrombosis, oral contraceptives can be continued as long as the patient is aware of the risk of unwanted pregnancy. For patients who are at moderate or high risk for venous thrombosis, oral contraceptives should be discontinued 6 weeks before surgery (Table 2) [17]. In addition, a pregnancy test

Table 1
Contraceptives

Estrogen plus progestin	Progestin only
Alesse	Micronor
Apri	Nor-QD
Aviane	Ovrette
Brevicon	Plan B
Demulen	Cerazette
Desogen	
Estrostep/Estrostep Fe	Norplant (implant)
Genora	Jadelle (implant)
Jenest	Progestasert (intrauterine)
Levlen/Tri-Levlen	Mirena (intrauterine)
Levlite	Implanon (implant)
Levora	Depo-Provera (injectable)
Lo/Ovral	Noristerat (injectable)
Loestrin/Loestrin Fe	
Ogestrel/Low-Ogestrel	
Microgestin/Microgestin Fe	
Mircette	
Modicon	
Necon	
Norinyl/Tri-Norinyl	
Nordette	
Ortho-Cept	
Ortho-Cyclen	
Ortho-Novum	
Ortho Tri-Cyclen	
Ovcon	
Ovral	
Seasonale	
Triphasil	
Trivora	
Yasmin	
Zovia	

preoperatively should be conducted in patients who have discontinued the oral contraceptives.

Hormone replacement therapy

Hormone replacement therapy (HRT) is used to counteract the long-lasting changes that influence the health and well being of postmenopausal women. These changes include an acceleration of bone loss, which in susceptible women may lead to vertebral, hip, and wrist fractures, and lipid changes, which may contribute to the acceleration of atherosclerotic cardiovascular disease noted in postmenopausal women [16]. Although the estrogen content of HRT preparations is much lower than that of oral contraceptives, these medications carry an increased risk of venous

Table 2
Thrombosis risk

Low	Medium	High
Travel >5 h	Age >50 y	Previous venous thromboembolism
	Heart failure	Malignancy
	Severe varicosities	Thrombophilia
	Chronic venous insufficiency	Cast immobilization
	Hormone use	Recent limb surgery
	Obesity	
	Pregnancy/post partum	

thromboembolism [18,19]. The risks associated with temporary discontinuation of HRT medications is minimal, and it is recommended that in women in whom a moderate to high risk of venous thromboembolism is expected, these medications be discontinued 4 to 6 weeks before surgery. Patients with a minimal risk of thrombosis can continue taking their HRT medications [17].

Selective estrogen receptor modulators

Selective estrogen receptor modulators (SERMs), which include tamoxifen and raloxifene, have proven extremely useful in the prevention and treatment of breast cancer, progesterone-resistant endometrial cancer, and osteoporosis. Nevertheless, this category of drugs is associated with an increased risk of venous thromboembolism, and, as such, the benefits of continuing this class of drugs versus the adverse effects of discontinuing them must be taken into account. For patients who are taking SERMs for breast cancer treatment, it is recommended that consultation with an oncologist be conducted [17]. In patients who are taking SERMs for the prevention of breast cancer and osteoporosis, there is less risk of harm to the patient if the medications are discontinued. If the patient carries a moderate to high risk for venous thrombosis, these medications should be discontinued for 4 weeks before surgery [17]. In patients with a low risk for thrombosis, the medication can be continued.

Hypolipidemic agents

Several drugs are used to decrease plasma low-density lipoprotein cholesterol. The three main classes of drugs used clinically are (1) HMG-CoA reductase inhibitors ("statins"), (2) bile acid resins, and (3) fibrates [20]. In addition, nicotinic acid and its derivatives can also be used. Studies have shown that these drugs carry a risk of myopathy and rhabdomyolysis, and that the risk is higher when they are used in combination [17,21–24]. Because these drugs are used for long-term reduction in vascular morbidity, it is suggested that they be discontinued 1 day before surgery; however, recent studies [25–28] have shown HMG-CoA reductase inhibitors to benefit patients by preventing vascular events through mechanisms other than cholesterol lowering (ie, plaque stabilization, reduction in inflammation, decreased thrombogenesis). It is recommended that this class of drugs be continued throughout the perioperative period [17].

Thyroid disease medications

Hypothyroidism affects many body systems that can influence perioperative outcome, including myocardial function, pulmonary ventilation, hemostasis, gastrointestinal motility, and free water balance. Currently, no randomized prospective studies are looking at hypothyroid patients versus controls. Previous opinion on perioperative management has been based on case studies reporting intraoperative hypotension, cardiovascular collapse, and extreme sensitivity to narcotics, sedatives, and anesthesia in undiagnosed hypothyroid patients [29,30]. For this reason, expert opinion has encouraged clinical and chemical euthyroidism to any surgery [4].

In the 1980s, two retrospective studies evaluated the hypothyroid patient undergoing surgery. One study by Weinberg and colleagues [31] revealed no difference in surgical outcome or perioperative complications, and it was concluded that there was no evidence to justify deferring needed surgery in patients with mild-to-moderate hypothyroidism, and insufficient evidence to make recommendations for patients with severe hypothyroidism. A study by Ladenson and colleagues [32] revealed a greater risk of intraoperative hypotension in noncardiac surgery and more postoperative gastrointestinal and neuropsychiatric complications; hypothyroid patients were also less likely to mount a fever with infection. Schiff and Welsh [4] suggest that patients with mild-to-moderate hypothyroidism may undergo urgent or emergent surgery without delay, and that patients with mild hypothyroidism can safely undergo elective surgery, with some risk of minor complications such as ileus, postoperative delirium, or infection without fever. They further state that elective surgery should be postponed in patients with moderate and severe hypothyroidism, for which thyroid replacement medications can be started with the same schedule in the outpatient setting. For patients with severe hypothyroidism who require emergent surgery, intravenous T3 and T4 and glucocorticoids should be initiated to bring the patient to a euthyroid level [4].

The effect of thyrotoxicosis on the heart carries perioperative risk for the hyperthyroid patient. T3 and T4 exert direct inotropic and chronotropic effects on cardiac muscle and can lead to limited cardiac reserves during surgery in the hyperthyroid patient [4]. The greatest risk to the perioperative thyrotoxic patient is thyroid storm, a rare but life-threatening complication that presents with fever, tachycardia, and confusion. Thyroid storm may quickly lead to cardiovascular collapse and death, which can occur in the inadequately treated or undiagnosed hyperthyroid patient during or soon after surgery [33,34]. Patients who have mild hyperthyroidism can undergo surgery with preoperative beta blockade with propranolol or other cardio-selective beta blockers [35]. Patients who have moderate-to-severe hyperthy-roidism should have elective surgery postponed until they are euthyroid. The thyrotoxic patient undergoing urgent or emergent surgery needs pre-medication with antithyroid agents (ie, thionamides, iodine, and iopanoic acid), beta blockade, and, possibly, corticosteroids [4].

Cardiovascular medications

Hypertension is the most common cardiovascular disease. The number of patients taking cardiovascular medications has increased greatly, as have the number of different medications. These patients include those with hyper-tension, mitral valve prolapse, and many other cardiac abnormalities. Sus-tained arterial hypertension damages blood vessels in the kidneys, heart, and brain and leads to an increased incidence of renal failure, coronary dis-ease, cardiac failure, and stroke [16]. Pharmacologic intervention to lower blood pressure has been shown to prevent damage to blood vessels and sub-stantially reduce morbidity and mortality rates. During the postoperative period, the risk of continuing these medications, possibly leading to signif-icant hypotension, must be weighed against the potential benefits of con-tinuing them.

The hypertensive patient may be treated with numerous drugs, which must be managed perioperatively. It is important to know what medications the patient is on and how to manage them accordingly. In the past, it was thought that medications for hypertension must be stopped days or even weeks before an elective surgical procedure; however, current practice is to continue patients on therapy by allowing them to take their medications with a small sip of water the morning of surgery [36].

The effectiveness of B-adrenergic receptor antagonists is dependant on the degree of sympathetic activity and is slight in subjects at rest. Beta blockers have beneficial effects when taken perioperatively. These character-istics become especially important during the perioperative period, which is associated with increased stress and catecholamine release. Beta blockers effectively reduce cardiac ischemia by reducing the myocardial oxygen demand. With this benefit in mind, and with the risk of withdrawal side effects, current practice is to continue patients on their beta-blocker regimen throughout the perioperative period. Several studies have shown that beta blockers reduce perioperative myocardial infarction and death, and recom-mendations suggest beginning beta blockers perioperatively in patients stratified as having a high risk for cardiovascular disease [17,37–39], espe-cially patients with diabetes (Table 3) [40]. Patients at high risk for cardio-vascular complications are advised to start B1-cardioselective beta blockers in the perioperative period to minimize the adverse pulmonary and periph-eral vascular effects mediated by B2-adrenergic receptors [17]. Patients should take their medications the morning of surgery and regularly when

Table 3
Cardiovascular risk factors

Nonmodifiable	Modifiable	Other factors
Increasing age	Tobacco use	Individual stress response
>65 y old	2–4 times more likely	Can exacerbate other conditions
Gender		
Male	High cholesterol	Alcoholism
Heredity		
African American	Hypertension	
Mexican American	Physical inactivity	
Hawaiian	Obesity	
Asian American	Diabetes mellitus	

permitted after surgery. Patients may be switched to an intravenous beta blocker if they are unable to take pills by mouth.

Centrally acting sympatholytics or alpha-2 agonists are also beneficial to the patient's cardiac health, but not as much research has been performed on these agents when compared with beta blockers. Centrally acting sympatholytics, which include methyldopa, guanabenz, and clonidine, reduce sympathetic outflow from vasopressor centers in the brain stem to exert their antihypertensive effect. Abrupt cessation of these drugs has been found to precipitate rebound hypertension [17]; therefore, these medications should be continued throughout the perioperative period. Alpha-2 agonists have some positive perioperative effects, including a decreased response to stress from intubation and the surgery itself. These drugs also reduce the amount of anesthetic required during surgery. They have been noted to possess sedative, anxiolytic, analgesic, and anti-shivering properties that are important during the induction and recovery phases of balanced anesthesia [41,42]. It is suggested that alpha-2 agonists be continued during the perioperative period owing to these effects and the possibility of withdrawal symptoms and rebound hypertension. Drugs such as clonidine may be changed to transdermal patches or intravenous administration for the patient taking nothing by mouth before surgery.

In addition to their anti-anginal and anti-arrhythmic effects, calcium channel blockers dilate peripheral arterioles and reduce blood pressure [16]. Calcium channel blockers exert their antihypertensive effect by inhibiting calcium influx into the arteriolar smooth muscle cells, reducing the caliber of the blood vessels. Due to this effect, concerns have been raised in the medical community of an increased risk of bleeding [43–45]; however, several studies have not substantiated these claims [46,47]. Because no serious interactions are noted with the concomitant use of this class of drugs and anesthetic agents, and because the evidence for the risk of bleeding is contradictory, it is recommended that these medications be continued throughout the perioperative period because the benefits of continued use outweigh the potentially hazardous effect of cessation. Few data suggest that these medications should be started in the perioperative period for added benefit, whereas beta blockers have substantial evidence for this claim.

Angiotensin-converting enzyme (ACE) inhibitors are drugs that are used later in the lineage of the course of the hypertensive patient. ACE inhibitors act by inhibiting the converting enzyme peptidyl dipeptidase that hydrolyzes angiotensin I to angiotensin II and inactivates bradykinin. The hypotensive activity results from an inhibitory action on the renin-angiotensin system and a stimulating action on the kallikrein-kinin system [16]. Studies have shown that continuation of ACE inhibitors results in prolonged hypotension owing to a blunting of the compensatory activation of the renin-angiotensin system during surgery [48,49].

The recommendations differ among patients based on the specific condition for which the medication is used. Current recommendations state that ACE inhibitors can be continued throughout the perioperative period, especially in patients taking them for the management of hypertension [17], unless the patient is hypotensive preoperatively. They work by altering the effect of renin in the renin-angiotensin system. The patient being treated with ACE inhibitors for hypertension should continue their normal regimen as long as the patient is not hypotensive preoperatively. On the other hand, in the patient taking ACE inhibitors for heart failure, one should hold their medication on the morning of surgery, especially if the baseline blood pressure is low, owing to the possibility of induction hypotension and postoperative hypertension [50].

Angiotensin receptor blockers exert a similar effect as ACE inhibitors; however, they have a mechanism of action downstream in the renin-angiotensin pathway. Angiotensin receptor blockers have been noted to cause significant hypotension, similar to that seen with use of ACE inhibitors, when continued throughout the perioperative period [24]. There are currently no definitive recommendations on the use of angiotensin receptor blockers throughout the perioperative period; therefore, it is recommended that they be discontinued on the day of surgery [17] and restarted postoperatively, as long as the patient is not hypotensive or renally impaired.

Many hypertensive patients are also placed on diuretics to maintain blood pressure and remove excess fluid from the body. The perioperative difficulty with this class of medication is the potential for hypovolemia and for hypokalemia with non–potassium sparing diuretics. It is recommended that diuretics be held the morning of surgery; they may be given intravenously during surgery, if necessary. The diuretic should be restarted when liquids are again tolerated by the patient postoperatively.

One should consider antibiotic therapy preoperatively for the prevention of endocarditis. According to the revised guidelines of the American Heart Association published in 1997, cardiac conditions for which antimicrobial prophylaxis is indicated before invasive dental or surgical procedures include the following: a prosthetic heart valve, prior history of infective endocarditis, cyanotic congenital heart defect, surgically constructed systemic or pulmonary conduit, hypertrophic cardiomyopathy, and mitral valve prolapse with regurgitation, valve thickening, or both [36]. Endocarditis prophylaxis is not recommended for the following: an atrial septal defect, surgically repaired ventricular septal defect, patent ductus arteriosus, isolated mitral valve prolapse, mild tricuspid regurgitation, previous rheumatic fever or Kawasaki disease without valvular dysfunction, cardiac pacemaker, and implantable defibrillator [36].

One must monitor and manage cardiac patients accurately to prevent myocardial ischemia and infarction. Patients on nitroglycerin should continue taking their medication in the usual dosage before surgery and continue the dosage intravenously after surgery until the medication can be taken by mouth.

Hemostasis effecting agents

Bleeding is a major concern in surgical patients. Compromise in the structural integrity of a vessel from surgical exploration results in most intraoperative and postoperative bleeding. Anticoagulant therapy further confounds the issue. Temporary interruption before surgery is required; otherwise, excessive operative bleeding may result. Many patients undergoing surgery are taking chronic medications that are intended to impair coagulation or take medications for another indication that have an unintended effect on hemostasis. Depending on the medication administered, its indication for use, and the risk for intraoperative bleeding and ischemic events, different approaches to perioperative medication management exist. Regardless of the approach to perioperative anticoagulation, patients need to have a normal or nearly normal state of coagulation during surgery; therefore, some increase in the risk of thromboembolism is unavoidable [51].

The risk of bleeding occurring with surgery in patients taking anticoagulant therapy is dependent upon patient age, the presence of other disease states, the type of surgery [52], the anticoagulant regimen and intensity, the length of warfarin therapy, the use of other drugs that affect hemostasis (especially heparin), the stability of anticoagulation, and the degree of monitoring [53–55].

Warfarin

Upon cessation of oral warfarin, it usually takes a few days for the international normalized ratio (INR) to fall to below 2.0. One study prospectively evaluated 22 patients with a baseline INR of 2.6 in whom it was deemed safe to discontinue warfarin [56]. The INR fell to 1.6 at 2.7 days and 1.2 at 4.7 days. For patients taking oral anticoagulants as thromboprophylaxis, the INR can be maintained around 1.5 before surgery. For patients with mechanical prosthetic valves, the preoperative INR should be maintained around 2.0. Once the INR is 2.0 or below, surgery can be performed with relative safety. Following surgery and after warfarin is restarted, it takes about 3 to 4 days for the INR to rise above 2.0. It is estimated that if warfarin is withheld for 4 days before surgery and treatment is started as soon as possible afterwards, patients would have a subtherapeutic INR for approximately 2 days before surgery and 2 days after surgery [51].

The risk of this short period of "under anticoagulation" is uncertain. A slight elevation of the INR to about 1.5 should theoretically provide partial protection against thromboembolism [57,58]. In support of this hypothesis, ultra–low dose warfarin (1 mg/day) has been used successfully to prevent thrombosis of central venous catheters and deep venous thrombosis in patients with malignancy in association with a marginal rise in the INR [57,58]. Furthermore, if the patient has been adequately anticoagulated for some time before the cessation of warfarin, it is generally assumed that almost any preexisting thrombus would have either resolved or endothelialized, thereby minimizing the risk of embolism [59]. Among patients with nonvalvular atrial fibrillation, more than 85% of thrombi resolve after 4 weeks of warfarin therapy as determined by transesophageal echocardiography [60].

In patients with an INR between 2.0 and 3.0 who are scheduled for elective surgery, warfarin should be withheld for 3 to 4 days to allow the INR to fall to a level of 1.5 to 2.0 before surgery [51,56,61]. Warfarin should be withheld for a longer period of time if the INR is normally maintained at a level greater than 3.0, or if it is necessary to reduce the INR to a lower level (eg, <1.5) [56]. If more rapid reversal of warfarin anticoagulation is required, warfarin should be withheld and a small dose (eg, 0.5 to 1.0 mg) of intravenous vitamin K1 administered.

Alternative preoperative or postoperative prophylaxis against thromboembolism with unfractionated heparin or low molecular weight heparin should be considered in high-risk patients for the period during which the INR is less than 2.0 [62,63]. In one retrospective study, use of the low molecular weight heparin enoxaparin was associated with lower total costs than use of unfractionated heparin [64]. This decrease was accomplished through the avoidance or minimization of inpatient care, with no increase in adverse events (eg, venous thromboembolism, major or minor bleeding).

Antiplatelet drugs

Because platelets have such a critical role in thromboembolic disease, antiplatelet drugs are potentially of immense therapeutic value [20]. Dipyridamole, ticlodipine, and clopidogrel all have antiplatelet activity, with dipyridamole also having additional vasodilator activity. Clopidogrel and ticlodipine are used most often in patients who have had previous cerebrovascular events, recent percutaneous cardiac procedures, or recent acute coronary syndromes, whereas dipyridamole is commonly used in patients with past stroke or transient ischemic attack [17,65]. There are limited data on which to base a decision to continue or hold these drugs in patients under-going noncardiac surgery [17], and the risk of intraoperative bleeding and ischemic events needs to be considered. Clopidogrel and ticlodipine reduce platelet aggregation by irreversibly inhibiting ADP from binding to its re-ceptor on platelets [16]. If this medicine needs to be stopped, it should be discontinued at least 7 to 10 days before surgery [17]. Dipyridamole, a phos-phodiesterase inhibitor, is discontinued at least 2 days before surgery if the decision is made to hold this drug [17].

Aspirin

Aspirin irreversibly inhibits platelet cyclooxygenase (COX) by irrevers-ible acetylation of this enzyme and prevents formation of the prostaglandin thromboxane A_2, inhibiting platelet aggregation and platelet degranulation. Because the average life span of a platelet is about 7 to 10 days, if the de-cision to discontinue aspirin is made, 5 to 7 days is sufficient for new func-tional platelet formation. Because the anuclear platelet cannot synthesize new proteins, it cannot manufacture new enzyme during its 10-day lifetime. The optimal perioperative management is uncertain, and significant prac-tice variations exists [66]. The decision to continue or withhold aspirin should reflect the balance of perioperative hemorrhage versus the risk of perioperative vascular complications [67]. In patients at high risk, in whom perioperative hemorrhage would result in minimal morbidity, aspirin should be continued. In high-risk patients in whom perioperative hemor-rhage would be catastrophic (ie, central nervous system surgery) or would impact surgical outcome, aspirin can be discontinued at only 3 to 5 days before surgery [67].

Non-steroidal anti-inflammatory drugs

Non-steroidal anti-inflammatory drugs (NSAIDs) block cyclooxygenase-1 (COX-1), cyclooxygenase-2 (COX-2), or nonspecifically both. Unlike aspi-rin, other salicylates and NSAIDs reversibly inhibit COX, which leads to decreased production of thromboxane A_2 and inhibition of platelet aggrega-tion. The duration of COX inhibition varies by agent and does not correlate well with the elimination half-life. For most NSAIDs, platelet function can be expected to normalize within 3 days of discontinuation [17]; therefore, it is acceptable to discontinue taking NSAIDs at least 3 days before surgery. NSAIDs are often prescribed for patients with rheumatic diseases as well as many other causes of inflammation. COX-1 inhibitors, such as aspirin, ibuprofen, naproxen sodium, and nabumetone, block the formation of thromboxane A_2, which impairs thromboxane-dependent platelet aggrega-tion and variably prolongs the bleeding time. The duration of action de-pends on the specific drug, dose, serum level, and half-life for these reversible NSAIDs. For a drug to clear the body, it takes approximately five times the half-life. It is recommended that ibuprofen be held for

1 day before surgery and naproxen sodium for 4 days owing to their half-lives of 2.5 hours and 16 hours, respectively [68]. The highly selective COX-2 inhibitor celecoxib (Celebrex) has no effect on platelet aggregation and hence no effect on bleeding time. Nevertheless, selective COX-2 inhibitors have the potential for renal toxicity and deleterious cardiovascular effects. It is recommended that this class of drugs be discontinued before surgery; however, for patients with dramatically decreased pain on COX-2 inhibitors, the agents can be continued [69].

Deep vein thrombosis prophylaxis

Within the first month after an acute episode of venous thromboembolism, each day without anticoagulation is associated with a 1% absolute increase in recurrence risk. Although postoperative intravenous heparin doubles the rate of bleeding, there is a net reduction in serious morbidity in such patients because the risk of postoperative recurrent venous thromboembolism is high. Heparin therapy is recommended both before and after surgery [51].

By 2 to 3 months after an acute episode of venous thromboembolism, the risk of recurrence is significantly reduced such that preoperative heparin therapy is probably not justified unless there are other risk factors for thromboembolism (see Table 2) [51]. Nevertheless, because of an expected 100-fold increase in the risk of venous thromboembolism after surgery, these patients should be treated postoperatively with heparin.

At more than 3 months after an episode of venous thromboembolism, preoperative anticoagulation is not needed, and postoperative intravenous heparin is also probably not necessary. In this setting, the bleeding associated with postoperative intravenous heparin offsets any beneficial effect from the prevention of major thromboembolic events [51]. Prophylactic measures that reduce the risk, such as subcutaneous low molecular weight heparin or compression stockings, are associated with a lower risk of bleeding than intravenous heparin and are safer alternatives [70].

Several recommendations can be made concerning the perioperative management of anticoagulation in patients with a history of venous thromboembolism. Elective surgery should be avoided in the first month after an acute episode of venous thromboembolism. If avoidance of elective surgery is not possible, warfarin should be withheld for 3 to 4 days, and intravenous heparin or low molecular weight heparin should be given before and after the procedure while the INR is below 2.0. The activated partial thromboplastin time (PTT) should be monitored during intravenous heparin use, and heparin should be continued until 6 hours before surgery [67].

If acute venous thromboembolism has occurred within 2 weeks, or if the risk of bleeding during intravenous heparin is high, a vena caval filter should be considered. Heparin or low molecular weight heparin should not be restarted postoperatively until at least 12 hours after major surgery and delayed longer if there is any evidence of bleeding.

If the patient has been receiving warfarin for more than 1 month but less than 3 months, preoperative intravenous heparin is probably not needed unless there are additional risk factors for recurrence. Postoperative intravenous heparin is recommended until warfarin therapy is resumed and the INR is above 2.0. The activated PTT should be checked 12 hours after restarting therapy to allow for a stable anticoagulation response and the dose of heparin adjusted accordingly.

If it has been 3 or more months since the last episode of acute venous thromboembolism and the patient has been taking warfarin, preoperative heparin is not necessary, but postoperative prophylaxis with subcutaneous heparin or low molecular weight heparin is recommended until oral anticoagulation is re-established.

Gastrointestinal agents

The stress of surgery can significantly increase the risk of stress-related mucosal damage. For this reason, gastrointestinal agents, namely, H_2 blockers and proton pump inhibitors, are continued throughout the perioperative period. These medications help prevent aspiration pneumonitis by controlling gastric acid acidity and volume. Because there are no known interactions between these medications and common anesthetic agents, continuation of these drugs is preferred [17]. It has been recommended to premedicate with an H_2 antagonist the evening before and the morning of surgery, with sodium citrate given immediately before induction in patients at high risk for aspiration pneumonitis [71]. For those patients who are unable to tolerate oral medications, intravenous formulations of these drugs exist. Of these agents, pantoprazole does not require any change in dosage because the bioavailability is the same as the oral dose [71].

Rheumatologic agents

Patients with rheumatologic conditions are usually treated with one drug or a combination of NSAIDs, glucocorticoids, and disease modifying antirheumatic drugs. Patients with rheumatic diseases are often prescribed glucocorticoids, usually for relatively long periods of time. The first surgical patient with iatrogenic adrenal insufficiency as a result of preoperative glucocorticoid withdrawal was reported in 1952 [72]. Current recommendations include individualization of supplementation based on the magnitude and involvement of the procedure, as well as the severity of the patient's condition. Salem and colleagues [73] published guidelines that related human cortisol production to the level of surgical intervention.

Side effects associated with the overwhelming administration of glucocorticoids include the possibility of hyperglycemia, hypertension, altered wound healing, and increased susceptibility to infections [74]. Patients on chronic glucocorticoids should receive their usual daily requirement throughout the perioperative period along with supplementation with a stress dose. Several studies have shown that a stress dose is needed only when the hypothalamic-pituitary-adrenal axis is suppressed. This suppression is often difficult to predict. General guidelines for increased risk with prednisone administration include patients taking 5 mg/day long-term, 7.5 to 10 mg/day for 1 month, more than 20 mg/day for 1 week, or high doses of other inhaled corticosteroids [75–77].

Perioperatively, hydrocortisone can be delivered intravenously or through intramuscular injection, in contrast to prednisone, which is commonly taken by mouth. Prednisone is approximately four times stronger than hydrocortisone. Most podiatric cases are considered to be minor or ambulatory in nature. When performing minor surgery, if a patient is on more than 10 mg/d of prednisone, 25 to 100 mg of hydrocortisone at induction is sufficient for a stress dose. Postoperatively, patients should resume the usual dose of corticosteroid the next day. When performing ambulatory procedures, one should administer 100 mg of hydrocortisone at discharge and prescribe a rapid taper of prednisone, or resume the patient's previous steroid dose [78–80].

Disease modifying anti-rheumatic drugs are composed of the traditional medications used, such as methotrexate, leflunomide, sulfasalazine, azathioprine, and hydroxychloroquine. Also included in this class of drugs are the biologic response modifiers that notably include the inhibitors of tumor necrosis factor (TNF)-[alpha] and interleukin-1 (IL-1). Methotrexate is a folic acid analogue that inhibits dihydrofolate reductase. It is one of the most common medications prescribed in the treatment of rheumatoid arthritis and many other rheumatologic conditions. Controversy exists regarding the stoppage or continuation of methotrexate in the perioperative period. Bridges and colleagues [78] published a small retrospective study looking at the perioperative effect of methotrexate in patients with rheumatoid arthritis who underwent elective orthopedic surgeries [78]. This study was the first to show an increase in perioperative complications when patients did not discontinue their methotrexate treatment before surgery. On the other hand, Grennan and colleagues [79] published a study of elective orthopedic surgical patients in which there was no increase in the number of infections or complications associated with continuation of methotrexate use. Due to its method of excretion, it is important to assess renal function in the patient on methotrexate. Excessive build up of methotrexate and its metabolites can lead to bone marrow suppression. It is recommended that methotrexate be held for 1 to 2 weeks before surgery in patients with renal impairment; however, there is no reason to stop perioperative methotrexate in the patient with sufficient kidney function [80].

Limited information is available on the use of other disease modifying anti-rheumatic drugs, including leflunomide, sulfasalazine, azathioprine, and hydroxychloroquine. Leflunomide is an antiproliferative agent that blocks pyrimidine, with a long half-life lasting weeks [82]. Because leflunomide has a predominant renal elimination, it is recommended that the drug be stopped for at least 2 weeks before surgery, with a restart a week after the procedure. Sulfasalazine and azathioprine have relatively short half-lives but have the same potential for bone marrow suppression as methotrexate [83,84]. Both of these medications have mostly a renal route for excretion; therefore, it is recommended that they be stopped at least a week before surgery and restarted approximately 1 week after surgery [81]. Hydroxychloroquine has minimal potential for toxicity with the low dosages used; therefore, continuation is not contraindicated.

The biologic response modifiers currently prescribed for rheumatoid arthritis include the anti–TNF-alpha agents etanercept, infliximab, and adalimumab, as well as the IL-1 antagonist anakinra. There are minimal data on the perioperative course of these medications. The minute amount of data that exists has been obtained in humans with Crohn's disease or studies in rats. Only infliximab has been studied in the perioperative period, and the information is derived from the manufacturer [82,85–87]. It is extremely difficult to advise podiatric patients about the continuation or discontinuation of these medications, and such recommendations are considered to be beyond the scope of this article. The IL-1 receptor antagonist modulator anakinra also suffers from a lack of hard data in relation to humans with rheumatoid arthritis. All of these medications would most likely cause flares of rheumatoid conditions if abruptly stopped; therefore, the conservative plan would be to stop the medications at least a week before surgery and to supplement the patient with other better understood medications [36]. Consultation with the patient's rheumatologist would be most prudent before prescribing a perioperative medication plan [36].

Pulmonary agents

Patients with pulmonary diseases are of particular importance when considering podiatric surgical intervention. In many podiatric procedures, the anesthesia of choice is monitored analgesia control sedation with locally infiltrated nerve blocks. With this type of anesthesia, the patient must be able to maintain their own airway without the assistance of intubation. In the patient with pulmonary disease, this consideration may sway the surgeon on the choice of procedure, patient positioning, and anesthesia to be used. Patients with pulmonary diseases, including asthma and chronic obstructive pulmonary disease, often take inhaled medications for treatment, including beta agonists and anticholinergic agents. These medications should be continued in the perioperative period for patients sustaining asthma and chronic obstructive pulmonary disease [88]. Inhaled medications decrease the breathing difficulties, such as bronchospasm, that may arise postoperatively.

Theophylline is another agent used for patients with pulmonary disorders. Theophylline is a methylxanthine drug that relaxes bronchial smooth muscle. It should be discontinued because it has severe toxicity at levels that are only slightly above therapeutic levels. Theophylline affects the heart and circulation by increasing the heart rate, heart contractility, and blood pressure. Other medications, such as corticosteroids and leukotrienes, are much safer and have less serious side effects when treating the patient in the perioperative setting. Patients with chronic pulmonary disease are often prescribed long-term doses of corticosteroids. These patients should continue taking these medications in the perioperative period so that their pulmonary condition does not worsen and they do not develop adrenal insufficiency. Short-term corticosteroids do not have an effect on wound healing or infection rates [89].

Asthma sufferers are usually prescribed leukotriene inhibitors as maintenance medications. Medications such as montelukast (Singulair), zafirlukast (Accolate), and zileuton (Zyflo) are the leukotriene inhibitors of choice for asthma. These drugs reduce the inflammatory response, reducing bronchospasm. Leukotrienes are approximately 100 times stronger than antihistamines. These medications have short half-lives with discontinuation but maintain effects for up to 3 weeks. These drugs do not have known detrimental side effects associated with stoppage, nor do they have an incidence of interference with anesthetic agents; therefore, it is recommended that they be continued throughout the perioperative period, including the morning of surgery and once the patient can tolerate oral medications.

Tobacco and alcohol

It is common to encounter patients who are candidates for podiatric procedures who either smoke tobacco products or drink alcoholic beverages on a regular basis. Chronic cigarette exposure produces profound changes in physiology and may alter responses to perioperative interventions and contribute to perioperative morbidity [90]. Given the variation among patients who are about to undergo podiatric surgery, it is important to differentiate between patients who are undergoing emergent surgery versus elective surgery. In the planning for surgery, time has an important role in the stoppage of tobacco use. A short abstinence period (12 to 72 hours) from tobacco products is sufficient to normalize several important cardiovascular parameters [91]. For smoking patients undergoing elective procedures, a minimum period of 4 to 6 weeks is appropriate to greatly influence postoperative respiratory morbidity and improve postoperative healing [92]. In the interim between consultation and surgery, a nicotine replacement therapy is often helpful for smoking patients [90].

As part of a good history taking process, the discovery of the patient's social history, including alcohol consumption, should be obtained. Alcohol is one of the most abused drugs in the United States today and is often a pertinent finding in the social history. In the presurgical phase, it is important to assess the patient who drinks in more depth. In addition to customary blood work, which may show alcoholic anemia or thrombocytopenia [93], liver testing should be performed to look for damage attributed to alcohol intake. It is also important to asses the hydration status of the patient, as well as their nutritional status. Additional tests to be ordered include total protein, albumin, globulin, alanine aminotransferase, and aspartate amino-transferase [93]. Also of interest is the prothrombin time, which will be pro-longed with liver damage [93]. Liver functionality is a factor when considering the type of anesthesia to be used, because lidocaine and bupiva-caine are both metabolized in the liver. Alternative local anesthetics, such as esters, may be used owing to their metabolism in the plasma. It is also im-portant for the anesthesiologist to be aware of the patient's alcohol history, because additional medications may be necessary during the induction of general anesthesia. It may be necessary for the patient with an extensive al-cohol history to see their primary care physician for counseling on cessation, replenishment of vitamins, and placement on a proper diet before clearing him or her for an elective surgical procedure. The patient with an addiction is a difficult customer to deal with perioperatively, especially with the avail-ability of the drug to which the person is addicted.

Summary

Podiatric surgical planning is a multifaceted endeavor that must include more than procedural planning. All of the medical conditions that the sur-gical candidate is experiencing must be addressed in the planning process. During the history and physical phase of patient care, it is vital to accu-rately obtain the patient's past medical history, surgical history, and current medications. These significant portions of the history can have an impact not only on the patient and procedure but also on other medical staff in-volved in a successful procedure, including the patient's other physicians, the anesthesiologist, and the nursing staff at the hospital or surgery center. It is also of great significance to assess the medicines used in a timely man-ner after surgery is decided upon as the course of action, because many medications must be altered or stopped days or weeks before surgery. Pre-operative testing may need to be performed for specific patients. Adequate planning must be done before surgery to enable the podiatric surgeon to ob-tain testing results in a timely manner and to permit adequate time to con-sult colleagues or fellow physicians, if deemed necessary. As physicians, podiatric surgeons, must be cognizant of the conditions affecting the health of the patient and must address each of these conditions before podiatric surgical intervention.

References

[1] Goldmann DR, Brown FH, Guarnieri DM. Perioperative medicine. 2nd edition. New York: McGraw-Hill, Inc; 1994.

[2] Merli GJ, Weitz HH. Medical management of the surgical patient. 2nd edition. Philadelphia: WB Saunders Company; 1998.

[3] Harris MI, Flegal KM, Cowie CC, et al. Prevalence of diabetes, impaired fasting glucose, and impaired glucose tolerance in US adults. Diabetes Care 1998;21:518–24.

[4] Schiff RL, Welsh GA. Perioperative evaluation and management of the patient with endocrine dysfunction. Med Clin North Am 2003;87(1):175–92.

[5] Hirsch IB, McGill JB. Role of insulin in management of surgical patients with diabetes mellitus. Diabetes Care 1990;13:980–91.

[6] Stagnaro-Green A. Perioperative glucose control: does it really matter? Mt Sinai J Med 1991; 58:299–304.

[7] Furnary AP, Zerr KJ, Grunkemeier GL. Continuous intravenous insulin infusion reduces the incidence of deep sternal wound infection in diabetic patients after cardiac surgical procedures. Ann Thorac Surg 1999;67:352–62.

[8] Pomposelli JJ, Baxter JK, Babineau TJ, et al. Early postoperative glucose control predicts nosocomial infection rate in diabetic patients. JPEN J Parenter Enteral Nutr 1998;22: 77–81.

[9] Scherpereel PA, Tavernier B. Perioperative care of diabetic patients. Eur J Anaesthesiol 2001;18:277–94.

[10] Hirsch IB, McGill JB, Cryer PE. Perioperative management of surgical patients with diabetes mellitus. Anesthesiology 1991;74:346–59.

[11] Gallacher SJ, Thomson G, Fraser WD, et al. Neutrophil bactericidal function in diabetes mellitus: evidence for association with blood glucose control. Diabet Med 1995;12:916–20.

[12] Golden SH, Peart-Vigilance C, Kao WHL. Perioperative glycemic control and the risk of infectious complications in a cohort of adults with diabetes. Diabetes Care 1999;22:1408–14.

[13] Van Den Berghe G, Wouters P, Weekers F, et al. Intensive insulin therapy in critically ill patients. N Engl J Med 2001;345:1359–67.

[14] Naito Y, Tamai S, Shingu K, et al. Responses of plasma adrenocorticotropic hormone, cortisol, and cytokines during and after upper abdominal surgery. Anesthesiology 1992;77: 426–31.

[15] Goschke H, Bar E, Girard J, et al. Glucagon, insulin, cortisol, and growth hormone levels following major surgery: their relationship to glucose and free fatty acid elevations. Horm Metab Res 1978;10:465–70.

[16] Katzung BG. Basic and clinical pharmacology. 9th edition. New York: Lange Medical Books/McGraw-Hill; 2004.

[17] Muluk V, Macpherson DS. Perioperative medication management. Up to Date; Available at: http://www.uptodate.com. 2006.

[18] Grady D, Wenger NK, Herrington D, et al. Postmenopausal hormone therapy increases risk for venous thromboembolic disease: The Heart and Estrogen/progestin Replacement Study [see comments]. Ann Intern Med 2000;132. p. 680–690.

[19] Miller J, Chan BK, Nelson HD. Postmenopausal estrogen replacement and risk for venous thromboembolism: a systematic review and meta-analysis for the US Preventive Services Task Force. Ann Intern Med 2002;136:680.

[20] Rang HP, Dale MM, Ritter JM, et al. Pharmacology. 5th edition. Edinburgh, Scotland: Churchill Livingstone Inc.

[21] Roizen MF. Anesthetic implications of concurrent diseases. In: Miller RD, editor. Anesthesia. Philadelphia: Churchill Livingstone; 2000. p. 903–1015.

[22] Farmer JA, Gotto AM. Dyslipidemia and other risk factors for coronary artery disease. In: Braunwald E, editor. A textbook of cardiovascular medicine. Philadelphia: WB Saunders; 1997. p. 1126.

[23] Hamilton-Craig I. Statin-associated myopathy. Med J Aust 2001;175:486.

[24] Shek A, Ferrill MJ. Statin-fibrate combination therapy. Ann Pharmacother 2001;35:908.

[25] Durazzo AE, Machado FS, Ikeoka DT, et al. Reduction in cardiovascular events after vascular surgery with atorvastatin: a randomized trial. J Vasc Surg 2004;39:967.

[26] Lindenauer PK, Pekow P, Wang K, et al. Lipid-lowering therapy and in-hospital mortality following major noncardiac surgery. JAMA 2004;291:2092.

[27] Poldermans D, Bax JJ, Kertai MD, et al. Statins are associated with a reduced incidence of perioperative mortality in patients undergoing major noncardiac vascular surgery. Circulation 2003;107:1848.

[28] Gertz K, Laufs U, Lindauer U, et al. Withdrawal of statin treatment abrogates stroke protection in mice. Stroke 2003;34:551.

[29] Abbott TR. Anaesthesia in untreated myxoedema. Br J Anaesth 1967;39:510–4.

[30] Kim JM, Hackman L. Anesthesia for untreated hypothyroidism: report of three cases. Anesth Analg 1977;56(2):299–302.

[31] Weinberg AD, Brennan MD, Gorman CA. Outcome of anesthesia and surgery in hypothyroid patients. Arch Intern Med 1983;143(5):893–7.

[32] Ladenson PW, Levin AA, Ridgway EC, et al. Complications of surgery in hypothyroid patients. Am J Med 1984;77(2):261–6.

[33] Strube PJ. Thyroid storm during beta-blockade. Anaesthesia 1984;39:343–6.

[34] McArthur JW, Rawson RW, Means JH, et al. Thyrotoxic crisis. JAMA 1947;132:868.

[35] Alderbeith A, Stenstrom G, Hasslegren PO. The selective beta-blocking agent metoprolol compared with antithyroid drugs as preoperative treatment of patients with hyperthyroidism: results from a preoperative randomized study. Ann Surg 1987;205:182–8.

[36] Eagle KA, Berger PB, Calkins H. ACC/AHA guideline update for perioperative cardiovascular evaluation for noncardiac surgery—executive summary: a report of the American College of Cardiology/American Heart Association Task Force on Practice Guidelines. Circulation 2002;105(10):1257–67.

[37] Yeager R, Moneta G, Edwards J, et al. Reducing perioperative myocardial infarction following vascular surgery. Arch Surg 1995;130:869.

[38] Mangano DT, Layug EL, Wallace A, et al. For the Multicenter Study of Perioperative Ischemia Research Group. Effect of atenolol on mortality and cardiovascular morbidity after noncardiac surgery. N Engl J Med 1996;335:1713.

[39] Poldermans D, Boersma E, Bax JJ, et al. The effect of bisoprolol on perioperative mortality and myocardial infarction in high-risk patients undergoing vascular surgery: Dutch Echocardiographic Cardiac Risk Evaluation Applying Stress Echocardiography Study Group. N Engl J Med 1999;341:1789.

[40] Gu W, Pagel PS, Warltier DC, et al. Modifying cardiovascular risk in diabetes mellitus. Anesthesiology 2003;98:774–9.

[41] Hayashi Y, Maze M. Alpha 2 adrenoceptor agonists and anaesthesia. Br J Anaesth 1993;71:108.

[42] Quintin L, Cicala R, Kent M, et al. Effect of clonidine on myocardial ischaemia: a double-blind pilot trial. Can J Anaesth 1993;40:85.

[43] Legault C, Furberg CD, Wagenknecht LE, et al. Nimodipine neuroprotection in cardiac valve replacement: report of an early terminated trial. Stroke 1996;27:593.

[44] Wagenknecht LE, Furberg CD, Hammon JW, et al. Surgical bleeding: unexpected effect of a calcium antagonist. BMJ 1995;310:776.

[45] Zuccala G, Pahor M, Landi F, et al. Use of calcium antagonists and need for perioperative transfusion in older patients with hip fracture: observational study. BMJ 1997;314:643.

[46] Effects of calcium antagonists on the risks of coronary heart disease, cancer and bleeding: Ad Hoc Subcommittee of the Liaison Committee of the World Health Organisation and the International Society of Hypertension. J Hypertens 1997;15:105.

[47] Grodecki-De Franco P, Steinhubl S, Taylor P, et al. Calcium antagonist use and perioperative bleeding complications: an analysis of 5157 patients. Circulation 1996;94(Suppl):476.

[48] Coriat P, Richer C, Douraki T, et al. Influence of chronic angiotensin-converting enzyme inhibition on anesthetic induction. Anesthesiology 1994;81:299.

[49] Pigott DW, Nagle C, Allman K, et al. Effect of omitting regular ACE inhibitor medication before cardiac surgery on haemodynamic variables and vasoactive drug requirements. Br J Anaesth 1999;83:715.

[50] Smith MS, Muir H, Hall R. Perioperative management of drug therapy, clinical considerations. Drugs 1996;51:238.

[51] Kearon K, Hirsch J. Current concepts: management of anticoagulation before and after elective surgery. N Engl J Med 1997;336(21):1506–11.

[52] Otley CC. Continuation of medically necessary aspirin and warfarin during cutaneous surgery. Mayo Clin Proc 2003;78:1392.

[53] Nieuwenhuis HK, Albada J, Banga JD, et al. Identification of risk factors for bleeding during treatment of acute venous thromboembolism with heparin or low molecular weight heparin. Blood 1991;78:2337.

[54] Levine MN, Raskob G, Landefeld S, et al. Hemorrhagic complications of anticoagulant treatment. Chest 1995;108:276S.

[55] Torn M, Rosendaal FR. Oral anticoagulation in surgical procedures: risks and recommendations. Br J Haematol 2003;123:676.

[56] White RH, McKittrick T, Hutchinson R, et al. Temporary discontinuation of warfarin therapy: changes in the international normalised ratio. Ann Intern Med 1995;122:40.

[57] Bern MM, Lokich JJ, Wallach SR, et al. Very low doses of warfarin can prevent thrombosis in central venous catheters: a randomized prospective trial. Ann Intern Med 1990;112:423.

[58] Levine M, Hirsh J, Gent M, et al. Double-blind randomised trial of a very-low-dose warfarin for prevention of thromboembolism in stage IV breast cancer. Lancet 1994;343:886.

[59] Loh E, St. John Sutton M, Wun CC, et al. Ventricular dysfunction and the risk of stroke after myocardial infarction. N Engl J Med 1997;336:251.

[60] Collins LJ, Silverman DI, Douglas PS, et al. Cardioversion of nonrheumatic atrial fibrillation: reduced thromboembolic complications with 4 weeks of pre-cardioversion anticoagulation are related to atrial thrombus resolution. Circulation 1995;92:160.

[61] Larson BJ, Zumberg MS, Kitchens CS. A feasibility study of continuing dose-reduced warfarin for invasive procedures in patients with high thromboembolic risk. Chest 2005;127:922.

[62] Spandorfer JM, Lynch S, Weitz HH, et al. Use of enoxaparin for the chronically anticoagulated patient before and after procedures. Am J Cardiol 1999;84:478.

[63] Kovacs MJ, Kearon C, Rodger M, et al. Single-arm study of bridging therapy with low-molecular-weight heparin for patients at risk of arterial embolism who require temporary interruption of warfarin. Circulation 2004;110:1658.

[64] Spyropoulos AC, Frost FJ, Hurley JS, et al. Costs and clinical outcomes associated with low-molecular-weight heparin vs unfractionated heparin for perioperative bridging in patients receiving long-term oral anticoagulant therapy. Chest 2004;125:1642.

[65] Diener HC, Cunha L, Forbes C, et al. European Stroke Prevention Study. 2. Dipyridamole and acetylsalicylic acid in the secondary prevention of stroke. J Neurol Sci 1996;143:1.

[66] Rustad H, Myhre E. Surgery during anticoagulant treatment: the risk of increased bleeding in patients on oral anticoagulant treatment. Acta Med Scand 1963;173:115.

[67] Lip GYH. Maneagment of anticoagulation before and after elective surgery. Up to Date; Available at: www.uptodate.com. 2006.

[68] Schafer AI. Effects of nonsteroidal anti-inflammatory drugs on platelet function and systemic hemostasis. J Clin Pharmacol 1995;35:209–19.

[69] Engelman RM, Hadji-Rousou I, Breyer RH, et al. Rebound vasospasm after coronary revascularization in association with calcium antagonist withdrawal. Ann Thorac Surg 1984;37:469.

[70] Kakkar VV, Cohen AT, Edmonson RA, et al. Low molecular weight versus standard heparin for prevention of venous thromboembolism after major abdominal surgery: the Thromboprophylaxis Collaborative Group. Lancet 1993;341:259.

[71] Pisegna JR. Switching between intravenous and oral pantoprazole. J Clin Gastroenterol 2001;32(1):27–32.

[72] Fraser CG, Preuss FS, Bigford WD. Adrenal atrophy and irreversible shock associated with cortisone therapy. JAMA 1952;149:1542–3.

[73] Salem M, Tainsh RE Jr, Bromberg J, et al. Perioperative glucocorticoid coverage: a reassessment 42 years after emergence of a problem. Ann Surg 1994;219:416–25.

[74] Shaw M, Mandell BF. Perioperative management of selected problems in patients with rheumatic diseases. Rheum Dis Clin North Am 1999;25:623–38.

[75] Cooper MS, Stewart PM. Corticosteroid insufficiency in acutely ill patients. N Engl J Med 2003;348:727–34.

[76] Coursin DB, Wood KE. Corticosteroid supplementation for adrenal insufficiency. JAMA 2002;287:236–40.

[77] Lamberts SW, Bruining HA, de Jong FH. Corticosteroid therapy in severe illness. N Engl J Med 1997;337:1285–92.

[78] Bridges SL Jr, Lopez-Mendez A, Han KH, et al. Should methotrexate be discontinued before elective orthopedic surgery in patients with rheumatoid arthritis? J Rheumatol 1991;18: 984–8.

[79] Grennan DM, Gray J, Loudon J, et al. Methotrexate and early postoperative complications in patients with rheumatoid arthritis undergoing elective orthopaedic surgery. Ann Rheum Dis 2001;60:214–7.

[80] Wluka A, Buchbinder R, Mylvaganam A, et al. Long-term methotrexate use in rheumatoid arthritis: 12 year follow-up of 460 patients treated in community practice. J Rheumatol 2000; 27:1864–71.

[81] Rozman B. Clinical pharmacokinetics of leflunomide. Clin Pharmacokinet 2002;41:421–30.

[82] Centocor Medical. Centocor Medical Information for Remicade (Infliximab). Rev. 1.3. Centocor Medical; Issue 26:2003.

[83] Howland WL. Methotrexate-associated bone marrow suppression following surgery. Arthritis Rheum 1988;31:1586–7.

[84] Kelley JT, Conn DL. Perioperative management of the rheumatic disease patient: Arthritis Foundation. Bull Rheum Dis 2002;51:58–75.

[85] Colombel JF, Loftus EV, Tremaine WJ, et al. Perioperative infliximab and/or immunomodulator therapy is not associated with increased postoperative complications in Crohn's disease. Presented at the Digestive Diseases Week. Orlando, May 18–21, 2003.

[86] Brzezinski A, Armstrong L, Del Real GA, et al. Infliximab does not increase the risk of complications in the perioperative period in patients with Crohn's disease [abstract no. 104783]. Presented at the Digestive Disease Week. San Francisco, May 19–22, 2002.

[87] Marchal L, D'Haens G, Van Assche G, et al. Infliximab does not increase postoperative rates in patients with Crohn's disease [abstract no. 100519]. Presented at the Digestive Diseases Week. Orlando, May 18–21, 2003.

[88] Stoller JK. Acute exacerbations of chronic obstructive pulmonary disease. N Engl J Med 2002;346:988–94.

[89] Kabalin C. Low complication rate of corticosteroid-treated asthmatics undergoing surgical procedure. Arch Intern Med 1995;155:1379–84.

[90] Warner DO. Perioperative abstinence from cigarettes: physiologic and clinical consequences. Anesthesiology 2006;104(2):356–67.

[91] Anderson ME, Belani KG. Short-term preoperative smoking abstinence. Am Fam Physician 1990;41(4):1191–4.

[92] Pearce AC, Jones RM. Smoking and anesthesia: preoperative abstinence and perioperative morbidity. Anesthesiology 1984;61(5):576–84.

[93] Albert SF. Elective foot surgery and the alcoholic. J Am Podiatry Assoc 1981;71(1):8–18.

ELSEVIER
SAUNDERS

Clin Podiatr Med Surg
24 (2007) 245–259

CLINICS IN
PODIATRIC
MEDICINE AND
SURGERY

Perioperative Nutrition and the Use of Nutritional Supplements

David H. Rahm, MD[a],*,
Jonathan M. Labovitz, DPM, FACFAS[b]

[a]VitaMedica Corporation, 1140 Highland Avenue, Suite 196,
Manhattan Beach, CA 90266, USA
[b]West Torrance Podiatrists Group, 3400 Lomita Boulevard,
#403, Torrance, CA 90505, USA

In the past 20 years, two major trends have emerged in the United States that may have a significant impact on elective surgery. The dietary habits and decreased activity levels of many Americans have led to an increased incidence of obesity [1,2]. The second trend is the aging population. Age-related health issues have increased that, coupled with an overweight society, have led to a declining health and nutritional status with increased susceptibility to chronic disease.

Optimal outcomes are desired by all surgeons. The podiatric surgeon affects the function of locomotion with each surgery, and some podiatric procedures can be considered to have a cosmetic component to them as well. The expectations of patients may sometimes exceed the goals and experience of the surgeon, increasing the necessity to optimize potential outcomes. Awareness of the subtle changes in the body during the perioperative period may aid in obtaining consistent surgical results. Nutritional insufficiencies remain one of the most reversible host factors that can render patients more susceptible to complications and impaired wound healing [3].

Obesity, aging, and nutrition

The extent of obesity and the prevalence of chronic disease have been well established. In fact, there is an exponential increase in mortality risk as weight increases [4–6]. Poorly nourished, obese, and especially diabetic patients are

---

* Corresponding author. VitaMedica Corporation, 1140 Highland Avenue, Suite 196, Manhattan Beach, CA 90266.
E-mail address: david@vitamedica.com (D.H. Rahm).

particularly prone to complications related to the perioperative period. Multisystemic effects on cardiovascular (coronary artery disease, hypertension, congestive heart failure), respiratory (pulmonary hypertension, sleep apnea, restrictive lung disease), endocrine (diabetes mellitus, thyroid disease), musculoskeletal, and even psychiatric systems need to be evaluated. There are reports of an increased risk of sudden death in patients with a body mass index (BMI) of greater than 35, and the risk of deep venous thrombosis is doubled with a BMI greater than 30. There is a 5% increased risk of sleep apnea with a BMI greater than 30 and three to four times the risk of respiratory depression from sedatives and analgesics with a BMI greater than 35. Poor healing and postoperative wound infections are also of significant concern in these patients. With these increased risks well known, ambulatory surgery centers are now placing limits on elective outpatient surgery based on a patient's BMI, where obesity is defined as a BMI greater than 30 and morbid obesity as a BMI greater than 35. Excluding the normal limitations of weight and operative table limits at many surgery centers, American Society of Anesthesiologists' (ASA) classes I, II, and III for obese patients and classes I and II for morbidly obese patients are becoming customary in the ambulatory surgical setting secondary to the potential for cardiovascular or respiratory sequelae. As the incidence of diabetes increases, this will have greater implications for care by the podiatric surgeon.

The National Health and Nutrition Examination Surveys (NHANES I, II, and III) are large-scale, government-sponsored studies evaluating the eating habits of Americans. NHANES III completed in 1994, reported that 64% of the United States population was overweight or obese [7]. In the past 20 years, obesity has more than doubled to 31% of Americans. Consequently, the incidence of diabetes mellitus has also risen dramatically. In 2001, diabetes accounted for the primary diagnosis at 27 million doctor visits. The survey also estimated an additional 5 million adults with diabetes who are undiagnosed.

Most Americans consume diets that are insufficient in the essential nutrients and high in caloric intake. More than 70% of adults do not meet two thirds of the Recommended Dietary Allowance for one or more nutrients [8–10]. The most notable area of deficiency revolves around a lack of fruits and vegetables [11,12]. Pre-packaged, processed, and instant type foods and meals are poor suppliers of the essential nutrients. These deficiencies result in a shortage of vitamins, minerals, and antioxidants that are important in the surgical patient to optimize tolerance of anesthesia, the stress of surgery, and wound healing.

The aging patient is also susceptible to an increase in perioperative complications. Poor nutrition in the elderly patient has been shown to lead to complications during hospitalization and increased mortality [13]. Wound healing complications may be the greatest concern in these patients secondary to the presence of chronic disease, medications, poor dentition, declining cognitive and functional status, and the environmental stress of poverty and isolation [13]. These factors may account for the more commonly seen delays in healing and an overall slower rate of recovery when aging patients are compared with younger patients. Aging also alters the normal regulatory functions of cell-mediated immunity. Decreased zinc, selenium, and vitamin B_6, prevalent in older patients, have been identified as micronutrients that alter immunity. The decrease in cell-mediated immunity, coupled with potential malnourishment and deficient levels of particular micronutrients, lead to an increased risk of postoperative infection.

Nutritional supplements in the United States

Americans have increased the use of alternative therapies to address health care needs. In an attempt to avoid pharmaceuticals, an increasing number of people are turning to herbal medicines. This use has provided an additional method of treating chronic disease that is difficult to control, although it may provide a less expensive treatment option. The readily accessible herbal medications available from nutrition stores, the Internet, and mail-order companies have greatly aided an explosion in the use of these treatments. Unfortunately, some of these compounds may have interactions with other supplements, with traditional medications, and with anesthetic agents.

A smaller segment of the population takes a multivitamin or other nutritional supplements for daily health maintenance. It has been recommended in the *Journal of the American Medical Association* to take a multivitamin daily [14,15]. This recommendation was made because the investigators concluded that daily multivitamins may help prevent the onset of heart disease and osteoporosis and may provide the basis for perioperative nutritional management [3,16].

Exclusion of supplements during the perioperative period

Particular nutritional supplements should be discontinued during the perioperative period. The list of supplements that should be stopped has been debated for several years [17–20]. All of the five most commonly used supplements (ginkgo biloba, St. John's wort, ginseng, garlic, echinacea) can have a negative impact during surgery [21,22]. It has become essential to have a detailed knowledge of the prescription medications, over-the-counter medications, and herbal supplements patients ingest.

Some herbal medications have been shown to cause complications such as prolonged bleeding, hypertension, tachycardia and other cardiovascular disturbances, drug interactions, and interference with anesthesia [22,23]. The ASA recommends discontinuing these herbal medications at least 2 weeks before surgery. Table 1 lists supplements that should be discontinued along with their respective potential adverse reactions.

Table 1
Supplements to exclude during the perioperative period

Supplement	Indication	Adverse effect
Bilberry	Antioxidant, visual acuity	Antiplatelet; inhibits clot formation; hypoglycemia
Dong quai	Menstrual cramps and menopausal disorder relief	May potentiate anticoagulant medications
Echinacea	Stimulates immune system	Hepatotoxicity; contraindicated with hepatotoxic drugs (eg, steroids, methotrexate)
Ephedra (ma-huang)[a]	CNS stimulant, appetite suppressant, anti-asthmatic, bronchodilator, nasal decongestant	HTN, tachycardia, cardiomyopathy, dysrhythmia, myocardial infarction
Feverfew	Migraines, allergies	May affect clotting; contraindicated with anticoagulant medications
Fish oil	Hypercholesterolemia, hyperlipidemia	Inhibits platelet adhesion and aggregation; excessive doses can inhibit wound healing
Garlic	Antispasmodic, antiseptic, HTN, antiviral, hypercholesterolemia	Contraindicated with anticoagulants, aspirin, NSAIDs
Ginger	Antinauseant, antispasmodic	Prolonged clotting time risk; contraindicated with anticoagulants, aspirin, NSAIDs
Ginkgo biloba	Antioxidant, vertigo, tinnitus, increased cerebral blood flow	Inhibits platelet activity factor; contraindicated with anticoagulants, aspirin, NSAIDs
Ginseng	Antioxidant; improves physical and cognitive performance	May interact with cardiac and hypoglycemic agents; contraindicated with anticoagulants, aspirin, NSAIDs
Goldenseal	Mild laxative; reduces inflammation	May worsen edema and HTN
Hawthorne	Ischemic heart disease, HTN, angina, chronic CHF	Potentiates actions of digitalis and other cardiac glycosides
Kava kava	Sedative, analgesic, anxiolytic, muscle relaxant	Potentiates CNS effects of barbiturates, antidepressants, antipsychotics, and general anesthesia
Licorice	Gastric and duodenal ulcers, gastritis, bronchitis	HTN, hypokalemia, edema
Melatonin	Insomnia, jet lag, seasonal affective disorder	Potentiates effects of general anesthesia and barbituates
Red clover	Menopausal symptoms	May potentiate anticoagulants
St. John's wort	Moderate antidepressant	Contraindicated with MAO inhibitors and SSRIs; many drug interactions; photosensitivity
Valerian	Mild sedative	Contraindicated with sedatives and anxiolytics
Vitamin E	Antioxidant, cardiovascular disease	Prolongs bleeding time

(*continued on next page*)

Table 1 (*continued*)

Supplement	Indication	Adverse effect
Yohimbe	Aphrodisiac, sexual stimulant	HTN; tachycardia; increases potency of anesthetic agents

Abbreviations: CHF, congestive heart failure; CNS, central nervous system; HTN, hypertension; MAO, monoamine oxidase; NSAIDs, non-steroidal anti-inflammatories; SSRIs, selective serotonin reuptake inhibitors.

[a] The Food and Drug Administration (FDA) regulates sales of ephedra because it has been abused by many dieters; the FDA maintains "ephedra is dangerous at any dose."

Perioperative nutrition

Recent statistics indicate a high likelihood of poor dietary habits in the surgical patient [8–10,12]. Although a complete history of the dietary habits of the surgical patient is not realistic, it is advisable to evaluate the patient's likelihood for malnutrition and to further question the nutritional status in potential malnourished patients. Short-term nutritional support may enhance patient satisfaction and surgical outcomes. Although it is not known whether enhancement of micronutrients in patients with normal nutritional status is beneficial, one prospective study evaluated macronutrient (protein, fat, and carbohydrate) supplementation in well-nourished patients undergoing major elective gastrointestinal surgery. The study concluded that pre- and postoperative high-energy, high-protein oral supplements provided no benefit in regards to wound healing, postsurgical infection, and length of hospital stay [24]. Table 2 lists the micronutrient supplements that are safe and potentially beneficial to use during the perioperative period, along with the recommend dosage.

Many podiatric surgical patients express concern that inactivity and potential limitations in weight-bearing status during the recovery period will cause weight gain. Nevertheless, decreasing caloric intake is not recommended during the perioperative period. Restricted caloric intake can reduce micronutrient ingestion necessary for adequate healing. Weight gain during the period of limited weight bearing and inactivity is also less likely than anticipated, because the body's metabolic requirements increase 10% to 100% secondary to cortisol release and the additional stress of surgery [25]. In addition, nutritional supplements are supposed to serve as an additional source of necessary nutrients while normal dietary intake provides the main source. Reduction of calories may translate to a reduction in the natural and best form of essential nutrients.

Perioperative supplementation

Perioperative supplementation may prove to be a simple way to increase potential outcomes in the surgical patient because changing dietary habits

Table 2
Supplements to include during the perioperative period

Nutrient	Mechanism of action	Dosage range
Vitamin A	Antioxidant; required for new cell growth, maintenance, and repair of epithelial tissue	15,000–25,000 IUs daily, (carotenoid and palmitate blend); limited use to 4 weeks
Vitamin C	Antioxidant; necessary for tissue growth and repair; primary role in collagen formation	500–750 mg daily in divided doses
B-complex vitamins (B_1, thiamin; B_2, riboflavin; B_3, niacin; B_6, pyroxidine; biotin; pantothenic acid; folic acid; B_{12}, cobalamin; choline, inositol)	Anti-stress	B-complex supplement
Zinc	Antioxidant; protein synthesis; collagen formation	15–21 mg daily
Selenium	Antioxidant; protects vitamin E; inhibits oxidation of fats	150–210 μg daily
Copper	Cross-linking of collagen and elastin; hemoglobin, red blood cell, and bone formation	1.5–2.0 μg daily
Arnica montana	Ecchymosis and edema	30X formula or higher TID postoperatively
Bromelain	Proteolytic enzyme minimizes inflammation and soft tissue injury	1500 mg per day; 2000–3000 MCUs per day taken TID starting 72 hours preoperatively
Flavonoids (quercetin and citrus biflavonoids)	Antioxidant; anti-inflammatory; prevents bruising and supports immune function with vitamin C	600–1500 mg daily

Abbreviations: IU, international unit; MCU, milk clotting unit.

and lifestyle is frequently a difficult task for many people. A surgical plan involving supplements to enhance (not replace) normal dietary habits may be the easiest for patient compliance. The suggestion of nutritional supplements may augment the micronutrient deficiencies that would otherwise potentially compromise surgical outcomes. Although there is no consensus on appropriate dosage of these supplements during the perioperative period, suggested dose ranges are provided in Table 2.

Oral nutritional supplementation can enhance surgical outcomes and reduce the risk of complications via four mechanisms: (1) promoting wound healing; (2) enhancing immunity; (3) reducing swelling, bruising, and inflammation; and (4) reducing oxidation caused by anesthetic agents and surgery.

Promoting wound healing

Wound healing is an organized process of inflammation, epithelialization, angiogenesis, and an accumulation of the cells involved in reorganization of the tissue. This process to restore the normal integrity of damaged tissue is usually successful; however, with the increase in chronic disease that may alter this normal process, wound healing may not progress as expected. A patient of poor health or nutritional status may not have the ability to supply the newly forming tissues with the essential nutrients necessary for angiogenesis and epithelialization.

Much has been written regarding nutritional deficiencies and wound healing with regard to diabetic patients and ulcer management. Mainly, the literature focuses on ulcer-related wound healing associated with macronutrient deficiencies. Protein and energy requirements are known to increase in these patients because there is an induction of metabolic stress causing an elevation of the metabolic state. The higher protein requirements and energy requirements are seen during the inflammatory and remodeling phases of wound healing. These findings are similar to the metabolic changes seen during surgery. The catabolic response in both scenarios causes a breakdown of skeletal muscle, decreased immunocompetence, and increased morbidity and mortality.

Changes in macronutrient requirements can also increase the severity of complications and postoperative infection [26]. The amino acid glutamine has a significant role in tissue function and in translocation of nitrogen to the wound, enhancing protein anabolism, and glutamine supplementation has been shown to aid in wound healing and to decrease hospital length of stay. Most of the studies involved parenteral glutamine administration; however, the nitrogen balance post elective surgery was also enhanced with oral administration [27].

Arginine is an essential amino acid that functions as the precursor of nitric oxide, which causes vasodilatation, antibacterial actions, and angiogenic activity. All of these properties can aid in wound healing, providing protection against postoperative infection. Arginine is also a substrate for cell proliferation, collagen synthesis, and protein synthesis. Daily oral arginine supplementation enhances the rate of collagen production when compared with that in control subjects [28].

Several vitamins and minerals display an effect on wound healing (see Table 2). Zinc is a trace mineral that has been reported in many studies to aid in wound healing. It serves as a cofactor for protein synthesis and is transported by albumin, demonstrating the importance of adequate protein intake. The role zinc has in protein synthesis affects DNA and RNA, fostering collagen synthesis and tissue growth and healing. Zinc also aids in vitamin A transport.

Zinc supplementation has been advocated in pressure ulcer management when zinc insufficiency is suspected. In fact, studies show that zinc does not accelerate wound healing unless the patient is deficient in zinc [29]. The National Pressure Ulcer Advisory Board notes that no substantial research supports zinc supplementation unless a deficiency is suspected [30]. When deficiency is suspected, zinc supplementation is advisable. Dosages below 40 mg/day (maximal dose) pose no risk for adverse effects. Excessive zinc intake can interfere with copper absorption and metabolism, which is another trace mineral important in wound healing because it is a cofactor for collagen cross-linking [31]. Zinc may also alter iron absorption, potentially leading to anemia.

Vitamin C is one of the most important nutrients for wound healing. Adequate vitamin C levels are required for collagen synthesis. More specifically, vitamin C allows for proper function of protocollagen hydroxylase, which produces collagen. One study demonstrated the need for supplementation of vitamin C to counter the deficient state. During World War II, British surgeons began administering 1000 mg of vitamin C per day for 3 days preoperatively and 100 mg per day during recovery secondary to the high volume of surgery from war casualties along with poor dietary intake, also as a result of the war. The incidence of wound healing complications decreased 76% upon supplementation [32]. In 1942, Hunt [33] confirmed the benefit of vitamin C supplementation with a study showing that 1000 mg per day during the postsurgical period led to increases in wound strength.

With these studies in mind, it is evident that vitamin C supplementation may be advisable in surgical patients because normal dietary intake is likely to be insufficient [3,32]. The need for supplementation is enhanced by the simple fact that vitamin C is water soluble; therefore, excess is excreted and not stored in fat. Ophthalmologists are routinely supplanting vitamin C in patients undergoing corneal transplants to optimize wound healing.

Diets supplementing macronutrients and micronutrients have been examined. Oral high-protein/high-energy diets supplemented with 9 g of arginine, 30 mg of zinc, and 500 mg of vitamin C have been studied; however, only one randomized, prospective, placebo-controlled study incorporated statistical analysis to determine the efficacy of the oral administration of the supplements. In 16 patients with pressure ulcers at stages 2, 3, or 4 and a BMI less than 28, supplementation accelerated the rate of ulcer healing nearly threefold in only 3 weeks [34]. In one study of orthopedic procedures, elective and emergent, patients were given postoperative high-energy and high-protein supplementation in a prospective fashion. Supplementation two times per day provided a significant decrease in major complications, including a reduction of postoperative infection (13.1% versus 21.6%) and bone fusion failure (0% versus 4.1%) [35].

Vitamin A is another nutrient that has been determined to be essential in regards to optimizing the intricate process of wound healing. Corticosteroids have been well known to impair wound healing via interference with the inflammatory process, fibroblast proliferation, collagen synthesis, and epithelialization. Vitamin A counters these functions by promoting re-epithelialization and restoring the inflammatory response. Vitamin A also promotes collagen synthesis [36]. The plastic surgery literature has documented the safety profile of vitamin A [22,36], determining that supplementation should be given for no more than 4 weeks during the perioperative period at a daily dose up to 25,000 international units (IUs) (see Table 2). Toxicity of vitamin A is rare, with fewer than 10 cases reported annually from 1976 to 1987. Toxic responses are reversible with cessation of the nutrient and usually occur after ingestion of 500,000 IU [37]. Mega-dose supplements have increased the prevalence of diarrhea and acute respiratory infections in children [38]. The main precaution is that vitamin A should not be used during pregnancy.

Enhancing immunity

Like aging, poor nutritional status effects cellular physiology and immune function. Cortisol release and stress, pain, and anesthesia can also affect immune function, potentially leading to a large number of negative factors affecting the immune system of the surgical patient. Obesity and diabetes mellitus have a role in cell-mediated immune status. Nearly every nutrient has a role in normal immune function, with deficient or excessive intake potentially having a negative impact. This crucial role clearly increases the potential susceptibility to pathogens during the postoperative period.

Malnourishment leading to a decreased ability to provide host protection can be caused by an insufficient intake of energy, macronutrients, or specific micronutrients. Obesity and excessive caloric intake can also compromise immune mechanisms. The normal aging process has a negative impact on immunity, which is likely enhanced by the frequent poor nutritional status in the elderly.

Particular nutrients are known to directly enhance immune status. Many of these nutritional factors have a role in reducing potential postoperative complications such as infection. One such nutrient is zinc, which, along with its role in wound healing, affects more than 300 enzymes that are involved in immune function. Because zinc facilitates T-lymphocyte development and activation, even a slight zinc deficiency may negatively impact immunity [39]. Zinc-deficient patients may experience an increased susceptibility to a host of pathogens via mechanisms ranging from the skin barrier to gene regulation of lymphocytes [40]. The effect zinc has on these various mediators of the immune system is based on its role in basic cellular function. Zinc is involved in DNA replication, RNA transcription, cell division, and cell activation. A small dose of zinc via supplementation is likely to boost immune function via T lymphocytes, reducing the potential incidence of postoperative infections and their sequelae.

Vitamin A also aids in immune function [41]. Animal studies involving vitamin A demonstrated an increase in cytokine expression and an increase in antibody production. In addition, vitamin A and related retinoids have a role in lymphopoiesis and white blood cell function. More specifically, vitamin A activates natural killer cells, lymphocytes, and macrophages. Patients undergoing surgery, persons with marginal nutrition, and elderly patients have all demonstrated a boost in immune function with vitamin A supplementation.

Other micronutrients are also immunoprotective. In addition to the wound healing benefits of arginine, it is a substrate for T-lymphocyte production and restoration of macrophage function [42]. Fish oils (omega-3 fatty acids) may be controversial during the postoperative period. The omega-3 fatty acids alter membrane fluidity and insulin sensitivity. They also modify production of leukotrienes, prostaglandins, and cytotoxin, decreasing the inflammatory and immunosuppressive mediators. More recently, it has been reported that arginine and fish oils work synergistically. A meta-analysis of 17 studies (n = 2305 patients) reported no adverse effects with pre- or postoperative supplementation of omega-3 fatty acids [42]; however, fish oils have been reported to delay wound healing in excessive quantities and may also have negative effects on coagulation (see Table 1).

One diet consisting of arginine, nucleotides in the form of RNA, and omega-3 fatty acids was given to patients postoperatively in a randomized prospective study. There was a significant reduction in infection and wound complications with major surgery (11% versus 37%) and a decreased length of hospital stay (16 versus 20 days) [43].

A meta-analysis was done evaluating this form of supplemented diet. Supplementation 5 to 7 days before surgery contributed to improved outcomes of morbidity in elective surgery patients. Significantly decreased postsurgical infection and a decreased length of hospital stay were noted, with the greatest benefit occurring with preoperative administration. Postoperative wound infection decreased 35% [42].

Large parenteral doses of glutamine also reduced the infection rate. It is likely glutamine will also reduce the infection rate when administered orally, because glutamine supplementation also expedites wound healing.

Reducing swelling, bruising, and inflammation

A novel approach to reducing the postsurgical inflammatory response is to treat the response before it is initiated. Frequently, podiatric surgeons use non-steroidal anti-inflammatory drugs (NSAIDs) pre- and postoperatively to reduce the inflammatory response; however, many studies have shown potential delays in bone healing, including non-unions when using selective and nonselective NSAIDs [44,45]. Esthetic surgeons are currently using alternative approaches to reduce inflammation, swelling, and bruising that naturally occur in the postoperative period [3].

Surgical dissection causes injuries to the tissues. These iatrogenic injuries involve release of pain-mediating chemicals and neurotransmitters and the release of vasoactive substances. This proinflammatory process can be attenuated by particular botanical compounds, such as bromelain, an enzyme derived from pineapple stems. Pre- and postoperative bromelain supplementation has been show to decrease bruising, swelling, pain, and healing time.

Several double-blind studies have verified the effectiveness of bromelain as an anti-inflammatory agent. The most common indication for bromelain involves treatment of inflammation and soft tissue injuries. Blonstein [46] confirmed acceleration of healing time from bruises and hematomas. Treatment of blunt injuries to the musculoskeletal system with bromelain supplementation results in a reduction of edema, tenderness, and pain at rest and with motion [47]. Acceleration of clinical signs of healing (pain and edema) has been observed with preoperative administration of bromelain [48,49]. One major advantage of bromelain supplementation is the low risk of side effects. Generally, bromelain is well tolerated, and in human clinical trials there is a low rate of toxicity. Cautions regarding bromelain include its use in cancer patients, because bromelain can increase the efficacy of 5-fluorouracil and vincristine. Bromelain may also potentiate the effects of oral antibiotics.

Healing of soft tissue injuries along with the reduction of pain and swelling can also be achieved with the use of a homeopathic formulation of *Arnica montana*. This medicinal herb has recently gained popularity with cosmetic surgeons [16]. Despite the ongoing debate in Western medicine regarding the use of herbal products, arnica has been deemed safe during the perioperative period, with toxicity being negligible [50,51]. Two reviews of the clinical use of arnica supplementation have been conducted on surgical and trauma patients. In a review of eight clinical trials, which mainly consisted of trauma patients, the efficacy of arnica was not comparable with the claims being made regarding its clinical use [52]. Nevertheless, Ludtke and Wilkins reviewed 37 clinical trials of arnica in trauma and surgical patients, concluding that arnica can be efficacious. Expanded research is necessary to further validate these claims [53].

Although *Arnica montana* may be safe and efficacious, case reports in the homeopathic literature have shown that some patients who take excessive arnica preoperatively may experience an increase in ecchymosis and edema [51]. It may be wise to refrain from arnica use preoperatively and to restrict its use to postoperative management. Clearly, this is a compound that needs further validation but may prove to be a beneficial adjunct in trauma patients and elective surgical patients.

Reducing oxidation

Oxidation of tissue is known to have detrimental effects on wound healing. The production of free radicals (a reactive form of oxygen) can have many deleterious effects, including disruption of normal cellular function, immune function suppression, increased cross-linking of tissues causing a loss of tissue flexibility, and increased lipid peroxidation. Many anesthetic agents and surgery itself cause an increase in cellular oxidation, having negative effects on wound healing and tissue quality.

In addition to acute and chronic diseases, surgery has been shown to decrease blood levels and tissue levels of several nutrients. At the same time, the increased oxidation caused by anesthetic agents may increase the normal requirements of these depleted vitamins and minerals. A decrease in the plasma concentration of vitamin C in the postoperative period often occurs and is associated with organ failure [54], such as end stage renal disease in diabetic patients. It has been postulated that the decreased vitamin C plasma concentrations are the result of free radical activity in response to surgical trauma. The nutrient deficiency may be exacerbated in the patient in a fasting state before surgery.

Beneficial antioxidants can deactivate the unstable free radical molecules produced by surgery and anesthetic agents, potentially reducing further tissue damage. The body attempts to produce its own antioxidant defense. Several enzymes such as catalase, superoxide dismutase, and glutathione peroxidase function as antioxidants. All three of these enzymes can be taken in oral supplement form; however, it is often easier to take supplements that enhance these natural enzymes than to consume the enzyme supplements directly [3,16].

When taken preoperatively, the administration of particular nutrients has been shown to protect against the potentially deleterious free radicals and oxidation from anesthesia and surgery [55,56]. Many vitamins and minerals act as antioxidants. Vitamins A and C, carotenoids, selenium, and bioflavonoids act as antioxidants. Although the specific requirements of the supplemental antioxidants are not well established, a few key points are commonly accepted. A combination of the antioxidants is recommended, because there are large variances in the specific antioxidant systems in different organs. Also, because large, mega-doses of specific nutrients are not recommended, smaller more measured doses of a broad spectrum are advised for antioxidant protection. It is advisable to consider an increased dose for patients who take antioxidants on a regular basis because there may be an increased daily requirement.

Summary

The importance of perioperative nutrition is growing in light of the rapidly increasing incidence of obesity and associated chronic illnesses such as diabetes mellitus, the advancing age of Americans, and the poor dietary habits of the population. Marginal or obvious deficiencies of particular nutrients can greatly impact the surgical patient, increasing the risk of complications. The podiatric surgeon should be aware of particular nutritional supplements and herbal supplements that can cause intraoperative complications. Although supplementation remains controversial, the research clearly demonstrates the need for vitamins and minerals perioperatively in patients with some degree of nutrient deficiency. Further research in elective surgical patients who are most likely to have a normal nutritional status is necessary, because it is unknown whether supplementation will provide additional benefit. Until more concrete evidence of clinical and economic efficacy is provided, widespread acceptance is unlikely. Regardless of the approach of the individual podiatric surgeon, the use of nutritional supplements in the surgical patient is not a panacea but a prudent adjunct to a comprehensive treatment plan.

References

[1] Must A, Spadano J, Coakley EH, et al. The disease burden associated with overweight and obesity. JAMA 1999;282(16):1523–9.
[2] Mokdad AH, Ford ES, Bowman BA, et al. Prevalence of obesity, diabetes, and obesity-related health risk factors, 2001. JAMA 2003;289(1):76–9.
[3] Rahm D. Perioperative nutrition and nutritional supplements. Plast Surg Nurs 2005;25(1): 21–8.
[4] Eckel RH, Kraus RM. American Heart Association call to action: obesity as a major risk factor for coronary heart disease. Circulation 1998;97:2099–100.
[5] Allison DB, Fontaine KR, Manson JE, et al. Annual deaths attributable to obesity in the United States. JAMA 1999;282:1530–8.
[6] Calle EE, Thun MJ, Petrelli BH, et al. Body-mass index and mortality in a prospective cohort of US adults. N Engl J Med 1999;341:1097–105.
[7] Kuczmarski RJ, Carroll MD, Flegal KM. Varying body mass index cutoff points to describe overweight prevalence among US adults: NHANES III (1988–1994). Obes Res 1997;5(6): 542–8.
[8] Block G. Dietary guidelines and the results of food consumption surveys. Am J Clin Nutr 1991;53:356S–7S.
[9] Kant AK, Schatzkin A. Consumption of energy-dense, nutrient poor foods by the US population: effect on nutrient profiles. J Am Coll Nutr 1994;13:285–91.
[10] Breslow RA, Subar AF, Patterson BH, et al. Trends in food intake: the 1987 and 1992 National Health Interview Surveys. Nutr Cancer 1997;28:86–92.
[11] Kant AK, Schatzkin A, Block G, et al. Food group intake patterns and associated nutrient profiles of the US population. J Am Diet Assoc 1991;91:1532–7.
[12] Van der Wielen RP, de Wild GM, de Groot LC, et al. Dietary intakes of energy and water-soluble vitamins in different categories or aging. J Gerontol A Biol Sci Med Sci 1996;51: B100–7.
[13] Kagansky N, Berner Y, Koren-Morag N, et al. Poor nutritional habits are predictors of poor outcome in very old hospitalized patients. Am J Clin Nutr 2005;82:784–91.
[14] Fairfield KM, Fletcher RH. Vitamins for chronic disease prevention in adults: scientific review. JAMA 2002;287(23):3116–26.
[15] Fletcher RH, Fairfield KM. Vitamins for chronic disease prevention in adults: clinical applications. JAMA 2002;287(23):3127–9.

[16] Rahm D. A guide to perioperative nutrition. Aesthetic Surg J 2004;24:385–90.

[17] O'Hara M, Kiefer D, Farrell K, et al. A review of 12 commonly used medicinal herbs. Arch Fam Med 1998;7(6):523–36.

[18] Miller LG. Herbal medicinals: selected clinical considerations focusing on known or potential drug-herb interactions. Arch Intern Med 1998;158(20):2200–11.

[19] Larkin M. Surgery patients at risk for herb-anaesthesia interactions. Lancet 1999;354(9187):1362.

[20] Cupp MJ. Herbal remedies: adverse effects and drug interactions. Am Fam Physician 1999;59(5):1239–45.

[21] Ernst E. The risk-benefit profile of commonly used herbal therapies: gingko, St. John's wort, ginseng, echinacea, saw palmetto, and kava. Ann Intern Med 2002;136:42–53.

[22] Petry JJ. Surgically significant nutritional supplements. Plast Reconstr Surg 1996;97(1):233–40.

[23] Ang-Lee NK, Moss J, Yuan CS. Herbal medicines and perioperative care. JAMA 2001;286(2):208–16.

[24] MacFie J, Woodcock NP, Palmer MD, et al. Oral dietary supplements in pre- and postoperative surgical patients: a prospective and randomized clinical trial. Nutrition 2000;16:723–8.

[25] White DA, Baxter M. Hormones and metabolic control. 2nd edition. London: Edward Arnold; 1994.

[26] Demling RH, DeSanti L. The stress response to injury and infection: role of nutritional support. Wounds 2000;12(1):3–14.

[27] Wilmore DW. The effect of glutamine supplementation in patients following elective surgery and accidental injury. J Nutr 2001;131:2543S–9S.

[28] Barbul A, Lazarou SA, Efron DT, et al. Arginine enhances wound healing and lymphocyte immune response in humans. Surgery 1990;108:331–7.

[29] Sandstead HH, Henriksen LK, Greger JL, et al. Zinc nutriture in the elderly in relation to taste acuity, immune response, and wound healing. Am J Clin Nutr 1982;35:1046–59.

[30] The National Pressure Ulcer Advisory Panel. Frequently asked questions: what is the role of nutritional support for patients in the prevention and treatment of pressure ulcers? Available at: http://www.npuap.org/faq.html.

[31] Thomas DR. The role of nutrition in prevention and healing of pressure ulcers. Med Clin North Am 1997;13:497–511.

[32] Bartlett MK, Jones FM, Ryan AE. The role of vitamin C in wound healing. Br J Surg 1941;28:436.

[33] Hunt AH. Vitamin C and wound healing. II. Ascorbic acid content and tensile strength of healing wounds in human beings. N Engl J Med 1942;226:474.

[34] Desneves KJ, Todorovic BE, Cassar A, et al. Treatment with supplementary arginine, vitamin C, and zinc in patients with pressure ulcers: a randomized controlled trial. Clin Nutr 2005;24:979–87.

[35] Lawson RM, Doshi MK, Barton JR, et al. The effect of unselected postoperative nutritional supplementation on nutritional status and clinical outcome of orthopedic patients. Clin Nutr 2003;22(1):39–46.

[36] Wicke C, Halliday B, Allen D, et al. Effects of steroids and retinoids on wound healing. Arch Surg 2000;135(11):1265–70.

[37] Bendich A, Langseth L. Safety of vitamin A. Am J Clin Nutr 1989;2:358–71.

[38] Stansfield SK, Pierre-Louis M, Lerebours G, et al. Vitamin A supplementation and increased prevalence of childhood diarrhea and acute respiratory infections. Lancet 1993;342:578–82.

[39] Beck FW, Prasad AS, Kaplan J, et al. Changes in cytokine production and T-cell subpopulations in experimentally induced zinc-deficient humans. Am J Physiol 1997;272:E1002–7.

[40] Shankar AH, Prasad AS. Zinc and immune function: the biologic basis of altered resistance to infection. Am J Clin Nutr 1998;68:447S–63S.

[41] Ross AC. Vitamin A and retinoids. In: Shiles ME, Olson J, Shike M, et al, editors. Modern nutrition in health and disease. 9th edition. Baltimore (MD): Wilkins and Wilkins; 2005.

[42] Waitzberg DL, Saito H, Plank LD. Postsurgical infections are reduced with specialized nutritional support. World J Surg 2006;30:1592–604.

[43] Daly JM, Lieberman MD, Goldfine J, et al. Enteral nutrition with supplemental arginine, RNA, and omega-3 fatty acids in patients after operation: immunologic, metabolic, and clinical outcome. Surg 1992;112(1):56–67.

[44] Simon AM, Manigrasso MB, O'Connor JP. Cyclo-oxygenase 2 function is essential for bone fracture healing. J Bone Miner Res 2002;17:963–76.

[45] Ro J, Sudmann E, Marton PF. Effect of indomethacin on fracture healing in rats. Acta Orthop Scand 1976;47:588–99.

[46] Blonstein JL. Control of swelling in boxing injuries. Practitioner 1969;203(214):206.

[47] Masson M. Bromelain in blunt injuries of the locomotor system: a study of observed applications in general practice. Fortschr Med 1995;113:303–6 [in German].

[48] Tassman GC, Zafran JN, Zayan GM. Evaluation of a plant proteolytic enzyme for the control of inflammation and pain. J Dent Med 1964;19:73–7.

[49] Tassman GC, Zafran JN, Zayan GM. A double-blind crossover study of a plant proteolytic enzyme in oral surgery. J Dent Med 1965;20:51–4.

[50] Lawrence WT. Arnica, safety and efficacy report. Plast Reconstr Surg 2003;15:1164–6.

[51] Riley D. *Arnica montana* and homeopathic dosing guidelines. Plast Reconstr Surg 2003; 112(2):693.

[52] Ernst E, Pittler MH. Efficacy of homeopathic arnica: a systematic review of placebo-controlled clinical trials. Arch Surg 1998;133(11):1187–90.

[53] Ludtke R, Wilkins J, Klinische. Wirksamkeitsstudien zu Arnica in homeoopathischen Zubereitungen. In: Albrecht H, Fruhwald M, editors. Jahrbach der karl und veronica carstens-stifung, band 5. Essen (Germany): KVC-Verlag; 1999. p. 97–112.

[54] Irvin TT. Vitamin C requirements in postoperative patients. Int J Vitam Nutr Res 1982; 23(Suppl):277–86.

[55] Nathans AB, Neff MJ, Jurkovich GJ, et al. Randomized, prospective trial of antioxidant supplementation in critically ill surgical patients. Ann Surg 2002;236(6):814–22.

[56] Kelly FJ. Use of antioxidants in prevention and treatment of disease. J Int Fed Clin Chem 1998;10(1):21–3.

ELSEVIER
SAUNDERS

Clin Podiatr Med Surg
24 (2007) 261–283

CLINICS IN
PODIATRIC
MEDICINE AND
SURGERY

Evaluating and Minimizing Cardiac Risk in Surgical Patients

Sondra Vazirani, MD, MPH[a],*,
Neil M. Paige, MD, MSHS[a],
Aksone Nouvong, DPM, FACFAS[b],
David Aungst, DPM[c]

[a]*Department of Medicine, VA Greater Los Angeles Healthcare System,
David Geffen School of Medicine-UCLA, 11301 Wilshire Boulevard, 10H1/111,
Los Angeles, CA 90073, USA*
[b]*Department of Medicine, VA Greater Los Angeles Healthcare System,
David Geffen School of Medicine-UCLA, Department of Surgery,
11301 Wilshire Boulevard, 10H2, Los Angeles, CA 90073, USA*
[c]*Department of Medicine, VA Greater Los Angeles Healthcare System, Olive View-UCLA
Medical Center, Department of Surgery, 11301 Wilshire Boulevard, 10H2,
Los Angeles, CA 90073, USA*

Cardiovascular complications are a major cause of postoperative morbidity and mortality. It is estimated that between 500,000 and 900,000 patients who undergo noncardiac surgery worldwide will suffer cardiac death, nonfatal myocardial infarction, or nonfatal cardiac arrest [1]. Physiologic factors associated with surgery predispose patients to myocardial ischemia or arrhythmia. Surgery may cause volume shifts, blood loss, and enhanced myocardial oxygen demand from elevations in heart rate and blood pressure secondary to stress from surgery. Interestingly, rather than supply and demand inequality, it is postulated that atherosclerotic plaque rupture is the major cause of perioperative myocardial infarction [2].

Cardiac risk associated with surgical procedures

The 2002 American College of Cardiology/American Heart Association (ACC/AHA) guidelines on perioperative cardiovascular evaluation for noncardiac surgery concluded that three elements must be assessed to determine the risk of cardiac events so that appropriate testing and therapeutic

---

* Corresponding author.
E-mail address: sondra.vazirani@med.va.gov (S. Vazirani).

0891-8422/07/$ - see front matter © 2007 Elsevier Inc. All rights reserved.
doi:10.1016/j.cpm.2006.12.005   *podiatric.theclinics.com*

measures can be undertaken to mitigate risk: (1) the surgery-specific risk of the planned operation, (2) the exercise (or functional) capacity of the patient, and (3) the patient-specific clinical variables that place the patient at increased operative risk [3].

Factors that determine the surgery-specific cardiac risk are the type of surgery performed and the hemodynamic stress associated with that procedure. The likelihood of perioperative cardiac events increases with the duration of and intensity of myocardial stressors. The ACC/AHA stratified the surgery-specific risk for noncardiac surgery into high, intermediate, and low (Box 1). High-risk surgery has a reported cardiac risk of greater than 5% and includes emergent major operations (especially in the elderly), aortic and other major vascular surgery (including peripheral vascular surgery but not carotid endarterectomy), and procedures that are prolonged or associated with significant fluid shifts or blood loss.

Low-risk procedures have a reported cardiac risk of less than 1%, whereas intermediate-risk procedures have a reported cardiac risk of less than 5% [3]. Podiatric surgery is not specifically listed in the ACC/AHA's surgery-specific list. Podiatric surgery performed under local anesthesia

---

Box 1. Cardiac risk[a] stratification for noncardiac surgical procedures [3]

High (reported cardiac risk often greater than 5%)
Emergent major operations, particularly in the elderly
Aortic and other major vascular surgery
Peripheral vascular surgery
Anticipated prolonged surgical procedures associated with large fluid shifts, blood loss, or both

Intermediate (reported cardiac risk generally less than 5%)
Carotid endarterectomy
Head and neck surgery
Intraperitoneal and intrathoracic surgery
Orthopedic surgery
Prostate surgery

Low[b] (reported cardiac risk generally less than 1%)
Endoscopic procedures
Superficial procedure
Cataract surgery
Breast surgery

---

[a] Combined incidence of cardiac death and nonfatal myocardial infarction.
[b] Do not generally require further preoperative cardiac testing.

would be considered a low-risk procedure, whereas a surgical case that involves more than minimal blood loss or that requires general or spinal anesthesia would qualify as intermediate risk.

Evaluating the patient's cardiac risk: risk indices

The most well-known risk index is the Goldman Cardiac Risk Index or Goldman Criteria. In 1977 Goldman and colleagues [4] prospectively evaluated 1001 patients aged more than 40 years who underwent major noncardiac surgery. Goldman identified nine independent factors that were correlated with cardiac complications: a preoperative third heart sound or jugular venous distention; myocardial infarction within 6 months; greater than five premature ventricular contractions per minute; rhythm other than sinus or premature atrial contractions on the preoperative electrocardiogram; age over 70 years; intraperitoneal, intrathoracic, or aortic operation; emergency surgery; significant aortic stenosis; and poor general medical condition. Each of these nine factors was assigned weighted points, and a patient could receive a maximal score of 53. Scores were then separated into four classes, each of which was assigned a different level of risk. Class 1 patients (those with 0 to 5 points) had a cardiac event rate of less than 1%, whereas class 4 patients (>25 points) had an event rate of 78%. The main limitations of using these criteria were (1) relatively few patients were studied and (2) the data came from the 1970s, predating advances in medical management and in anesthesia and surgical improvements. In 1986 Detsky and colleagues [5] updated and modified the Goldman Criteria by adding variables including angina and pulmonary edema. The American College of Physicians (ACP) used the Detsky index in their preoperative evaluation position statement in 1997 [6].

In 1999 Lee and colleagues [7] derived and validated an index to predict cardiac risk in major noncardiac surgery known as the Revised Cardiac Risk Index (RCRI). Six independent risk factors for cardiac complications were identified: high-risk surgery (defined as intraperitoneal, intrathoracic, or suprainguinal vascular surgery), a history of ischemic heart disease, a history of congestive heart failure, a history of cerebrovascular disease, diabetes treated with insulin, and a preoperative creatinine level greater than 2.0 mg/dL. Among the 1422 patients in the validation cohort with zero, one, two, or greater or equal to three RCRI risk factors, the rate of complications was 0.4%, 0.9%, 7%, and 11%, respectively. The performance of the RCRI was superior to that of the Goldman and Detsky indices.

Preoperative guidelines today

Currently, the most widely used and accepted guidelines are that developed by the ACC/AHA [3]. These guidelines rely on evidence as well as the expert opinion of the 12 committee members. The ACC/AHA has defined perioperative cardiac risk as the risk of myocardial infarction, heart failure, or death. Emergent cases and asymptomatic patients who have undergone coronary revascularization within 5 years should proceed to the operating room. For all other patients, clinical predictors of cardiac risk should be determined (Box 2).

Major clinical predictors of risk include unstable coronary syndromes (acute or recent myocardial infarction as defined as less than 1 month or class III or IV angina), decompensated heart failure, significant arrhythmias, or severe valvular disease. Patients with these major clinical predictors should be evaluated extensively and should not undergo nonemergent surgery until that evaluation is complete.

Intermediate clinical predictors for perioperative cardiac risk include mild angina, prior myocardial infarction (by history or EKG; myocardial infarction beyond 30 days), a history of congestive heart failure, diabetes mellitus, and renal insufficiency as defined as a creatinine level greater than 2.0 mg/dL. Because these patients have an increased pretest probability of coronary disease, functional status should be assessed. Patients who can exceed 4 metabolic equivalents (METS) of activity (Box 3) and who are scheduled for an intermediate- or low-risk surgery may proceed to the operating room. For intermediate-risk patients who cannot exceed 4 METS or who are undergoing high-risk surgery, noninvasive stress testing is recommended for further risk stratification.

Minor clinical predictors are defined as age greater than 70 years, an abnormal EKG (eg, nonspecific T-wave abnormalities, old bundle-branch block, left ventricular hypertrophy), rhythm other than sinus, low functional capacity, a history of stroke, and uncontrolled hypertension. Unless such patients are scheduled to have a high-risk surgical procedure and have poor functional status, it is acceptable for them to proceed to the operating room. The guidelines recommend noninvasive testing even for patients with minor clinical predictors who are to undergo high-risk surgeries.

A patient's functional status can predict his or her perioperative risk. Traditionally, patients are assessed on their ability to attain 4 METS. Can they walk 4 mph on level ground for two blocks, climb one flight of stairs, climb a hill, or carry 25 lbs of groceries from the store to the car (Box 3)? In a study by Reilly and colleagues [8], patients reporting poor exercise tolerance had more perioperative complications (20.4% versus 10.4%; $P<.001$). Specifically, they had more myocardial ischemia ($P = .02$) and more cardiovascular ($P = .04$) and neurologic ($P = .03$) events. Poor exercise tolerance predicted a risk for serious complications independent of all other patient characteristics, including age (adjusted odds ratio, 1.94; 95% confidence interval, 1.19–3.17). The likelihood of a serious complication occurring was inversely related to the number of blocks that could be walked ($P = .006$) or flights of stairs that could be climbed ($P = .01$).

Although poor exercise tolerance has been associated with an increased risk of postoperative complications and myocardial ischemia, the positive

Box 2. Clinical predictors of increased perioperative cardiovascular risk (myocardial infarction, heart failure, death) [3]

Major
Unstable coronary syndromes
    Acute or recent myocardial infarction[a] with evidence of important
        ischemic risk by clinical symptoms or noninvasive study
    Unstable or severe[b] angina (Canadian class III or IV)[c]
Decompensated heart failure
Significant arrhythmias
    High-grade atrioventricular block
    Symptomatic ventricular arrhythmias in the presence of underlying
        heart disease
    Supraventricular arrhythmias with uncontrolled ventricular rate
Severe valvular disease

Intermediate
Mild angina pectoris (Canadian class I or II)
Previous myocardial infarction by history or pathologic Q waves
Compensated or prior heart failure
Diabetes mellitus (particularly insulin dependent)
Renal insufficiency

Minor
Advanced age
Abnormal ECG (left ventricular hypertrophy, left bundle-branch block,
    ST-T abnormalities)
Rhythm other than sinus (eg, atrial fibrillation)
Low functional capacity (eg, inability to climb one flight of stairs with
    a bag of groceries)
History of stroke
Uncontrolled systemic hypertension

---

[a] The American College of Cardiology National Database Library defines recent myocardial infarction as greater than 7 days but less than or equal to 1 month (30 days); acute myocardial infarction is within 7 days.
[b] May include "stable" angina in patients who are unusually sedentary.
[c] Campeau L. Grading of angina pectoris. Circulation 1976;54:522–3.
Modified from ACC/AHA Guidelines for the Perioperative Cardiovascular Evaluation for Noncardiac Surgery. J Am Coll Cardiol 1996:27:910–48. © 1996 The American College of Cardiology Foundation and American Heart Association, Inc. Permission granted for one time use. Further reproduction is not permitted without permission of the ACC/AHA. This material is the exclusive property of and is provided by ACC/AHA and is protected under U.S. Copyright and international laws. Any use of this material, including downloading or copying from this web site [or CD ROM] for your personal use, will indicate your consent and agreement to the terms stated in this notice. No right, title or interest in the material is conveyed to you as a result of any such downloading or copying, and such downloaded or copied material may not be used for any commercial purpose.

Box 3. Estimated energy requirements for various activities [3]

1 MET
　　Can you take care of yourself?
　　Eat, dress, or use the toilet?
　　Walk indoors around the house?
　　Walk a block or two on level ground at 2 to 3 mph or
　　　　3.2 to 4.8 km/h?

4 METs
　　Do light work around the house like dusting or washing dishes?
　　Climb a flight of stairs or walk up a hill?
　　Walk on level ground at 4 mph or 6.4 km/h?
　　Run a short distance?
　　Do heavy work around the house like scrubbing floors or
　　　　lifting or moving heavy furniture?
　　Participate in moderate recreational activities like golf, bowling,
　　　　dancing, doubles tennis, or throwing a baseball or football?

Greater than 10 METs
　　Participate in strenuous sports like swimming, singles tennis,
　　　　football, basketball, or skiing?

_____

From Eagle KA, et al. ACC/AHA guideline update for perioperative cardiovascular evaluation for noncardiac surgery - executive summary: a report of the American College of Cardiology/American Heart Association Task Force on Practice Guidelines (Committee to Update the 1996 Guidelines on Perioperative Cardiovascular Evaluation for Noncardiac Surgery), J Am Coll Cardiol 2002;39(3):542–53. © 2002 The American College of Cardiology Foundation and American Heart Association, Inc. Permission granted for one time use. Further reproduction is not permitted without permission of the ACC/AHA.

predictive value of poor exercise tolerance is low [8]. Cardiopulmonary complaints associated with exertion certainly require further evaluation. True functional status may be difficult to assess in patients with foot pain or abnormalities of the lower extremities. In this situation, the cardiac risk may be overestimated [9]. For these patients, the ACC/AHA guidelines would recommend noninvasive stress testing for an intermediate-risk patient, even if the reason for poor exercise tolerance is foot pain or abnormality of the lower extremity.

Evaluating the patient's cardiac risk: history and physical

The history

To determine cardiac risk, a detailed past medical and surgical history should be obtained. All patients should be asked about chest pain, shortness of breath or dyspnea on exertion, orthopnea, syncope, and lower extremity edema, which may indicate the presence of significant heart disease. Determining functional capacity or exercise tolerance is a crucial element of the history. During the history, the clinician should inquire about several specific diseases as described in the following sections [9a].

Coronary artery disease

Does the patient have a history of heart disease, myocardial infarction, or heart attack? Has the patient recently had chest pain or dyspnea with exertion? How frequent are the episodes? Have symptoms been occurring more frequently or do they occur with less exertion? Do the episodes occur at rest? Has the patient needed to use more nitroglycerin in the recent past? Has he or she had prior cardiac evaluations including stress tests, echocardiography, coronary angiography, coronary angioplasty, or bypass surgery? How recent was the evaluation done and what was found?

Valvular and congenital heart disease

Does the patient have a history of a murmur, valvular disease, or a congenital abnormality? Has the patient ever been advised to take an antibiotic for endocarditis prophylaxis for a dental or surgical procedure? Has the patient had heart valve surgery or replacement? Inquire about the patient's most recent echocardiogram as understanding the nature of the abnormality or structure and position of affected valves is necessary to determine which patients will need antibiotics for endocarditis prophylaxis or perioperative anticoagulation. Endocarditis prophylaxis and perioperative anticoagulation will be discussed later in this text.

Congestive heart failure (CHF)

Does the patient have a history of congestive heart failure or symptoms of dyspnea on exertion, orthopnea, paroxysmal nocturnal dyspnea, cough, or lower extremity edema? Has the patient had a recent echocardiogram to evaluate the ejection fraction or for evidence of diastolic dysfunction? In order to undergo surgery, patients with a history of CHF should be stable and well compensated.

Dysrhythmias and pacemakers

Does the patient have a history of an arrhythmia or symptoms such as palpitations or syncope? Has an arrhythmia been documented on prior EKGs or holter monitor? Does the patient take anticoagulation or antiplatelet medication? Warfarin is commonly given to patients with atrial fibrillation in order to reduce the risk of stroke. Does the patient have a pacemaker or an automatic implantable cardioverter defibrillator (AICD)? Often this information is found on a card that the patient carries in his or her wallet. If so, when was it implanted and when was it last checked? Although remote and mild electrocautery (such as in the eye) may not interfere with pacemaker functioning, pacemakers generally require reprogramming before surgery to eliminate electrocautery interference.

Cerebrovascular disease

Has the patient ever had a stroke or transient ischemic attack? Symptoms can include one-sided weakness or numbness, inability to speak, or word finding difficulty. What evaluation did the patient have and was the cause of the stroke identified? Did the patient have an irregular heart beat or atrial fibrillation? Is the patient taking anticoagulation medicine such as aspirin, aspirin/dipyridamole (Aggrenox), clopidogrel, or warfarin?

Peripheral vascular disease

Does the patient have claudication when walking a specific distance or number of blocks? If so, when does it come on, and does it go way with rest? Patients with severe claudication often have concomitant atherosclerotic disease including coronary artery disease.

Diabetes mellitus

Does the patient have history of diabetes mellitus? Symptoms of polyuria, polydipsia, and polyphagia may signify poorly controlled diabetes or a new onset of diabetes. In a patient with a history of diabetes, inquire about recent blood sugar control, medication use, and schedule. If the patient uses insulin, ask about the types of insulin, schedule, and doses? Insulin and other diabetic medication will need to be adjusted in the perioperative period.

Kidney disease

Does the patient have a history of chronic kidney disease or renal insufficiency? Inquire as to the cause if the patient knows it. Preoperative renal insufficiency (creatinine level >2.0 mg/dL) is an intermediate cardiac risk factor. Has the patient been on dialysis in the past? Has his or her renal function been stable?

Medications

A detailed medication history should be obtained including the patient's use of over-the-counter and herbal remedies. A patient's medications may provide further insight into his or her medical history and often has implications for perioperative management.

Patients will be asked to take nothing my mouth after midnight of the morning of surgery to minimize gastric filling and the risk of aspiration. It is the responsibility of the preoperative consultant to determine which medications the patient should take on the morning of surgery. Most chronic cardiac medications should be continued through the perioperative period. For example, beta blockers have been shown to reduce cardiovascular complications in intermediate- to high-risk patients undergoing high-risk surgery. If the patient is taking a beta blocker, it should always be continued throughout the perioperative period. Beta-blocker withdrawal can lead to tachycardia, hypertension, and increased cardiac demand. This topic is explored further in the section on risk reduction. Continuing certain cardiac medications (eg, angiotensin-converting enzyme [ACE] inhibitors and angiotensin II receptor blockers) on the morning of surgery is controversial. These agents have been associated in certain populations with intraoperative hypotension and should be held in patients with baseline low blood pressure, such as those with heart failure [10]. Continuing diuretic medication is also controversial because these agents can potentially cause hypokalemia and hypovolemia, but there is no true consensus among experts on this issue [11]. Generally in a stable outpatient who has had a thorough preoperative examination with normal laboratory studies, diuretics may be continued.

The use of aspirin, warfarin, and non-steroidal anti-inflammatory drugs (NSAIDs) should be evaluated closely for risk versus benefit. Each drug increases the risk of bleeding from the surgery; however, if stopped, patients will lose the protective effect of aspirin with regard to myocardial infarction and cardiovascular mortality. Generally, aspirin (and NSAIDs) are stopped at the request of the surgeon. Perioperative anticoagulation is discussed in more detail later in this article. Herbal remedies should generally be discontinued, and many are contraindicated during the perioperative period [12]. Ginkgo biloba is an herbal remedy that patients often take to improve memory. It may increase the risk of bleeding in the perioperative period, as can garlic and ginseng, and should be discontinued at least 1 week before surgery.

In patients with diabetes, medications need to be adjusted during the perioperative period. Generally, oral agents are held on the morning of surgery, and insulin is reduced to one half of the dose with use of a dextrose drip and monitoring of sugars in the holding area [13].

Social history and habits

Smoking is a well-known risk factor for perioperative complications, including respiratory complications during anesthesia and an increased risk of postoperative cardiopulmonary complications, infections, and impaired wound healing. All patients should be asked if they smoke and should be advised to curtail their smoking for at least 6–8 weeks before their scheduled elective surgery [14].

An alcohol and drug history is also important to ascertain. Alcohol and drug use have implications for anesthesia, as well introducing the possibility of drug or alcohol withdrawal in the perioperative period.

Physical examination

A thorough physical examination is a necessary component of the preoperative evaluation. The clinician should evaluate the patient's vitals signs, including blood pressure, heart rate, and the regularity of rhythm, the rate and ease of respiration, and temperature. Severe hypertension can signify serious underlying disease or be a risk factor for perioperative complications.

The patient should be evaluated for cardiovascular disease. One should listen to the heart to determine whether the patient has a murmur, which may indicate valvular disease. One should note whether the patient's heart rhythm is irregular, which may signify atrial fibrillation. Look for signs of heart failure, which may include elevated jugular venous pressure, pedal edema, or an S_3 gallop. Carotid, abdominal, and femoral bruits may indicate atherosclerotic disease. Asymptomatic carotid bruits do not necessarily need to be evaluated before surgery, because they do not increase the stroke risk for patients undergoing general surgery [15]. A pulmonary examination is also critical, listening for equal breath sounds or the presence of wheezes, crackles, or rhonchi.

Generally, new and abnormal physical findings warrant further evaluation before surgery.

Evaluating the patient's cardiac risk: laboratory testing, chest radiography, and electrocardiography

Should all patients have a set of specific "routine" laboratory studies as part of their routine preoperative evaluation? The answer is not necessarily, but most physicians and surgeons will order a battery of tests before surgery based on the policy of the hospital where they practice (including medicolegal issues), as well as to detect unsuspected abnormalities that may impact the perioperative period [16,17]. Which preoperative laboratory studies to order should be based on the age and comorbidities of the patient. For example, for a patient with hypertension and a history of chronic kidney disease, a complete blood count, serum electrolytes, and creatinine should be obtained.

Complete blood count

A complete blood count should be obtained if more than minimal blood loss from the procedure is expected. A complete blood count should be obtained in all patients with a history of systemic disease, including chronic kidney disease, chronic lung disease, malignancy, congestive heart failure, woman who are still menstruating, and in any patient who has a history of, or symptoms and signs of anemia (ie, increased lethargy, shortness of breath, or conjunctival pallor).

Serum chemistries (electrolytes, creatinine, glucose)

Serum chemistries, which in many hospitals are often referred to as a "Chem 7" or "SMA-7," should be obtained in all patients aged more than 45 years, or if the patient has a history of anemia, diabetes mellitus, cardiac or renal disease, malignancy, or thyroid disease. Serum electrolytes, especially serum potassium, should be obtained for patients with hypertension or who are taking medications that are likely to alter electrolyte balance, including diuretics and ACE inhibitors. This group also includes patients who have recently had chemotherapy. Measuring creatinine is also important, because it is an intermediate cardiac risk factor.

Coagulation studies

Coagulation studies (prothrombin time/international normalized ratio [INR], partial thromboplastin time) should not be routinely ordered; rather, these studies are indicated for patients with a personal or family history suggesting a bleeding diathesis or thrombophilia. In patients who are currently on or have been on anticoagulation medication or who have a history of liver disease or malnutrition, coagulation studies should be evaluated. Coagulation studies have also been advised in complex surgical cases when large blood loss is anticipated.

Other preoperative tests

Electrocardiography
An EKG is not indicated for asymptomatic subjects undergoing low-risk procedures. An EKG should be obtained in all patients with prior coronary revascularization procedures, patients with a prior hospitalization for heart disease, patients with a history of diabetes, and asymptomatic male patients older than 45 years or female patients older than 55 years. It is used as a screening test for coronary artery disease in the latter two groups. If on history, a patient is identified to have a recent episode of chest pain or shortness of breath, an EKG is also warranted. Additionally, a baseline study is useful for patients at increased risk for cardiac complications so that a comparison is available if chest pain or EKG changes occur after surgery.

Chest radiography
Chest radiography is indicated for all patients with respiratory symptoms or abnormalities on examination, and for all patients with a history of and current symptoms of congestive heart failure, valvular heart disease, or cardiac shunts. Patients aged more than 50 years should also have a chest radiograph as part of their preoperative evaluation [17].

Evaluating the patient's cardiac risk: cardiac studies

The ACC/AHA guidelines recommend a stepwise (algorithmic) approach to determining which patients will need or not need further cardiac testing. Several important points, especially as they apply to podiatric surgery, are as follows [3]:

Some emergent surgeries may not allow time for preoperative cardiac evaluation. In this situation, the need for surgery typically outweighs the risk of perioperative complications. Postoperative risk stratification may be appropriate.

In patients with unstable coronary disease, decompensated heart failure, or severe valvular disease, elective surgery should be postponed until the issues have been sufficiently addressed.

Patients without recurrent cardiac symptoms who have had a coronary revascularization procedure in the past 5 years generally do not need further cardiac testing.

If a patient has had a coronary evaluation in the past 2 years and the findings were favorable, it is usually not necessary to repeat testing unless the patient has experienced a change or new symptoms of coronary ischemia.

Patients with intermediate risk factors and moderate or excellent functional capacity can generally undergo intermediate-risk surgery with little likelihood of perioperative cardiac complications. On the other hand, noninvasive testing should be considered in patients with poor functional capacity.

Noninvasive testing should be considered for patients with poor functional capacity.

Noninvasive testing is often used to determine the need for coronary angiography. Noninvasive cardiac studies include an exercise treadmill test, myocardial perfusion (radionucleotide study) with exercise stress, myocardial perfusion (radionucleotide study) with pharmacologic stress, and functional echocardiography with exercise or pharmacologic stress. Which test to order depends on the standard of practice in the community or hospital in which one works and the functional capacity of the patient. Generally, if a patient is able, exercise stress testing is preferred to pharmacologic stress [18]. Because many patients needing podiatric surgery will be unable to walk on a treadmill, tests using pharmacologic stress may be warranted.

An exercise treadmill or exercise tolerance test is an effective and inexpensive modality that can provide electrocardiographic data on the presence or absence of ischemia during exercise. It can provide information on the patient's functional capacity as well. The exercise tolerance test has a much higher sensitivity for detecting three-vessel or left main coronary artery disease than for detecting milder abnormalities. The treadmill EKG is less accurate in women owing to the lower pretest probability of coronary artery disease. Medications (eg, beta blockers and calcium channel blockers) that attenuate the heart's response to exercise may also make the test less sensitive. Functional echocardiography detects wall motion abnormalities indicating myocardium at risk during exercise, but its interpretation can also be affected by the patient's medications and the expertise of the operator.

Radionucleotide imaging with exercise stress should be considered in women, in patients with baseline left bundle branch block, and in patients who cannot stop their cardiac medications. The patient is injected with a nuclear tracer such as thallium or sestamibi. Serial images are obtained during exercise and then several hours later. Comparisons are made between the exercise images and the rest images. Regions that demonstrate perfusion during rest but not during exercise are considered to be ischemic or areas of risk. Regions that do not demonstrate perfusion during exercise or rest are considered to be scar or nonviable myocardium. If a patient is unable to exercise, a pharmacologic agent can be given that mimics stress by causing coronary vasodilatation, which can lead to hypoperfusion in areas supplied by stenotic coronary arteries [18].

Each of these tests has excellent sensitivity for detecting severe coronary artery disease. The choice should be guided by the patient's gender, baseline EKG, current medications and whether they can be held, the patient's ability to walk (exercise), and cost (radionucleotide imaging is three to four times more expensive).

Rest echocardiography is useful in determining left ventricular function, detecting valvular stenosis or regurgitation. It is generally not useful in detecting coronary artery disease. Patients with depressed left ventricular function or wall motion abnormalities may warrant further evaluation for coronary artery disease with a functional echocardiogram or radionucleotide study.

Lowering cardiac risk

Identifying patients at increased cardiac perioperative cardiac risks allows one to intervene to minimize that risk. From a cardiac perspective, optimization of medical therapies and coronary revascularization are possible interventions.

Beta blockers

Beta blockers have been studied to reduce cardiac risk perioperatively. Physiologically, beta blockers slow the heart rate, prolonging coronary artery diastolic filling time. They also dampen the postoperative sympathetic drive, which may prevent arrhythmias and rupture of an atheromatous plaque [19]. Atheromatous plaque rupture has been postulated to be the mechanism of perioperative myocardial infarction [2].

Several randomized trials investigating the use of perioperative beta blockade have been performed. Early studies suggested that patients taking beta blockers preoperatively had reduced myocardial ischemia [20,21], rates of myocardial infarction [22], and mortality at 6 and more months postoperatively [21]; however, other more recent trials using perioperative beta blockers have not shown these benefits [23,24]. A subsequent meta-analysis of all randomized beta-blocker trials found insufficient evidence to recommend widespread use of perioperative beta blockers [25].

A recent large retrospective nonrandomized trial investigated the benefits of perioperative beta blockers in 600,000 patients undergoing noncardiac surgery at community hospitals. Subjects in the study group were enrolled if they were on beta blockers on the first 2 days of admission, and controls were matched based on their RCRI score [7]. Patients with congestive heart failure were excluded, because this could be a potential contraindication to beta blocker use. All of the patients were followed up until hospital discharge.

The results suggested that beta blockers reduced mortality for patients at intermediate and high cardiac risk, defined as an RCRI score of 2 or greater. The study also concluded that in patients considered to be at low risk for cardiac events (RCRI score of 0 or 1), perioperative beta blockers may have a deleterious effect [26]. Given the limitations of a retrospective study, this study further added to the uncertainty of widely using perioperative beta blockers for all patients undergoing noncardiac surgery.

The ACC/AHA published guidelines in 2006 addressing the use of perioperative beta blockers in noncardiac surgery [27]. They addressed the many limitations of evidence, including the conflicting conclusions, heterogeneity of studies, and inadequately powered trials. Notably, practical issues such as how, when, and how long perioperative beta blockers should be used have not been well delineated.

The guidelines recommend several indications. Class I indications (evidence or general agreement that the treatment is beneficial) include continuing ongoing beta blockers in patients already taking them for cardiovascular disease and for patients at high cardiac risk as found on preoperative testing. Class IIa indications (conflicting evidence but in favor of usefulness) for initiating perioperative beta blockers include patients undergoing vascular surgery or intermediate- or other high-risk surgery with known coronary artery disease or with multiple clinical predictors of risk (see Box 2). Patients with only a single clinical predictor for cardiac risk undergoing intermediate- or high-risk surgery can be considered for initiation of beta blockers (Class IIb recommendation, usefulness less well established).

In their review of the evidence, Auerbach and Goldman [9] suggest using perioperative beta blockers in patients with two or more risk factors on the RCRI. This recommendation is in line with those mentioned previously, because the RCRI is similar to the intermediate clinical predictors list developed by the AHA/ACC guidelines. Perioperative beta blockade is also recommended for all patients who have long-term indications, including patients post myocardial infarction, with acute coronary syndromes, and with left ventricular dysfunction. In patients with vascular disease or diabetes, there are conflicting data on the use of beta blockers, but the evidence appears to favor their use [28].

If a patient is determined to be a high-risk patient who would benefit from perioperative beta blockade, beta blockers should be started days to weeks before the procedure, and the dose should be titrated to a target heart rate of 50 to 60 beats per minute at rest. Although studies have stopped perioperative beta blockade at the time of discharge, it is reasonable to continue beta blockers for 7 days postoperatively or indefinitely if there is a long-term indication.

Other medications

Other medications have been used to reduce cardiac risk in the perioperative period, including calcium channel blockers, nitroglycerin, alpha-2-agonists, and HMG-coenzyme A reductase inhibitors (or "statins"). Stevens and others [29] performed a systematic review of randomized trials that used medications to offer perioperative cardiac protection. There was no benefit from calcium channel blockers or nitroglycerin, although there were only three randomized studies with calcium channel blockers and one with nitroglycerin.

In the same meta-analysis, the alpha-2-agonists (both clonidine and mivazerol in 614 patients) decreased ischemia during surgery but had no effect on myocardial infarction. Although the alpha-2-agonists decreased the risk of cardiac death, the benefit was small; 83 patients need to be treated with this medicine to prevent one death. Another meta-analysis that evaluated the use of alpha-2-agonists to decrease perioperative cardiovascular complications found that these agents did reduce mortality and myocardial infarction after vascular surgery; however, this trend was not significant for other surgeries [30]. Wallace and colleagues [31] performed a randomized, placebo-controlled trial using prophylactic clonidine among veteran patients with coronary artery disease undergoing noncardiac surgery. Patients were given a loading dose of oral clonidine and then received a transdermal patch for 4 days. There was a significant reduction in perioperative myocardial ischemia and death; however, when patients who also received preoperative or intraoperative beta blockers were excluded, the mortality benefit diminished. Currently, an alpha-2-agonist such as clonidine can be considered as an alternative in patients who cannot tolerate beta blockers.

Several studies have suggested that statins such as simvastatin or atorvastatin can reduce perioperative mortality in patients undergoing vascular surgery [32,33]. In patients undergoing noncardiac surgery, Lindenauer and colleagues [34] performed a retrospective cohort study on a large national database and found that statin use reduced the risk of in-hospital mortality. Dunkelgrun and colleagues [35] recently completed a review and concluded that "perioperative statin therapy improves short and long-term cardiac outcome following noncardiac surgery. This cardiovascular protection has been attributed to the so-called pleiotropic effects, which have a positive effect on plaque stability." Further research on the use of perioperative statins to decrease the risk of cardiovascular complications in noncardiac surgery is needed before formal guidelines on their use can be offered.

Revascularization

Patients with a recent history of cardiac chest pain or a positive stress test or functional study are referred for angiography before their elective surgery. The purpose of angiography is to determine whether the patient is a candidate for a revascularization procedure. These procedures can include a percutaneous coronary intervention (PCI), which is also known as angio-plasty or angioplasty with intraluminal stenting, or coronary artery bypass grafting (CABG).

The notion that preoperative CABG could reduce perioperative cardiac events was based largely on retrospective data [36]. The Coronary Artery Surgery Study Registry found that patients who had CABG before elective noncardiac surgeries, when compared with medically treated patients, had fewer detrimental cardiovascular events, including decreased operative mortality and nonfatal myocardial infarction [37,38]. Retrospective data also suggested that preoperative PCI before noncardiac surgery also reduced cardiac events [39].

Proposing revascularization, by definition, will require delaying surgery to allow for recovery time and subjects patients to the risk of the revascular-ization process itself. CABG carries an overall 1% to 2% perioperative mortality rate [40] and is associated with perioperative myocardial infarction and stroke. Although PCI may seem like a "quicker" alternative to CABG preoperatively, the stents associated with PCI may complicate matters as well. Drug-eluding stents used to prevent restenosis are now commonly used but have an increased risk of in-stent thrombosis for a longer duration of time when compared with bare metal stents [41]. The US Food and Drug Administration (FDA) recommends continuation of aspirin and clopidogrel for 3 to 6 months depending on the drug-eluting stent used; however, reports of late thrombosis associated with drug-eluting stents have led the ACC/AHA to recommend continuing aspirin and clopidogrel for up to 12 months [28]. Surgery will be delayed for up to 1 year if antiplatelet agents cannot be stopped for the surgical procedure. Alternatively, if surgery needs to be done in a shorter time frame and PCI is deemed necessary, balloon angioplasty or bare metal stents can be considered, because they require shorter periods of antiplatelet agents.

The 2002 ACC/AHA guidelines made recommendations regarding pre-operative revascularization based mainly on expert opinion [3]. With respect to CABG, the guidelines suggest that only a small subset of high-risk patients would require CABG to "get them through" surgery. Patients who should undergo revascularization before intermediate- or high-risk surgeries are those who have high-risk coronary anatomy and would derive a long-term benefit from the CABG. The 2004 ACC/AHA guidelines on the indications for CABG provide a detailed discussion on the topic [42].

Since the proposal of the 2002 ACC/AHA guidelines, a randomized study has been published that supports the recommendation against "prophylactic" revascularization. The coronary artery revascularization prophylaxis (CARP) trial attempted to measure the benefit of coronary artery revascular-ization in veteran patients before elective vascular surgery [43], a high-risk surgery. Patients with at least one vessel with 70% or more stenosis on angiography were randomized to CABG or PCI versus medical therapy. There was no difference in postoperative myocardial infarction rates and no improvement in mortality at 30 days postoperatively and at 2.7 years after randomization. Both groups were treated with intensive medical therapy. It was concluded that revascularization in this patient population conferred no benefit. The study had many limitations. It included only veteran patients with stable cardiac symptoms and without an urgent need for surgery. Only 9% of patients screened were eligible for the study. Additionally, revascularization, both PCI and CABG, were done based on anatomy rather than symptoms. Fifty-one percent of patients had an RCRI score of less than 2, implying a relatively low cardiac complication risk.

Management of perioperative anticoagulation

Patients taking medications that impact hemostasis have an increased risk of perioperative bleeding. Surgeons often provide patients with a list of medications to stop before surgery. These medications typically include aspirin, NSAIDs, warfarin, clopidogrel, vitamin E, and herbal medications. Generally, patients are advised to stop these agents 7 to 10 days before surgery; however, patients may be able to continue medications longer into the preoperative period. The medical consultant should review the patient's medication list and give advice on timing to start and stop such medications. The following sections review the recommendations for the use of antiplatelet agents and warfarin during the perioperative period.

Aspirin and non-steroidal anti-inflammatory drugs

Aspirin and NSAIDs affect platelet aggregation by inhibiting prostaglandin synthesis and reducing the production of thromboxane A_2. Although NSAIDs cause reversible inhibition of platelet cyclooxygenase, aspirin is an irreversible inhibitor. Most NSAIDs can be discontinued 3 days before surgery and some as short as 1 day to minimize bleeding risk [44]. In a recent in vitro study of healthy volunteers taking ibuprofen, normalization of platelet function occurred within 24 hours of cessation [45].

Because aspirin irreversibly inhibits platelets, it needs to be stopped 7 to 10 days before surgery. Checking bleeding times to assess bleeding potential after aspirin cessation is no longer recommended because the test is subjective, and because it is an inaccurate predictor of perioperative bleeding [46].

The reason why the patient is taking daily aspirin must be determined. The medical consultant may need to confer with the patient's surgeon and subspecialist if he or she is uncertain whether aspirin cessation would cause more harm than benefit. For example, a cardiologist may request that aspirin may be continued perioperatively in patients with unstable angina. Additionally, aspirin withdrawal of greater than 5 days duration has been associated with an increased risk of acute coronary syndrome or stroke in patients with known cardiovascular disease [47,48]. It is reasonable to recommend continuing aspirin if bleeding risk is low and the risk of acute cardiovascular disease is high.

Clopidogrel

Clopidogrel is also an antiplatelet agent, but its mechanism of action is different than that of aspirin and NSAIDs in that it inhibits platelet aggregation by selectively and irreversibly inhibiting binding of ADP to its platelet receptor. It is approved by the FDA for many uses, including stroke prophylaxis, acute coronary syndromes, myocardial infarction, peripheral vascular disease, and after coronary artery stent placement [49]. To achieve normal platelet function, clopidogrel should be stopped at least 7 days before surgery [49]. As is true for aspirin, it is important for the preoperative consultant to know the indication for clopidogrel and to ensure it is safe to stop the medication preoperatively. Patients having PCI can undergo a range of procedures, including transluminal balloon angioplasty, bare metal stent placement, or drug-eluding stent placement. Drug-eluding stents have delayed epithelialization, and the FDA initially recommended that patients continue clopidogrel and aspirin for 3 to 6 months (for sirolimus and paclitaxel stents, respectively) to prevent in-stent thrombosis. However, the ACC/AHA recommends continuing the agents for up to 12 months [28]. If urgent surgery and vascular intervention are necessary, one could consider angioplasty alone or a bare metal stent to shorten the duration of antiplatelet therapy. If drug eluding stents are placed, elective surgery should ideally be deferred for one year.

Warfarin

Long-term warfarin therapy is indicated to prevent stroke in patients with atrial fibrillation or mechanical heart valves and to prevent recurrent venothromboembolic disease. In nearly all cases, surgeons will request that warfarin be discontinued before nonemergent surgery and that the INR return to normal or near normal. One exception is that ophthalmologists may perform cataract surgery on patients taking warfarin. Determining which patients can safely stop warfarin during the perioperative period and who will require "bridging" anticoagulation to minimize the risk of thromboembolism is an important task of the medical consultant who must weigh the risks of bleeding versus thrombosis.

Kearon and Hirsh [50] developed mathematical models to determine the risk of thromboembolism and major bleeding using various strategies for perioperative anticoagulation. In one strategy, warfarin was stopped and the INR was allowed to drift down to baseline. In the other, warfarin was stopped and intravenous heparin was given for 2 days before and 2 days after surgery. In both strategies, warfarin was stopped 4 days before surgery and restarted 1 day after surgery. It was concluded that surgery should be postponed if possible in patients who have had a venous thromboembolism or arterial embolism within 1 month of the scheduled surgery. If this is not possible, heparin bridging is indicated. In patients who have had a venous thromboembolism in the preceding 3 months, postoperative heparin is recommended.

In patients with nonvalvular atrial fibrillation or mechanical heart valves, Kearon and Hirsh's models suggested that heparin bridging conferred an excess risk of major bleeding and death, and was not justified. A criticism of their report is that they used a straight 8% complication rate of thrombotic events for patients with mechanical heart valves without taking into account the position or type of valve.

The American College of Chest Physicians (ACCP) in 2004 published guidelines regarding perioperative management of the vitamin K antagonists, including warfarin [51]. The guidelines recommend stopping warfarin 4 days preoperatively and resuming postoperatively. For patients at low risk of thromboembolism (ie, patients >3 months out from a previous venous thromboembolism, a history of average-risk atrial fibrillation, or a bi-leaflet aortic valve replacement), warfarin can be stopped and resumed postoperatively; however, the guidelines give an option of using pre- and postoperative prophylactic heparin (unfractionated heparin or low molecular weight heparin). For patients at intermediate risk of thromboembolism, prophylactic heparin is recommended pre- and postoperatively. For patients at high risk (venous thromboembolism at <3 months, older aortic valve replacements, and all mitral valve replacements), therapeutic doses of heparin are recommended approximately 2 days preoperatively and prophylactic doses of heparin postoperatively.

Despite the recommendations, the ACCP guidelines are difficult to strictly apply clinically for several reasons. First, the recommendations are based on observational data. Second, other alternatives may be equally reasonable, but the guidelines do not provide guidance on when to use optional therapy [52].

If a heparin bridge is used, a decision must be made to use unfractionated heparin versus low molecular weight heparins. Unfractionated heparin requires hospital admission and continuous intravenous administration with frequent laboratory monitoring. It is a preferable agent when anticoagulation requires faster reversal given its shorter half-life and is also more reliably reversible with protamine. The low molecular weight heparins have the advantage that they can be given subcutaneously; therefore, they can be administered to outpatients. Dosing is generally weight based, but special considerations are needed in obese patients, given the discrepancy between actual and ideal body weights, and in patients who have renal failure, because the drug is renally excreted. Although using the low molecular weight heparins as a bridge is not an approved FDA indication, their use is widespread and is considered an acceptable standard of care.

Endocarditis prophylaxis

Although uncommon, endocarditis is associated with significant morbidity and mortality, and preventative measures should be used when appropriate [53]. Endocarditis usually occurs in the setting of patients with structural heart disease when bacteremia develops with endocarditis-causing organisms. There are no randomized clinical controlled trials to support the recommendations made by the AHA in 1997; rather, these recommendations are based on available literature and expert opinion. Endocarditis prophylaxis is recommended in patients who are at increased risk for endocardial infection based on structural defects and in whom such infection would be associated with a high likelihood of morbidity and mortality.

The classic types of surgery that require endocarditis prophylaxis owing to bacteremia-producing potential are dental, respiratory, gastrointestinal, and genitourinary procedures. Most elective and outpatient podiatric surgeries are performed through surgically scrubbed skin and are unlikely to produce bacteremia; however, bacteremia can result from incision and drainage of infected tissues, which is common in patients with diabetes. In this case, patients defined as high or moderate risk from a cardiac standpoint should have prophylaxis based on the suspected pathogen [53]. Examples of high-risk patients include those with prosthetic heart valves, prior bacterial endocarditis, and complex cyanotic congenital heart disease. Moderate-risk patients include those with other uncorrected congenital conditions (such as bicuspid aortic valves or ventricular septal defects), acquired valvular disease, hypertrophic cardiomyopathy, and mitral valve prolapse with regurgitation.

Summary

Cardiovascular complications are a major cause of postoperative morbidity and mortality, but proper assessment of risk and subsequent interventions can help diminish these complications. Often, surgeons request medical "clearance" for patients before scheduling them for surgery. The term *clearance* is a misnomer because it applies no risk, and stating that a patient is "clear for surgery" provides no information regarding his or her medical status.

Assessing the patient's risk is based on the type of surgery performed and on individual patient characteristics. The latter can be established with a thorough history and physical, laboratory testing, risk indices, and cardiology studies. This risk factor assessment or preoperative evaluation has five components: (1) assessing the current medical status of the patient, (2) providing risk stratification, (3) suggesting interventions to optimize the patient's medical status and reduce cardiac risk, (4) providing specific recommendations for proper perioperative care, and (5) educating the patient about medication use perioperatively.

References

[1] Devereaux PJ, Goldman L, Cook DJ, et al. Perioperative cardiac events in patients undergoing noncardiac surgery: a review of the magnitude of the problem, the pathophysiology of the events and methods to estimate and communicate risk. CMAJ 2005;173(6):627–34.

[2] Dawood MM, Gupta DK, Southern J, et al. Pathology of fatal perioperative myocardial infarction: implications regarding pathophysiology and prevention. Int J Cardiol 1996;57(1): 37–44.

[3] Eagle KA, Berger PB, Calkins H, et al. ACC/AHA guideline update for perioperative cardiovascular evaluation for noncardiac surgery—executive summary: a report of the American College of Cardiology/American Heart Association Task Force on Practice Guidelines (Committee to Update the 1996 Guidelines on Perioperative Cardiovascular Evaluation for Noncardiac Surgery). J Am Coll Cardiol 2002;39(3):542–53.

[4] Goldman L, Caldera DL, Nussbaum SR, et al. Multifactorial index of cardiac risk in noncardiac surgical procedures. N Engl J Med 1977;297(16):845–50.

[5] Detsky AS, Abrams HB, Forbath N, et al. Cardiac assessment for patients undergoing noncardiac surgery: a multifactorial clinical risk index. Arch Intern Med 1986;146(11): 2131–4.

[6] Guidelines for assessing and managing the perioperative risk from coronary artery disease associated with major noncardiac surgery. American College of Physicians. Ann Intern Med 1997;127(4):309–12.

[7] Lee TH, Marcantonio ER, Mangione CM, et al. Derivation and prospective validation of a simple index for prediction of cardiac risk of major noncardiac surgery. Circulation 1999;100(10):1043–9.

[8] Reilly DF, McNeely MJ, Doerner D, et al. Self-reported exercise tolerance and the risk of serious perioperative complications. Arch Intern Med 1999;159(18):2185–92.

[9] Auerbach A, Goldman L. Assessing and reducing the cardiac risk of noncardiac surgery. Circulation 2006;113(10):1361–76.

[9a] LeBlond RF, DeGowin RL, Brown DD. DeGowin's Diagnostic Examination, Eighth Edition, New York: McGraw-Hill Publishing, 2004. p. 903–14.

[10] Smith MS, Muir H, Hall R. Perioperative management of drug therapy, clinical considerations. Drugs 1996;51(2):238–59.

[11] Kroenke K, Gooby-Toedt D, Jackson JL. Chronic medications in the perioperative period. South Med J 1998;91(4):358–64.

[12] Ang-Lee MK, Moss J, Yuan CS. Herbal medicines and perioperative care. JAMA 2001; 286(2):208–16.

[13] Schiff RL, Welsh GA. Perioperative evaluation and management of the patient with endocrine dysfunction. Med Clin North Am 2003;87(1):175–92.

[14] Moller A, Tonnesen H. Risk reduction: perioperative smoking intervention. Best Pract Res Clin Anaesthesiol 2006;20(2):237–48.

[15] Blacker DJ, Flemming KD, Link MJ, et al. The preoperative cerebrovascular consultation: common cerebrovascular questions before general or cardiac surgery. Mayo Clin Proc 2004; 79(2):223–9.

[16] Pasternak LR. Preoperative laboratory testing: general issues and considerations. Anesthesiol Clin North America 2004;22(1):13–25.

[17] Smetana GW, Macpherson DS. The case against routine preoperative laboratory testing. Med Clin North Am 2003;87(1):7–40.

[18] Lee T. Cardiac noninvasive testing. In: Goldman L, Braunwald E, editors. Primary cardiology. Philadelphia: WB Saunders; 1998. p. 44–56.

[19] Cruickshank JM. Beta-blockers continue to surprise us. Eur Heart J 2000;21(5):354–64.

[20] Stone JG, Foex P, Sear JW, et al. Myocardial ischemia in untreated hypertensive patients: effect of a single small oral dose of a beta-adrenergic blocking agent. Anesthesiology 1988; 68(4):495–500.

[21] Mangano DT, Layug EL, Wallace A, et al. Effect of atenolol on mortality and cardiovascular morbidity after noncardiac surgery: Multicenter Study of Perioperative Ischemia Research Group. N Engl J Med 1996;335(23):1713–20.

[22] Poldermans D, Boersma E, Bax JJ, et al. The effect of bisoprolol on perioperative mortality and myocardial infarction in high-risk patients undergoing vascular surgery: Dutch

Echocardiographic Cardiac Risk Evaluation Applying Stress Echocardiography Study Group. N Engl J Med 1999;341(24):1789–94.

[23] Brady AR, Gibbs JS, Greenhalgh RM, et al. Perioperative beta-blockade (POBBLE) for patients undergoing infrarenal vascular surgery: results of a randomized double-blind controlled trial. J Vasc Surg 2005;41(4):602–9.

[24] Juul AB, Wetterslev J, Gluud C, et al. Effect of perioperative beta blockade in patients with diabetes undergoing major non-cardiac surgery: randomised placebo controlled, blinded multicentre trial. BMJ 2006;332(7556):1482.

[25] Devereaux PJ, Beattie WS, Choi PT, et al. How strong is the evidence for the use of perioperative beta blockers in non-cardiac surgery? Systematic review and meta-analysis of randomised controlled trials. BMJ 2005;331(7512):313–21.

[26] Lindenauer PK, Pekow P, Wang K, et al. Perioperative beta-blocker therapy and mortality after major noncardiac surgery. N Engl J Med 2005;353(4):349–61.

[27] Fleisher LA, Beckman JA, Brown KA, et al. ACC/AHA 2006 guideline update on perioperative cardiovascular evaluation for noncardiac surgery: focused update on perioperative beta-blocker therapy. A report of the American College of Cardiology/American Heart Association Task Force on Practice Guidelines (Writing Committee to Update the 2002 Guidelines on Perioperative Cardiovascular Evaluation for Noncardiac Surgery): developed in collaboration with the American Society of Echocardiography, American Society of Nuclear Cardiology, Heart Rhythm Society, Society of Cardiovascular Anesthesiologists, Society for Cardiovascular Angiography and Interventions, and Society for Vascular Medicine and Biology. Circulation 2006;113(22):2662–74.

[28] Smith SC Jr, Allen J, Blair SN, et al. AHA/ACC guidelines for secondary prevention for patients with coronary and other atherosclerotic vascular disease: update endorsed by the National Heart, Lung, and Blood Institute. Circulation 2006;113(19):2363–72.

[29] Stevens RD, Burri H, Tramer MR. Pharmacologic myocardial protection in patients undergoing noncardiac surgery: a quantitative systematic review. Anesth Analg 2003;97(3):623–33.

[30] Wijeysundera DN, Naik JS, Beattie WS. Alpha-2 adrenergic agonists to prevent perioperative cardiovascular complications: a meta-analysis. Am J Med 2003;114(9):742–52.

[31] Wallace AW, Galindez D, Salahieh A, et al. Effect of clonidine on cardiovascular morbidity and mortality after noncardiac surgery. Anesthesiology 2004;101(2):284–93.

[32] Schouten O, Kertai MD, Bax JJ, et al. Safety of perioperative statin use in high-risk patients undergoing major vascular surgery. Am J Cardiol 2005;95(5):658–60.

[33] Ward RP, Leeper NJ, Kirkpatrick JN, et al. The effect of preoperative statin therapy on cardiovascular outcomes in patients undergoing infrainguinal vascular surgery. Int J Cardiol 2005;104(3):264–8.

[34] Lindenauer PK, Pekow P, Wang K, et al. Lipid-lowering therapy and in-hospital mortality following major noncardiac surgery. JAMA 2004;291(17):2092–9.

[35] Dunkelgrun M, Schouten O, Feringa HH, et al. Beneficial effects of statins on perioperative cardiovascular outcome. Curr Opin Anaesthesiol 2006;19(4):418–22.

[36] Wesorick DH, Eagle KA. The preoperative cardiovascular evaluation of the intermediate-risk patient: new data, changing strategies. Am J Med 2005;118(12):1413.

[37] Foster ED, Davis KB, Carpenter JA, et al. Risk of noncardiac operation in patients with defined coronary disease: the Coronary Artery Surgery Study (CASS) registry experience. Ann Thorac Surg 1986;41(1):42–50.

[38] Eagle KA, Rihal CS, Mickel MC, et al. Cardiac risk of noncardiac surgery: influence of coronary disease and type of surgery in 3368 operations. CASS Investigators and University of Michigan Heart Care Program: Coronary Artery Surgery Study. Circulation 1997;96(6):1882–7.

[39] Hassan SA, Hlatky MA, Boothroyd DB, et al. Outcomes of noncardiac surgery after coronary bypass surgery or coronary angioplasty in the Bypass Angioplasty Revascularization Investigation (BARI). Am J Med 2001;110(4):260–6.

[40] Peterson ED, Coombs LP, DeLong ER, et al. Procedural volume as a marker of quality for CABG surgery. JAMA 2004;291(2):195–201.

[41] Babapulle MN, Joseph L, Belisle P, et al. A hierarchical Bayesian meta-analysis of randomised clinical trials of drug-eluting stents. Lancet 2004;364(9434):583–91.

[42] Eagle KA, Guyton RA, Davidoff R, et al. ACC/AHA 2004 guideline update for coronary artery bypass graft surgery: summary article. A report of the American College of Cardiology/American Heart Association Task Force on Practice Guidelines (Committee to Update the 1999 Guidelines for Coronary Artery Bypass Graft Surgery). Circulation 2004;110(9): 1168–76.

[43] McFalls EO, Ward HB, Moritz TE, et al. Coronary-artery revascularization before elective major vascular surgery. N Engl J Med 2004;351(27):2795–804.

[44] Spell NO 3rd. Stopping and restarting medications in the perioperative period. Med Clin North Am 2001;85(5):1117–28.

[45] Goldenberg NA, Jacobson L, Manco-Johnson MJ. Brief communication: duration of platelet dysfunction after a 7-day course of Ibuprofen. Ann Intern Med 2005;142(7):506–9.

[46] Peterson P, Hayes TE, Arkin CF, et al. The preoperative bleeding time test lacks clinical benefit: College of American Pathologists' and American Society of Clinical Pathologists' position article. Arch Surg 1998;133(2):134–9.

[47] Ferrari E, Benhamou M, Cerboni P, et al. Coronary syndromes following aspirin withdrawal: a special risk for late stent thrombosis. J Am Coll Cardiol 2005;45(3):456–9.

[48] Sibon I, Orgogozo JM. Antiplatelet drug discontinuation is a risk factor for ischemic stroke. Neurology 2004;62(7):1187–9.

[49] Clopidogrel: Drug information, L-C, Inc. Copyright 1978–2006. Available at: http://uptodate online.com/utd/content/topic.do?topicKey=drug_a_k/2193&type=A&selectedTitle=5~51. Accessed October 2, 2006.

[50] Kearon C, Hirsh J. Management of anticoagulation before and after elective surgery. N Engl J Med 1997;336(21):1506–11.

[51] Ansell J, Hirsh J, Poller L, et al. The pharmacology and management of the vitamin K antagonists: the Seventh ACCP Conference on Antithrombotic and Thrombolytic Therapy. Chest 2004;126(3 Suppl):204S–33S.

[52] Guyatt G, Schunemann HJ, Cook D, et al. Applying the grades of recommendation for antithrombotic and thrombolytic therapy: the Seventh ACCP Conference on Antithrombotic and Thrombolytic Therapy. Chest 2004;126(3 Suppl):179S–87S.

[53] Dajani AS, Taubert KA, Wilson W, et al. Prevention of bacterial endocarditis: recommendations by the American Heart Association. Clin Infect Dis 1997;25(6):1448–58.

ELSEVIER
SAUNDERS

Clin Podiatr Med Surg
24 (2007) 285–309

CLINICS IN
PODIATRIC
MEDICINE AND
SURGERY

An Infectious Disease Update on Antibiotics: Emerging Resistance

John S. Steinberg, DPM[a],*, Paul J. Kim, DPM[b],
Mark R. Abbruzzese, MD[c]

[a]*Department of Plastic Surgery, Georgetown University School of Medicine, 3800 Reservoir Road NW, Main Bldg. 1st Floor, Limb Center, Washington, DC 20007-2113, USA*
[b]*Arizona Podiatric Medicine Program, Midwestern University Division of Dental and Medical Education, Midwestern University College of Health Sciences, 19555 North 59th Ave., Glendale, AZ 85308, USA*
[c]*Georgetown University School of Medicine, 3800 Reservoir Road NW, Main Bldg. 1st Floor, Limb Center, Washington, DC 20007-2113, USA*

With the rise in antibiotic resistance, the appropriate selection of antibiotics has become a focus of attention in podiatric practice. A variety of antibiotics is available to the podiatric physician in the treatment of bacterial soft tissue and bone infections encountered in the lower extremity (Table 1). It is unrealistic, irresponsible, and unacceptable to treat all bacterial infections of the lower extremity with a single broad-spectrum antibiotic. The appropriate and judicious use of antibiotics specifically targeting the offending organism is necessary to slow down the growing concerns of bacterial resistance [1–4].

Proper assessment and interpretation of clinical signs and symptoms is the obvious starting point to diagnose an active infection. For soft tissue infections, the classic signs include rubor (redness), tumor (swelling), dolor (pain), calor (heat), and function laesa (loss of function). The assessment of a superficial infection (cellulitis) should include marking a line of demarcation as a reference for advancing or receding infection (Fig. 1). When an open wound is present, wound depth should be probed using a sterile instrument, which enables the clinician to fully examine the extent of the wound and may aid in the diagnosis of infection of the bone [5]. Any odor or drainage emanating from an open wound should be noted. In the presence of aggressive infection, the patient may report fever, flu-like symptoms, malaise,

---

* Corresponding author. Georgetown University Hospital, 3800 Reservoir Road, 1-Main-West, Center for Wound Healing, Washington, DC 20007-2113.
E-mail address: steinberg@usa.net (J.S. Steinberg).

Table 1
Clinical syndromes and initial treatment options

Syndrome	Description	Organism	Initial treatment options
Cellulitis	An acute spreading infection of the skin and connective tissue	Most often G+ but can be any skin flora organism	PO: penicillins, cephlasporins, clindamycin, macrolides IV: penicillins, cephlasporins, clindamycin, vancomycin
Paronychia	Infection about a nail border	G+ cocci	PO: penicillins, cephlasporins, clindamycin, macrolides
Erythrasma	Superficial interdigital bacterial infection of the skin characterized by well-defined but irregular reddish brown patches Coral-red fluorescence on Woods lamp	Corynebacterium	Erythromycin
Ecythyma	Greenish-yellow crusted, punched-out lesions	G+ cocci	PO: penicillins, cephlasporins, clindamycin, erythromycin, macrolides
Clostridial cellulitis	Infection of devitalized subcutaneous tissue due to trauma or surgery Gas seen on plain films	G+ rods	IV: penicillins, imipenem/cilastin
Nonclostridial anaerobic cellulitis	Similar to clostridial cellulitis Diabetes may be an underlying factor	Polymicrobial including aerobic and anaerobic	IV: imipenem/cilastin, ticarcillin/clavulanic acid, piperacillin/tazobactam, ampicillin/sulbactam
Necrotizing fasciitis	Acute, rapidly progressive infection involving superficial and/or deep tissue A strong probability of systemic toxicity Gas seen on plain films	Polymicrobial, pseudomonads, G+ cocci, G−	IV: empiric treatment, radical debridement a must

Synergistic necrotizing fasciitis	Similar to necrotizing fasciitis but also involves muscle	Polymicrobial, pseudomonads, G+ cocci, G−	IV: empiric treatment, radical debridement a must
Clostridial myonecrosis	Acute, rapidly progressive infection involving muscle Muscle undergoes necrosis A strong probability of systemic toxicity Gas and crepitus present	G+ bacilli	IV: empiric treatment (penicillin, clindamycin), radical debridement a must
Nonclostridial myonecrosis	Less acute and less systemic toxicity than clostridial myonecrosis	Mixed flora	IV: treat isolated organism(s)
Infected vascular gangrene	Associated with peripheral vascular disease and diabetes	G+, G−	IV: piperacillin/tazobactam, ticarcillin/clavulanic acid, ampicillin/sulbactam
Acute osteomyelitis	Infection of bone typically seen in children and adolescents Associated with constitutional symptoms (fever, chills, malaise) Usually a single organism	G+, G−	IV: treat isolated organism(s)
Osteomyelitis secondary to a contiguous focus or direct extension	Direct inoculation of bone	Polymicrobial but usually G+	IV: clindamycin, imipenem/cilastin, piperacillin/tazobactam, amoxicillin/clavulanic acid, ampicillin/sulbactam
Osteomyelitis secondary to vascular insufficiency	Results from inadequate blood supply to tissues Associated with diabetic patients	Polymicrobial	IV: empiric treatment, address ischemia
Open fractures	Results from bacterial contamination at fracture sites	G+ most common	IV: penicillins, aminoglycosides
Puncture wounds	Superficial or deep infection typically of soft tissue	G+, pseudomonads	PO/IV: treat isolated organism(s)

(continued on next page)

Table 1 (*continued*)

Syndrome	Description	Organism	Initial treatment options
Bite wounds	Animal and human bite causes inoculation of bacteria present in oral cavity of offender	G+, G−, *Pasteurella* (dog and cat)	PO: amoxicillin/clavulanic acid IV: ampicillin/sulbactam, carbapenems
Burn wounds	Note liquefaction and necrosis	G+, pseudomonads	PO/IV: treat isolated organism(s)
Diabetic foot infections	Can present as acute or chronic wounds	Polymicrobial but usually G+, aerobic, anaerobic	PO/IV: depending on severity of infection, initial treatment should be broad spectrum (augmentin, piperacillin/tazobactam, carbapenems, ticarcillin/clavulanic acid, ampicillin/sulbactam), then treat isolated organisms

Abbreviations: G+, gram positive; G−, gram negative; IV, intravenous; PO, by mouth.

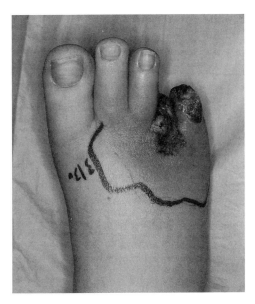

Fig. 1. Drawn line of demarcation for purpose of tracking infection progression/regression.

nausea, vomiting, or diarrhea. In many immune-compromised patients, however, these systemic factors present with a lesser frequency because the patient is unable to mount a significant systemic response to the infection.

Gram stain, culture, and sensitivity are valued tools to aid in the diagnosis and treatment of infection (Box 1). If a culture is warranted, both aerobic and anaerobic cultures should be taken. Culture and sensitivity reports guide the clinician to prescribe appropriate antibiotics. Deep tissue and bone cultures are best taken in the operating room. Swab cultures of drainage, purulence, or open wound surfaces should be reserved for wounds that have a high index of suspicion for infection. This selective use of cultures is of key importance because superficial swab cultures often grow normal skin flora and nonpathogenic wound contaminants. Overaggressive prescribing based on surface culture results contributes to the growing antibiotic resistance.

Ancillary tests can also assist the clinician in diagnosing an infection. Laboratory tests are of particular importance in patients who have soft tissue infections that show signs and symptoms of systemic toxicity including fever or hypothermia, tachycardia (heart rate > 100 beats per minute), and hypotension (systolic blood pressure < 90 mm Hg or 20 mm Hg below baseline) [6]. These laboratory tests include blood cultures, complete blood cell count (CBC) with differential, creatinine, bicarbonate, creatine phosphokinase, and C-reactive protein levels [6]. An elevated white blood cell (WBC) count can indicate an aggressive infectious process. Immature polymorphonuclear leukocytes (bands) may also be an important indicator of

Box 1. Bacterial infectious pathogens encountered in the lower extremity

Gram-positive cocci
  Staphylococcus aureus
  Staphylococcus epidermidis
  Streptococcus pyogenes
  Streptococcus pneumoniae
  Enterococcus faecalis
  Enterococcus faecium
  Methicillin-resistant *Staphylococcus aureus*
  Methicillin-resistant *Staphylococcus epidermidis*
  Vancomycin-resistant *Enterococcus*
  Vancomycin-intermediate *Staphylococcus aureus*
  Erythromycin-resistant *Streptococcus pyogenes*

Gram-positive bacilli
  Corynebacterium diptheria
  Corynebacterium jeikeium
  Bacillus anthracis
  Bacillus cereus
  Clostridium difficile
  Clostridium septicum
  Clostridium perfringens
  Clostridium histolyticum
  Listeria monocytogenes
  Erysipelothrix rhusiopathiae

Gram-negative cocci
  Neisseria meningitides
  Neisseria gonorrhoeae
  Actinobacter calcoaceticus
  Kingella
  Moraxella

Gram-negative rods
  Pseudomonas aeruginosa
  Ekinella corrodens

Gram-negative bacilli
  Escherichia coli
  Shigella dysenteriae
  Salmonella choleraesuis

Klebsiella pneumoniae
Enterobacter cloacae
Serratia marcescens
Proteus mirabilis
Proteus vulgaris
Yersinia pestis
Morganella morganii

Other important bacteria
Vibrio vulnificus
Mycobacterium marinum
Aeromonas hydrophilia
Pasteurella multocida

infection. An increase in bands occurs with acute infections when the production of mature WBCs cannot keep up with the demand. This process is referred to as a "left shift." When a high WBC count or fever is present, blood cultures should be ordered. Blood cultures (two sets) are drawn 20 minutes apart and from different sites. Erythrocyte sedimentation rate and C-reactive protein may also be markers of infection; however, these values are nonspecific to infection and are more reflective of general inflammatory conditions. It should also be noted that an immunocompromised patient may not exhibit a robust response to infection. Patients who are immunocompromised are often more likely to have infections that are polymicrobial or contain atypical bacterial pathogens.

Radiographic modalities may also be helpful in the diagnosis of infection. Standard plain-film radiographs can assist in the diagnosis of bone infection (osteomyelitis) or the presence of gas in the soft tissue planes (Fig. 2). Some

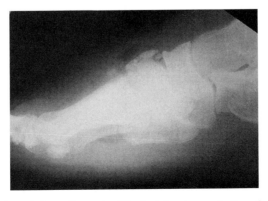

Fig. 2. Plain-film lateral view radiograph of the foot showing gas in the soft tissue with significant infection present.

radiographic markers of bone infection include periosteal elevation, cortical erosions, sequestrum, and involucrum. There may be a delay in these radiographic findings of bone infection; hence, follow-up radiographs over several weeks may be helpful. When there is suspicion for osteomyelitis on plain-film radiographs, MRI may be used for a more definitive diagnosis. An MRI may also be used to look for soft tissue infections such as abscess located in the deeper layers of tissue (Fig. 3). CT may be used to visualize changes in the cortical bone due to infection. Nuclear medicine bone scans reflect changes in metabolic activity of bone and are very sensitive but often are nonspecific for bone infections. The indium 111 WBC–labeled and the technetium 99m WBC–labeled (exametazime) scans are more specific for infection than traditional bone scans. These types of scans have been reported to yield comparable levels of sensitivity and specificity as histopathologic evaluations of bone specimens for the diagnosis of osteomyelitis [7].

When the diagnosis of an infection is made, the specific bacteria are identified through culture and sensitivity, and therapeutic intervention is started. Laboratory markers are important to monitor antibiotic treatment. Renal function, as measured by creatine clearance; hepatic function, as measured by aspartate aminotransferase, alanine aminotransferase, alkaline phosphatase, and bilirubin; and bone marrow function, as measured by CBC are useful measures to adjust antibiotic doses and to monitor for antibiotic-related toxicities. Figs. 4 and 5 provide further examples of podiatric infections.

The following section discusses selected antibiotics more commonly used in podiatric practice and new important research pertaining to growing resistance to certain antibiotics. Newer antibiotics less familiar to the podiatric physician are also discussed. The reader is referred to Table 2 for more information regarding commonly used antibiotics in the treatment of lower-extremity infections.

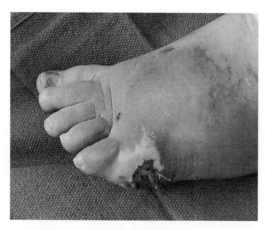

Fig. 3. Forefoot infection in a patient who has diabetes. Note extensive soft tissue involvement and underlying osteomyelitis of fifth toe and metatarsal.

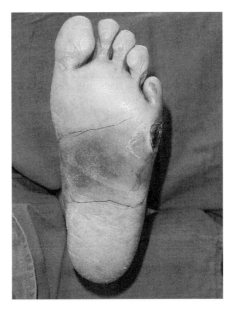

Fig. 4. Infected ulceration with proximal tracking into plantar soft tissue space.

Discussion of selected antibiotics

Penicillins

The penicillins have been the mainstay for the treatment of complicated soft tissue and bone infections in the lower extremity. These drugs encompass the subclasses of the natural penicillins, aminopenicillins, semisynthetic penicillins, and penicillin/β-lactamase inhibitors. The mechanism of action for these antibiotics is in the inhibition of bacterial cell wall synthesis.

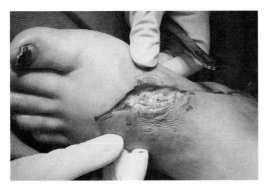

Fig. 5. Intraoperative photograph demonstrating purulence in deep fascial tissue of dorsal mid-foot requiring aggressive debridement.

Table 2
Antibiotics overview

Drug	Dose	Route	Clinical indications	Comments
Natural penicillins				
Penicillin G	2.4 million U q 4 h	IV	Skin and skin structure infections caused by *Staphylococcus* and *Streptococcus* (group A, B, C, G) Treatment of choice for erysipelas, gonococci, *Clostridium*, *Actinomyces israelii*, *Peptostreptococcus*, *Viridans*, *Bartonella bacilliformis*, *Treponema pallidum*	Renal dosing
	1.2 million U/d	IM	—	—
Penicillin V	250–500 mg qid	PO	See penicillin G	Renal dosing
Aminopenicillins				
Ampicillin	250–500 mg	PO	G– infections (*Escherichia coli*, *Proteus mirabilis*, *Ekinella corrodens*), *Enterococcus*	Renal dosing Empty stomach
	0.5–2g q 6 h	IM/IV	—	—
Amoxicillin	250–500 mg tid	PO	See ampicillin	Renal dosing Amoxicillin has better bioavailability than ampicillin
Semisynthetic penicillins (penicillinase resistant)				
Nafcillin	1–2 g q 4–6 h	IM/IV	Staphylococcal infections (bone and joint, septicemia, skin and soft tissue)	Hepatic and renal dosing
Dicloxacillin	250–500 mg qid	PO	Skin and soft tissue infections, *Staphylococcus*, *Streptococcus*	Hepatic and renal dosing Should be taken on empty stomach
	500 mg–1 g qid for severe infections	PO		

Drug	Route	Dose	Indications	Notes
Penicillin/β-lactamase inhibitor				
Amoxicillin/clavulanic acid (Augmentin)	PO	500–875 mg bid	Animal and bite wounds, less severe diabetic foot infections that can be treated on outpatient basis, skin and soft tissue infections with mixed flora, subcutaneous abscess, *Enterococcus*	Renal dosing; Clavulanic acid is always 125 mg; Take with food/water to prevent gastrointestinal effects
Ampicillin/sulbactam (Unasyn)	IM/IV	1.5–3 g q 6 h	Skin and soft tissue infections, animal or human bites, mild-to-moderate diabetic foot infections, *Enterococcus*	Renal dosing
Piperacillin/tazobactam (Zosyn)	IV	3.375–4.5 g q 4–6 h	Diabetic foot infections, empiric therapy for aerobic and anaerobic infections, bite wounds Covers *Pseudomonas aeruginosa*, *Enterococcus*	Renal dosing
Cephalosporins				
First generation				
Cefazolin (Ancef)	IM/IV	1–2 g q 8 h	Surgical prophylaxis, skin infections, traumatic wounds. *Staphyloccus*, *Streptococcus*	Renal dosing
Cephalexin (Keflex)	PO	250–500 bid–qid	Skin and skin structure infections, G+ infections	Renal dosing
Cefadroxil (Duricef)	PO	500 mg q 12 h or 1 g q 24 h	Similar to cephalexin	Renal dosing
Second generation				
Cefuroxime (Ceftin)	IV	1.5 g q 8 h	Skin/soft tissue infections, cellulitis, septic arthritis, osteomyelitis	—
	PO	250–500 mg bid	—	—

(continued on next page)

Table 2 (*continued*)

Drug	Dose	Route	Clinical indications	Comments
Third generation				
Ceftriaxone (Rocephin)	1–2 g q 12–24 h	IM/IV	Gonococcal infections; bacteria septicemia; bone, joint, and skin and skin structure infections	Biliary excretion Good drug for renal-impaired patients
Ceftazidime (Fortaz)	1 g q 8 h	IM/IV	Skin and skin structure infections	—
	2 g q 12 h	IM/IV	Bone and joint infections; coverage of *Pseudomonas aeruginosa*; septicemia	—
Cefdinir (Omnicef)	300 mg bid	PO	Uncomplicated skin and soft tissue infections	—
Fourth generation				
Cefepime (Maxipime)	1–2 g q 12 h	IV	Cellulitis, skin and skin structure infections that include *Pseudomonas aeruginosa, Staphylococcus aureus,* Enterobacteriaceae	Renal dosing
Next generation				
Ceftobiprole	—	—	Currently in phase 3 studies at the time of submission	—
Carbapenem				
Imipenem/cilastin (Primaxin)	500 mg q 6–8 h	IV	Used in severe limb and life-threatening conditions	Renal dosing

Drug	Dose	Route	Uses/Comments	Notes
Ertapenem (Invanz)	1 g q 24 h	IV	Diabetic foot infections, animal or human bites, complicated skin and skin structure infections	Renal dosing
Fluoroquinolones				
Ciprofloxacin (Cipro)	400 mg q 12 h 500–750 mg bid	IV PO	G– organisms including *Pseudomonas aeruginosa*; osteomyelitis (G–): can be used in synergy with clindamycin for diabetic foot infections	Renal dosing
Levofloxacin (Levaquin)	500–750 mg q 24 h 750 mg for severe infections	PO/IV	Better G+ coverage than ciprofloxacin, complicated skin and skin structure infections	Renal dosing
Moxifloxacin (Avelox)	400 mg q 24 h	PO/IV	Uncomplicated and complicated skin and skin structure infections; better G+ activity than ciprofloxacin; anaerobic G– coverage (*Bacteroides fragilis*)	—
Monobactam				
Aztreonam (Azactam)	1–2 g q 8h	IV	Covers only G– organisms; can be used in penicillin- or cephalosporin-allergic patients	Renal dosing

(continued on next page)

Table 2 (*continued*)

Drug	Dose	Route	Clinical indications	Comments
Aminoglycosides				
Gentamicin	5–7 mg/kg q 24 h	IV	G− infections; used in antibiotic beads; used in synergy with β-lactams for G+ infections (1 mg/kg IV q 8 h); skin, bone, and soft tissue infections; burns The topical form of gentamicin cream is used also for burns, wounds with *Pseudomonas aeruginosa* and other G− organisms	Renal dosing
Tobramycin	5–7 mg/kg q 24 h	IV	G− infections; septicemia; bone, skin, and skin structure infections Used in antibiotic beads	Renal dosing
Amikacin	15 mg/kg q 24 h	IV	G− infections, septicemia, bone and joint infections, skin and soft tissue infections, burns	Renal dosing
Sulfonamides				
Trimethoprim/ sulfamethoxazole (Bactrim)	80/400–160/800 mg bid	PO	MRSA; can be used in synergy with rifampin; used in penicillin-allergic patients; G−; staphylococcal infections; osteomyelitis	Needs renal dosing 160 mg trimethoprim/800 mg sulfamethoxazole
Macrolides				
Erythromycin	250–500 mg qid	PO	Can be used in penicillin-allergic patients for staphylococcal and streptococcal infections Can be used topically for treatment of erythrasma	—
Azithromycin (Zithromax)	250–500 mg q 24 h	PO/IV	Can be used in penicillin-allergic patients for streptococcal infections, skin and skin structure infections, cat-scratch disease	Drug tends to stay in body for up to 10 d

	Dose	Route	Uses	Comments
Tetracyclines				
Tetracycline	250–500 mg qid	PO	Madura foot; Lyme disease; can be used in penicillin-allergic patients for staphylococcal and streptococcal infections; *Clostridium tetani*; MRSA	Take on empty stomach; Can cause photosensitivity reaction; Aluminum, calcium, magnesium, and iron can impair absorption
Doxycycline	100 mg q 12 h	PO/IV	MRSA; Lyme disease; can be used in penicillin-allergic patients for staphylococcal and streptococcal infections	Aluminum, calcium, magnesium, and iron can impair absorption
Minocycline	100 mg q 12 h	PO/IV	MRSA; can be used in synergy with rifampin; can be used in penicillin-allergic patients for staphylococcal and streptococcal infections	Aluminum, calcium, magnesium, and iron can impair absorption
Oxazolidinone				
Linezolid (Zyvox)	600 mg q 12 h	PO/IV	MRSA, VRE, *Enterococcus*	Need weekly CBC, caution with SSRIs
Streptogramin				
Quinupristin/dalfopristin (Synercid)	7.5 mg/kg q 8–12 h	IV	VRE, MRSA, complicated skin and skin structure infections caused by *Staphylococcus aureus*, *Streptococcus pyogenes*, *Enterococcus faecium*	—
Lipopeptide				
Daptomycin (Cubicin)	4 mg/kg q 24 h	IV	Complicated skin and skin structure infections (mostly G+ organisms), MRSA, VRE, *Enterococcus*	Renal dosing; Can cause myopathy; Need to monitor creatine kinase

(continued on next page)

Table 2 (*continued*)

Drug	Dose	Route	Clinical indications	Comments
Glycopeptide				
Vancomycin (Vancocin)	1 g q 12 h	IV	MRSA, MRSE, bone and joint infections, septicemia, surgical prophylaxis in penicillin-allergic patients and when using implants Can be used in penicillin-allergic patients for G+ organisms; can be used in antibiotic beads; *Enterococcus*	Renal dosing IV form needs to be infused over 60 min to prevent "red man" syndrome
Dalbavancin	500–1000 mg/wk	IV	G+ infections including MRSA, corynebacterium	Safety profile similar to linezolid
Teicoplanin (Targocid)	6–12 mg/kg/d	IM/IV	G+ infections, MRSA	See vancomycin
Glycylcyclines				
Tigecycline (Tygacil)	50–100 mg q 12 h	IV	For complicated skin and skin structures infections including G+, G−, MRSA	—
Other				
Metronidazole (Flagyl)	500 mg q 6 h 250–500 mg tid	IV PO	Anaerobic infections (almost all G− organisms), skin and skin structure infections, septicemia, bone and joint infections Drug of choice for pseudomembranous colitis caused by *Clostridium difficile*	Renal dosing Has antiabuse effects with alcohol
Clindamycin (Cleocin)	300–900 mg q 8 h 150–450 mg qid	PO/IV PO	Penicillin- and cephalosporin-allergic patients, anaerobic infections, osteomyelitis, septicemia, skin and soft tissue infections, surgical prophylaxis, diabetic ulcers	Hepatic dosing Need to take oral form with full glass of water Associated with *Clostridium difficile* colitis

Rifampin	300 mg bid	PO	Can be used in synergy with a quinolone for diabetic foot infections
			Has high bone penetration
			Used in combination with other drugs (trimethoprim/sulfamethoxazole, ciprofloxacin, vancomycin, minocycline) to prevent rapid development of resistance
			Used alone for mycobacteria infections
			Causes red discoloration of bodily fluids

Abbreviations: G+, gram positive; G−, gram negative; IM, intramuscular; IV, intravenous; MRSA, methicillin-resistant *Staphylococcus aureus*; PO, by mouth; SSRIs, selective serotonin reuptake inhibitors; VRE, vancomycin-resistant *Enterococcus*.

This class is considered bactericidal. Generally, these antibiotics have been used for the treatment of gram-positive infections in the lower extremity; however, the extended-spectrum penicillins are effective against gram-negative organisms including *Pseudomonas aeruginosa*. The addition of chemical derivatives such as clavulanate (clavulanic acid), sulbactam, and tazobactam has extended the spectrum of penicillins by inhibiting β-lactamases. Penicillin/β-lactamase inhibitors have been shown to be effective against bacteria commonly encountered in diabetic foot wounds [8–10]. Methicillin resistance, however, has spurred the development of other antibiotics that are discussed in the following sections.

Cephalosporins

The cephalosporins are a large group of antibiotics with four distinct generations. Cephalosporins are similar to the penicillins in that they act to inhibit cell wall synthesis and are considered bactericidal. The difference in the generations is based on their spectrum of activity. The first-generation cephalosporins are generally effective against gram-positive organisms, with activity against selected gram-negative organisms. This class includes the commonly used antibiotics in podiatric practice, cefazolin and cephalexin. The second-generation cephalosporins have increased gram-negative coverage and some have anaerobic coverage. The third-generation cephalosporins have improved gram-negative coverage compared with the second-generation cephalosporins, with selected activity against *Pseudomonas aeruginosa*. The third- and fourth-generation cephalosporins have extended coverage against *Escherichia coli*, *Klebsiella pneumoniae*, *Proteus mirabilis*, *Enterobacter*, *Serratia*, and *Morganella* [11,12].

Carbapenems

The carbapenem group includes imipenem/cilastin, meropenem, and ertapenem. The carbapenems have a broad spectrum of activity including coverage of gram-positive and some gram-negative bacteria. They act to inhibit bacterial cell wall synthesis. Their clinical usage in the lower extremity involves the treatment of moderate-to-severe diabetic foot infections without osteomyelitis, animal or human bites, and complicated skin and skin structure infections [9,13,14]. One advantage of ertapenem is that it uses once-daily dosing, making it a cost effective drug and useful in the outpatient setting [15]. A limitation of ertapenem is that it does not cover *Pseudomonas aeruginosa*, methicillin-resistant *Staphylococcus aureus* (MRSA), or *Enterococcus*.

Fluoroquinolones

The advanced-generation fluoroquinolones (quinolones) consist of ciprofloxacin, levofloxacin, gatifloxacin, and moxifloxacin. Their mechanism of action is to inhibit DNA synthesis. Ciprofloxacin can be effectively used to treat gram-negative organisms including *Pseudomonas aeruginosa*. This antibiotic can also be used in combination with clindamycin for polymicrobial diabetic foot infections. Of note to the lower-extremity specialist is that ciprofloxicin has been reported to contribute to Achilles and other tendon ruptures/tenosynovitis [16,17]. Ciprofloxacin also is known to cause hypoglycemia in patients taking oral sulfonylureas such as glyburide [18]. It is believed that most of these effects (tendopathy, hypoglycemia, and so forth) are class related and not necessarily specific to ciprofloxacin. The bioavailability of all quinolones is significantly decreased by antacids containing magnesium or aluminum and other products containing calcium, iron, or zinc [19,20]. Levofloxacin has better gram-positive coverage than ciprofloxacin and can therefore be used for complicated skin and skin structure infections. Levofloxacin, however, has also been implicated in causing hypoglycemic states in diabetic patients [21]. Moxifloxacin offers anaerobic gram-negative coverage (*Bacteroides fragilis*) and has better gram-positive activity than ciprofloxacin. Moxifloxacin has been reported to be as effective as extended-spectrum penicillins for the treatment of skin and skin structure infections [22].

Monobactam

Aztreonam belongs to the monobactam (β-lactamase) class of antibiotics. Aztreonam inhibits bacterial cell wall synthesis with activity against gram-negative bacteria including Enterobacteriaceae and *Pseudomonas aeruginosa*. Aztreonam has also been shown to be effective for the treatment of *Pseudomonas aeruginosa* septic arthritis and osteomyelitis [23]. Aztreonam has been effectively used for the treatment of some multiresistant gram-negative bacteria and some antimicrobial-resistant strains of *Pseudomonas aeruginosa* [24,25]; however, other investigations have revealed that there are a growing number of aztreonam-resistant strains of *Pseudomonas aeruginosa* [26].

Aminolgycosides

The aminoglycosides (gentamicin, tobramycin, amikacin) are most often used for severe gram-negative infections. They have significant adverse side effects that include nephrotoxicity (reversible), ototoxicity (irreversible), and neuromuscular blockade (reversible). It is therefore important to monitor peaks and trough levels 24 hours after initiation of therapy and every 2 to 3 days to maximize the efficacy of aminoglycosides while minimizing their potential adverse effects. Dosing of aminoglycosides should be calculated using the Sarrubi and Hull [27] calculation, which takes into account serum creatinine, lean body weight, age, and sex. Trough samples should be drawn 30 minutes before the next dose, whereas peak levels should be drawn 15 to 30 minutes after completion of intravenous (IV) treatment. The aminoglycosides can be given in multiple or single daily doses. In an attempt to decrease the nephrotoxic effect, a once-daily pulse dosing regimen has been advocated. This dosing regimen is purported to decrease the potential for nephrotoxicity [28–30]. A synergistic effect has also been reported when aminoglycosides are used in combination with penicillins or cephalosporins against aminoglycoside-resistant strains of *Pseudomonas aeruginosa* [31].

Sulfonamides

Trimethoprim and sulfamethoxazole work synergistically to inhibit bacterial DNA synthesis in gram-positive and gram-negative organisms. Studies have also reported that trimethoprim/sulfamethoxazole is often effective against community-acquired, uncomplicated MRSA infections [4,32]; however, there has been increasing concern about bacterial resistance to trimethoprim/sulfamethoxazole [33].

Macrolides

Erythromycin, clarithromycin, and azithromycin make up the macrolide class of antibiotics. The macrolide class is effective in treating gram-positive organisms and has been used in the treatment of pneumococcal infections. These antibiotics inhibit protein assembly and are bactericidal to some pathogens and bacteriostatic to others. Erythromycin has a poor tolerability profile with a likelihood of causing gastrointestinal distress. There has also been some concern about erythromycin-resistant strains of *Streptococcus pyogenes* [34].

Tetracyclines

Tetracycline, doxycycline, and minocycline are members of the tetracycline antibiotic class and work to inhibit protein synthesis. Tetracyclines are broad-spectrum antibiotics with bacateriostatic effects against gram-positive and gram-negative organisms. Doxycycline and minocycline have been effectively used in the treatment MRSA infections of skin and soft tissue structures [35,36].

Glycylcyclines

Tigecycline, a glycylcycline, is similar to the tetracyclines in that it inhibits bacterial protein synthesis. This is a relatively new antibiotic with a wide spectrum of activity including activity against multidrug-resistant gram-positive and gram-negative organisms [37]. This new antibiotic has shown favorable results against MRSA isolates [11]. The tolerability of this drug appears to be similar to that of other antibiotics, but because of its relatively new introduction to the market, the potential adverse effects are still being investigated.

Rifampin

Rifampin has a narrow spectrum of activity and targets gram-positive and acid-fast bacillus. This agent works by inhibiting protein synthesis. Rifampin is a drug of choice for the treatment of mycobacterial infections but is also effective against MRSA infections [4]. Rifampin has been used in combination with other antibiotics including ciprofloxacin and trimethoprim/sulfamethoxazole for the treatment of MRSA infections [38,39]; however, there has been a growing concern of bacterial resistance to rifampin in combination drug therapy [38,39].

Oxazolidinone

Linezolid is in the class of antibiotics known as the oxazolidinones. This antibiotic inhibits bacterial protein synthesis. Linezolid has been set apart from other antibiotics due to its efficacy against resistant bacteria including MRSA and vancomycin-resistant *Enterococcus* (VRE). Linezolid has been reported to be as effective as aminopenicillin/β-lactamase inhibitors for the treatment of diabetic foot infections and potentially more effective than teicoplanin in the treatment of MRSA [40,41]. Linezolid can be administered parenterally and orally with comparable efficacy [40], which allows for easy transition from IV therapy to oral therapy for long-term administration. A weekly CBC should be drawn for patients taking linezolid due to the possibility of thrombocytopenia. There is also a potential for a drug interaction with serotonergic agents including selective serotonin reuptake inhibitors, which may result in developing serotonin syndrome [42,43]. Symptoms of serotonin syndrome include cognitive dysfunction, hyperpyrexia, hyper-reflexia, incoordination, confusion, and delirium.

Streptogramin

Quinupristin and dalfopristin are combined into one formulation, which allows them to have improved bactericidal activity. They act by inhibiting bacterial protein synthesis. Quinupristin/dalfopristin has demonstrated activity against MRSA and VRE [44]. Quinupristin/dalfopristin is effective against gram-positive bacteria encountered in complicated skin and skin structure infections but is not superior to cefazolin, oxacillin, or vancomycin [45].

Lipopeptide

Daptomycin is in the class of antibiotics known as the cyclic lipopeptides. Daptomycin inhibits bacterial protein synthesis and has bactericidal effects. This antibiotic has wide gram-positive bacterial coverage. More important, daptomycin can be used against resistant strains including VRE and MRSA with a high safety profile [46,47]. In vitro evidence suggests that daptomycin is effective against gram-positive isolates less susceptible to linezolid and quinupristin/dalfopristin [48].

Glycopeptides

Vancomycin, teicoplanin, and dalbavancin are part of the glycopeptides class of antibiotics. Vancomycin is effective against gram-positive bacteria and works by inhibiting bacterial cell wall synthesis. Historically, vancomycin has been used for the treatment of MRSA or for patients who have a penicillin allergy. The monitoring of peak and trough serum levels has been questioned in the literature [49–53]. Some advocate for the monitoring of only trough serum levels [51]. These trough serum levels should be drawn within 30 minutes of the next dose.

Teicoplanin and dalbavancin are lesser-recognized antibiotics in the glycopeptides class. Teicoplanin has been shown to be as effective as cefazolin for the treatment of gram-positive bacterial infections but not as effective as linezolid for the treatment of MRSA infections [41,54]. One potential advantage of teicoplanin is that it can be administered intramuscularly, with similar efficacy as with IV administration [55].

The clinical use of dalbavancin is relatively new. This antibiotic inhibits bacterial cell wall synthesis and has been reported to be more effective than vancomycin against most gram-positive strains in vitro. In addition, dalbavancin is as effective as linezolid in the treatment of complicated skin and skin structure MRSA infections [56,57]. Once-weekly dosing makes this antibiotic a convenient option.

Tetanus prophylaxis

Vaccine-preventable infectious diseases have a significant effect on the health of adults and children. This effect is especially demonstrable in the setting of foot injury and infection. Tetanus vaccine (booster) should be administered to patients who have not been boosted within 10 years or when the clinical situation dictates. Clinicians should always ask about the immunization status of their patients.

Summary

This article reviews some of the important antibiotics available for use in the podiatric clinical practice. Newer generations of "older" drugs and new, biosynthesized agents continue to come on the market. The older antibiotics continue to be effective for most cases of infections involving the lower extremity. They will likely continue to be effective in the future with greater clinical knowledge of the infectious process and specific targeting of the offending organism.

Although the antibiotic choices available appear to be plentiful, a cautious and systematic evaluation of the infectious process, with the isolation of the offending organism or organisms, is necessary to curtail the growing bacterial resistance encountered in podiatric practice. Selective antibiotic use is essential for the appropriate treatment of infections and is of particular importance given the number of years that it takes for new drug research and development. Appropriate consultation with an infectious disease specialist will help to ensure that the best possible treatment plan is implemented and will help to maintain antibiotic efficacy into the future.

References

[1] Barrett TW, Moran GJ. Update on emerging infections: news from the centers for disease control and prevention [commentary]. Ann Emerg Med 2004;43:45–7.

[2] Chambers HF. The changing epidemiology of Staphylococcus aureus. Emerg Infect Dis 2001;7:178–82.

[3] Cohen PR, Kurzrock R. Community-acquired methicillin-resistant Staphylococcus aureus skin infection: an emerging clinical problem. J Am Acad Dermatol 2004;50:277–80.

[4] Moran GJ, Krishnadasan A, Gorwitz RJ, et al. EMERGEncy ID Net Study Group. Methicillin-resistant S. aureus infections among patients in the emergency department. N Engl J Med 2006;355(7):666–74.

[5] Grayson ML, Gibbons GW, Balogh K, et al. Probing to bone in infected pedal ulcers: a clinical sign of underlying osteomyelitis in diabetic patients. J Am Med Assoc 1995;273:721–3.

[6] Stevens DL, Bisno AL, Chambers HF, et al. Infectious Diseases Society of America. Practice guidelines for the diagnosis and management of skin and soft-tissue infections. Clin Infect Dis 2005;41:1373–406.

[7] Ertugrul MB, Baktiroglu S, Salman S, et al. The diagnosis of osteomyelitis of the foot in diabetes: microbiological examination vs. magnetic resonance imaging and labeled leukocyte scanning. Diabet Med 2006;23(6):649–53.

[8] Zeillemaker AM, Veldkamp KE, van Kraaij MG, et al. Piperacillin/tazobactam therapy for diabetic foot infection. Foot Ankle Int 1998;19:169–72.

[9] Lipsky BA, Berendt AR, Deery HG, et al. Infectious Diseases Society of America. Diagnosis and treatment of diabetic foot infections. Clin Infect Dis 2004;39:885–910.

[10] Lipsky BA, Armstrong DG, Citron DM, et al. Ertapenem versus piperacillin/tazobactam for diabetic foot infections (SIDESTEP): prospective, randomised, controlled, double-blinded, multicentre trial. Lancet 2005;366(9498):1695–703.

[11] Denis O, Deplano A, Nonhoff C, et al. In vitro activities of ceftobiprole, tigecycline, daptomycin, and 19 other antimicrobials against methicillin-resistant Staphylococcus aureus strains from a national survey of Belgian hospitals. Antimicrob Agents Chemother 2006; 50(8):2680–5.

[12] Goldstein EJC, Citron DM, Merriam CV, et al. In vitro activity of ceftobiprole against aerobic and anaerobic strains isolated from diabetic foot infections. Antimicrob Agents Chemother 2006;50(11):3959–62.

[13] Gesser RM, McCarroll KA, Woods GL. Efficacy of ertapenem against methicillin-susceptible Staphylococcus aureus in complicated skin/skin structure infections: results of a double-blind clinical trial versus pipercillin-tazobactam. Int J Antimicrob Agents 2004;23(3):235–9.

[14] Grayson ML, Gibbons GW, Habershaw GM, et al. Use of ampicillin/sulbactam versus imipenem/cilastatin in the treatment of limb-threatening foot infections in diabetic patients. Clin Infect Dis 1994;18:683–93.

[15] Tice AD. Ertapenem: a new opportunity for outpatient parenteral antimicrobial therapy. J Antimicrob Chemother 2004;53(Suppl 2):ii83–6.

[16] van der Linden PD, van de Lei J, Nab HW, et al. Achilles tendinitis associated with fluoroquinolones. Br J Clin Pharmacol 1999;48:433–7.

[17] van der Linden PD, Sturkenboom MCJM, Herings RMC, et al. Fluoroquinolones and risk of Achilles tendon disorders: case-control study. BMJ 2002;324:1306–7.

[18] Roberge RJ, Kaplan R, Frank R, et al. Glyburide-ciprofloxacin interaction with resistant hypoglycemia. Ann Emerg Med 2000;36(2):160–3.

[19] Kara M, Hasinoff BB, McKay DW, et al. Clinical and chemical interactions between iron preparations and ciprofloxacin. Br J Clin Pharmacol 1991;31(3):257–61.

[20] Frost RW, Lasseter KC, Noe AJ, et al. Effects of aluminum hydroxide and calcium carbonate antacids on the bioavailability of ciprofloxacin. J Antimicrob Chemother 1992;36(4):830–2.

[21] Wang S, Rizvi AA. Levofloxacin-induced hypoglycemia in a nondiabetic patient. Am J Med Sci 2006;331(6):334–5.

[22] Giordano P, Song J, Pertel P, et al. Sequential intravenous/oral moxifloxacin versus intravenous pipercillin-tazobactam followed by oral amoxicillin-clavulanate for treatment of complicated skin and skin structure infection. Int J Antimicrob Agents 2005;26(5):357–65.

[23] Conrad DA, Williams RR, Couchman TL, et al. Efficacy of aztreonam in the treatment of skeletal infections due to Pseudomonas aeruginosa. Rev Infect Dis 1991;S7:S634–9.

[24] Scully BE, Neu HC. Use of aztreonam in the treatment of serious infections due to multiresistant gram-negative organisms, including Pseudomonas aeruginosa. Am J Med 1985;78(2):251–61.

[25] Rodriguez CN, Rodriguez-Morales AJ, Garcia A, et al. Antimicrobial resistance of Pseudomonas aeruginosa strains isolated from surgical infections in a 7-year period at a general hospital in Venezuela. Surg Infect 2006;7(3):269–73.

[26] Tomasoni D, Gattuso G, Chiarelli C, et al. Epidemiological surveillance of multi-drug resistant Pseudomonas aeruginosa in Montova hospital Italy. Infez Med 2006;14(2):85–91.

[27] Sarrubi FA, Hull JW. Gentamicin serum concentrations: pharmacokinetic predictions. Ann Intern Med 1976;85:183–9.

[28] Verpooten GA, Giuliano RA, Verbist L, et al. Once-daily dosing decreases renal accumulation of gentamicin and netilmicin. Clin Pharmacol Ther 1989;45:22–7.

[29] Preston SL, Briceland LL. Single daily dosing of aminoglycosides. Pharmacotherapy 1995;15:297–316.

[30] Ferriols-Lisart R, Alos-Alminana M. Effectiveness and safety of once-daily aminoglycosides: a meta-analysis. Am J Health Syst Pharm 1996;53(10):1141–50.

[31] Baltch AL, Bassey C, Hammer MC, et al. Synergy with cefsulodin or piperacillin and three aminoglycosides or aztreonam against aminoglycoside resistant strains of Pseudomonas aeruginosa. J Antimicrob Chemother 1991;27(6):801–8.

[32] Kaka AS, Rueda AM, Shelburne SA, et al. Bactericidal activity of orally available agents against methicillin-resistant Staphylococcus aureus. J Antimicrob Chemother 2006;58(3):680–3.

[33] Huovinen P. Increases in rates of resistance to trimethoprim. Clin Infect Dis 1997;24(Suppl 1):S63–6.

[34] Capoor MR, Nair D, Deb M, et al. Resistance to erythromycin and rising penicillin mic in Streptococcus pyogenes in India. Jpn J Infect Dis 2006;50(5):334–6.

[35] Ruhe JJ, Monson T, Bradsher RW, et al. Use of long-acting tetracyclines for methicillin-resistant Staphylococcus aureus infections: case series and review of the literature. Clin Infect Dis 2005;40(10):1429–34.

[36] Carter MK, Ebers VA, Younes BK, et al. Doxycycline for community-associated methicillin-resistant Staphylococcus aureus skin and soft-tissue infections. Ann Pharmacother 2006;40(9):1693–5.

[37] Doan TL, Fung HB, Mehta D, et al. Tigecycline: a glycylcycline antimicrobial agent. Clin Ther 2006;28(8):1079–106.

[38] Peterson LR, Quick JN, Jensen B, et al. Emergence of ciprofloxacin resistance in nosocomial methicillin-resistant Staphylococcus aureus isolates. Resistance during ciprofloxacin plus rifampin therapy for methicillin-resistant S aureus colonization. Arch Intern Med 1990; 150(10):2151–5.

[39] Walsh TJ, Standiford HC, Reboli AC, et al. Randomized double-blinded trial of rifampin with either novobiocin or trimethoprim-sulfamethoxazole against methicillin-resistant Staphylococcus aureus colonization: prevention of antimicrobial resistance and effect of host factors on outcome. Antimicrob Agents Chemother 1993;37(6):1334–42.

[40] Lipsky BA, Itani K, Norden C. Linezolid Diabetic Foot Infections Study Group. Treating foot infections in diabetic patients: a randomized, multi-center, open-label trial of linezolid versus ampicillin-sublactam/amoxicillin-clavulanate. Clin Infect Dis 2004;38(1): 17–24.

[41] Cepeda JA, Whitehouse T, Cooper B, et al. Linezolid versus teicoplanin in the treatment of gram-positive infections in the critically ill: a randomized, double-blind, multicentre study. J Antimicrob Chemother 2004;53:345–55.

[42] Lavery S, Ravi H, McDaniel WW, et al. Linezolid and serotonin syndrome. Psychosomatics 2001;42:432–4.

[43] Wigen CL, Goetz MB. Serotonin syndrome and linezolid. Clin Infect Dis 2002;34:1651–2.

[44] Allington DR, Rivey MP. Quinupristin/daltopristin: a therapeutic review. Clin Ther 2001; 23(1):24–44.

[45] Nichols RL, Graham DR, Barriere SL, et al. Syndercid Skin and Skin Structure Infection Group. Treatment of hospitalized patients with complicated gram-positive skin and skin structure infections: two randomized, mutlicentre studies of quinupristin/dalfopristin versus cefazolin, oxacillin or vancomycin. J Antimicrob Chemother 1999;44: 263–73.

[46] Tally FP, Zeckel M, Wasilewski MM, et al. Daptomycin: a novel agent for gram-positive infections. Expert Opin Investig Drugs 1999;8(8):1223–38.

[47] Carpenter CF, Chambers HF. Daptomycin: another novel agent for treating infections due to drug-resistant gram-positive pathogens. Clin Infect Dis 2004;38:994–1000.

[48] Anastasiou DM, Thorne GM, Luperchio SA, et al. In vitro activity of daptomycin against clinical isolates with reduced susceptibilities to linezolid and quinupristin/dalfopristin. Int J Antimicrob Agents 2006;28(5):385–8.

[49] Freeman CD, Quintiliani R, Nightingale CH. Vancomycin therapeutic drug monitoring: is it necessary? Ann Pharmacother 1993;27:594–8.

[50] Cantu TG, Yamanaka-Yuen NA, Lietman PS. Serum vancomycin concentrations: reappraisal of their clinical value. Clin Infect Dis 1994;18:533–43.

[51] Saunders NJ. Why monitoring peak vancomycin concentrations? Lancet 1994;344:1748–50.

[52] Shalansky S. Rationalization of vancomycin serum concentrations monitoring. Can J Hosp Pharm 1995;48:17–24.

[53] Creekmore F. Vancomycin levels: to draw or not to draw. S D J Med 1998;51:195–6.

[54] Stevens DL. Teicoplanin for skin and soft tissue infections: an open study and a randomized, comparative trial versus cefazolin. J Infect Chemother 1999;5(1):40–5.

[55] Chirurgi VA, Edelstein H, Oster SE, et al. Randomized comparison trial of teicoplanin i.v., teicoplanin i.m., and cefazolin therapy for skin and soft tissue infections caused by gram-positive bacteria. South Med J 1994;87(9):875–80.

[56] Goldstein EJC, Citron DM, Merriam CV, et al. In vitro activities of dalbavancin and nine comparator agents against anaerobic gram-positive species and corynebacteria. Antimicrob Agents Chemother 2003;47(6):1968–71.

[57] Jauregui LE, Babazadeh S, Seltzer E, et al. Randomized, double-blind comparison of once-weekly dalbavancin versus twice-daily linezolid therapy for the treatment of complicated skin and skin structure infections. Clin Infect Dis 2005;41:1407–15.

ELSEVIER
SAUNDERS

Clin Podiatr Med Surg
24 (2007) 311–332

CLINICS IN
PODIATRIC
MEDICINE AND
SURGERY

Osteoporosis: Pathogenesis, New Therapies and Surgical Implications

Jonathan M. Labovitz, DPM, FACFAS[a,b,c,*], Kate Revill[d]

[a]Private Practice, 3400 Lomita Boulevard, #403, Torrance, CA 90505, USA
[b]West Los Angeles-Veterans Administration Medical Center, Los Angeles, CA, USA
[c]Baja Project for Crippled Children, Torrance, California, USA
[d]Samuel Merritt College of Podiatric Medicine, 370 Hawthorne Avenue, #613, Oakland, CA 94609, USA

Many developments have occurred in the realm of bone healing in the past few years. Genetic discoveries, new proteins affecting bone health, and new treatments have all steered our treatment of traumatic and iatrogenic fractures in a number of new avenues during this explosion of new research; however, a seemingly simple and potentially major pathologic force we encounter daily may be affecting our outcomes more than originally anticipated. With the aging baby boomer population and the inevitable increase in patients with osteoporosis, increased awareness will become mandatory.

Osteoporosis strikes many subsets of the world population, including women, the elderly, and those suffering from arthritis, auto-immune diseases, HIV, and the immunocompromised. This disease predisposes people to an increased risk of low trauma and fragility fractures. The baby boomer generation and an increasing lifespan may burden the economy by creating such a large group susceptible to such a potentially devastating disease. The novel treatments and coping with the potentially challenging surgical implications will aide the podiatric physician in both medical and surgical management of osteoporosis.

Epidemiology

Osteoporosis, the most common bone disorder, effects more than 10 million people in the United States; it will likely effect 14 million over the

* Corresponding author. 3400 Lomita Boulevard, #403, Torrance, CA 90505.
E-mail address: dr_labovitz@feetandankles.com (J.M. Labovitz).

age of 50 by 2020 [1]. Around the world, 200 million women alone are estimated to have osteoporosis, and this is one of the most common diseases in developed countries.

More than 1.5 million hip fractures alone are reported in the United States per year, increasing to an estimated 6.3 million by 2050 [1]. There is a significant increase in mortality or loss of independence after sustaining hip fractures in the elderly. Less than one third of the remaining patients ever regain their prefracture state of physical activity [1]. Osteoporotic fractures of the vertebrae also have a high rate of disability. In the realm of podiatric medicine, insufficiency fractures of the foot and ankle have been reported in numerous studies of postmenopausal women; these were likely related to pathomechanics and postural abnormalities [2].

Each year approximately $17 billion is spent on osteoporotic fractures in the United States. It is projected that the cost will rise to $50 billion by 2040. This cost surpasses that of breast cancer, strokes, lung disease, or diabetes mellitus. This trend is seen throughout the world, with the rate of expenditures rising faster than the national inflation rate [1]. This cost analysis fails to include the economic burden of nursing home care, convalescent care, rehabilitation, and disability following the fractures.

High-risk groups include those with low estrogen levels, prior history of fracture, immunosuppressant, or steroid therapy, long-term secondary amenorrhea, low body mass index, and maternal history of hip fracture or osteoporosis [3]. Other activities that have been linked to osteoporosis are smoking, alcohol, and low dietary consumption of calcium and vitamins D and K. These dietary insufficiencies are especially influential during childhood and adolescence. In older patients, risk factors also include poor eyesight, sensorimotor deficiency, and anything that can increase the likelihood of falls (Box 1).

Pathogenesis

Osteoporosis is caused by an imbalance of bone metabolism, with the equilibrium favoring osteoclast function. An increase in the porosity of the bone, measured by the bone mineral density (BMD) occurs via three seemingly unrelated pathways; however, as research has progressed, these pathways seem to encompass a number of other disease states and are likely to be more related than originally thought.

It is now understood that bone remodeling is a physiologic process that maintains bone mass and skeletal integrity, with bone resorption independent from bone formation [4]. There is a constant renewal of bone matrix with osteoblasts and osteoclasts functioning while trying to achieve an equilibrium. It appears that the three main regulating pathways affecting bone metabolism—endocrine/paracrine regulation, central nervous system (CNS) regulation, and mechanical stress, all influence the RANK/RANKL/OPG system.

Box 1. Risk factors

Major risk factors
Personal history of fracture as adult
History of fragility fracture in first-degree relative
Low body weight (<127 lbs.)
Current tobacco use
Use of corticosteroids >3 months

Minor risk factors
Impaired vision
Estrogen deficiency at <45 years old
Dementia
Poor health/frailty
Recent falls
Low calcium
Low physical activity
Alcohol consumption >2 drinks/day

Receptor activated of nuclear factor-κB (RANK) is a receptor found on the surface of osteoclast progenitors, mature osteoclasts, chondrocytes, and some epithelial tumor cell lines [5]. RANKL is the RANK ligand, which binds to RANK on the cell surface, activating mature osteoclasts. RANKL is produced by activated T-cells and is directly involved in osteoclast maturation. Osteoprotegerin (OPG) is a tumor necrosis factor receptor, which serves as a decoy receptor for RANKL, thus decreasing osteoclastogenesis and inhibiting bone resorption. Therefore, the paracrine role of this cytokine system has become essential for skeletal biology, with alterations in the RANKL/OPG ratio being responsible for many metabolic bone diseases.

Endocrine/paracrine regulation

Estrogen is commonly considered to be a primary regulator of bone metabolism because of its role as a protective agent for preventing osteoporosis in women. Estrogen appears to be involved in anabolic and anticatabolic means of regulating bone turnover. The hormone acts through the estrogen receptor α (ERα) when mediating skeletal effects. Activation of the ERα increases the expression of numerous growth factors and cytokines, such as tumor growth factor-β (TGF-β), causing a direct effect accelerating osteoclast apoptosis and having a role in bone formation. It has been noted, however, that the protective effects of estrogen may also involve suppression of interleukin-1 (IL-1), interleukin-6 (IL-6), and tumor necrosis factor-α (TNFα), which are factors that enhance bone resorption and the genesis of osteoclasts. Increased levels of these cytokines were noted in women who underwent oopherectomy and did not receive estrogen replacement, whereas women receiving estrogen replacement therapy failed to have elevated levels [6].

The RANK/RANKL/OPG system is affected by estrogen. RANKL directly correlates to bone resorption levels and inversely proportional to 17-β estradiol serum levels. RANKL expression was two to three times higher than normal for postmenopausal women not taking estrogen replacement [7]. Estrogen and phytoestrogens up-regulate the transcription of osteoblastic-derived OPG. A positive correlation between serum estradiol levels and OPG exists in men and women. In a study of 180 postmenopausal women, a significant positive relationship was discovered between serum OPG and BMD at total body, total hip, and the femoral neck [8].

Parathyroid hormone (PTH) controls bone turnover via calcium and vitamin D regulation. PTH usually increases serum calcium, thereby possibly decreasing the calcium content within the bone. PTH increases RANKL levels and down-regulates OPG, thus stimulating osteoclastogenesis [6,7,9]. Additionally, Seck and colleagues [10] showed that levels of human PTH are inversely proportional to OPG levels.

Whereas continuous PTH exposure has been reported to increase the RANKL/OPG ratio up to 25 fold, intermittent PTH exposure has been shown to be anabolic, encouraging bone growth secondary to an increase in insulinlike growth factor-1 (IGF-1) [7]. Vitamin D3, similar to prostaglandin E2 and glucocorticoids, also down-regulates the expression of OPG on stromal cells.

Nutritional aspects may be involved too. Essential fatty acids (EFAs) and metabolites such as γ-linoleic acid, eicosapentaenoic acid, and docosahexaenoic acid, have been reported to have a beneficial action in osteoporosis [11]. It has been noted that an increase in the EFAs causes enhanced calcium absorption and decreased calcium excretion. EFAs may also inhibit IL-1, IL-2, and TNF-α, and regulate bone metabolism via blocking 3-hydroxy-3-methylglutaryl coenzyme A (HMG-CoA) reductase activity. Lastly, EFAs may increase bone morphogenic protein (BMP) production [11]. Similarly, statins, which are HMG-CoA reductase inhibitors, may also regulate cytokines, increase BMP production, and directly cause osteoclast apoptosis.

Whereas the cytokine regulation may define the role of estrogens, EFA, and statins, it has been proposed that nitrous oxide (NO) is the link between these compounds and the RANK/RANKL/OPG system. All three of these compounds can increase the production of constitutive or endothelial NO [6]. In addition, PTH and vitamin D up-regulate nitric oxide synthetase and osteoblasts produce NO synthetase [6,9].

NO is formed by converting L-arginine to NO by nitric oxide synthetase. The two known pathways involve the endothelial pathway (eNOS) and the inducible pathway (iNOS). The endothelial pathway provides NO used for normal osteoblast function, which responds to exogenous estrogen and mechanical stress. Raloxifene, an estrogen receptor modulator effective in postmenopausal osteoporosis prevention, triggers a dose-dependent release of endothelial NO, which inhibits osteoclast activity [6]. Nitroglycerin ointment, an NO donor, increased serum osteocalcin and bone-specific alkaline phosphatase levels. In addition, nitroglycerin ointment is as effective as estrogen replacement therapy in preventing bone loss in postmenopausal women [12]. The inducible pathway causes an increase in cytokine formation such as IL-1, thus effecting bone resorption [13]. Levy and colleagues [14] showed that eNOS knockout mice have reduced bone mass and volumes with abnormal maturation of osteoblasts. Afzal and coworkers [15] reported that endolthelial NO plays a role in coordinating osteoblast differentiation and bone mineralization.

Fan and colleagues [9] claim that NO potently suppresses RANKL expression in stromal cells, which are precursors to osteoclasts, and up-regulates OPG expression. This directly alters the RANKL/OPG equilibrium generated by the stromal cells, reducing osteoclastic potential. Although these findings seem to indicate that NO has an anabolic function, the findings are dose-dependent. Low concentrations of NO contribute to the anabolic effects on bone; however, high concentrations induce greater bone resorption and inhibit osteoblast proliferation, possibly via a negative feedback mechanism [6].

Some interesting research now indicates that dietary habits effect bone metabolism as well. Animal studies have shown increased frequency of small meals results in prolonged bone turnover suppression and a net gain in bone mass [16]. In addition, parenteral feeding results in bone loss, indicating that enteric hormones may play a role in regulating bone mass [17]. These enteric hormones directly modulate osteoblast and osteoclast function and maturation. They may also provide an indirect role through monocyte and T-lymphocyte function.

Central nervous system regulation

The neurologic regulation of bone metabolism is centrally controlled via a hypothalamic axis. Leptin, a hormone located within the brain, binds to the ventromedial nuclei of the hypothalamus. This initiates a neuronal signaling cascade involving the sympathetic nervous system, causing norepinephrine to stimulate β_2-adrenergic receptors on the osteoblast surface, thus reducing bone formation.

Leptin may be a key component in the central regulation of a number of other pathologies. The involvement of the sympathetic nervous system may explain the osteopenia associated with chronic regional pain syndromes. In fact, β-blockers such as propanolol may inhibit the catabolic effect the sympathetic nervous system has on bone, thus blocking up-regulation of RANKL [18,19].

Leptin is also considered the anti-obesity hormone. Low levels of leptin or leptin resistance are associated with obesity, possibly serving as the link between increased body weight and low incidence of reduced BMD and osteoporosis. The obesity effects of leptin, however, involve neuro-peptides functioning along a different pathway in the CNS, independent of the anti-osteogenic effects [19].

Other CNS regulators have also been implicated in reducing BMD. Anticonvulsants and opiates are associated with a decreased BMD. The anticonvulsants may cause this effect secondary to increased catabolic effects on vitamin D and PTH, with phenobarbitol causing the greatest reduction in BMD of the anticonvulsants. Opiates are likely to affect BMD by suppressing the endocrine system. Opiates may decrease serum levels of the sex-related hormones [20]. Lastly, depression is known to involve the CNS and also BMD. Depression stimulates IL-6 production and leads to inactivity, effecting bone metabolism [20].

Mechanical stress

It is widely accepted that low BMD is associated with significant weight loss or low body weight. In fact, malnutritional states (eg, anorexia nervosa) and malabsorption syndromes are also associated with low BMD. Mechanical stress may be one cause of this relationship.

The stress from the body weight on the bones effects the internal architecture of the bones via the trabecular pattern. In an unpublished study involving patients on 90 days of strict bed rest at 6° head-down tilt, patients developed a loss of BMD each month, independent of gender. The decreased BMD ranged from 1.9% to 2.9%, depending on the anatomical site measured by CT. Postural control was also decreased, which may account for an increased risk of falls. (C. Rubin, personal communication, 2006). In a microgravity environment in space, a 2% to 3% loss in BMD occurs on a monthly basis, also validating the effects of a loss of mechanical stress on the skeleton to maintain BMD [21].

The RANK/RANKL/OPG system is also involved with mechanical stress, increasing OPG levels and lowering serum RANKL levels, whereas long periods of immobilization have the opposite effect [7]. In animal models, administering OPG to immobilized subjects mitigated the negative effects of long-term immobilization on bone metabolism.

Treatment options

Prevention

The most important treatment is prevention. As clinicians, we need to be attentive to the high-risk patient. One of the more commonly undiagnosed classes is men. In a study of 363 patients, Lin and Lane [22] showed that only 27% of men received treatment, whereas 71% of women were treated for osteoporosis. For those patients who are at a high risk of fractures, Delaney [23] recommended cessation of tobacco, reduction of alcohol consumption, strengthening and weight-bearing exercises, and visual correction to decrease fall risk. Although low impact exercise is unlikely to effect BMD, it is likely to reduce fall risk. Fall risk has been reduced 47.5% from tai chi chuan [22]. Other exercises have also been studied. Post-menopausal women who participated in a jumping regimen in a weighted vest three times per week had a 1.54% increased BMD of the femoral neck after 5 years [22].

Dietary considerations are important when evaluating prevention of osteoporosis. One of the major factors effecting BMD is peak bone mass. The most important time for osseous development is during childhood and adolescence. A diet rich in calcium and vitamin D is essential for microarchitectural development of the bone [22]. Adequate calcium intake is considered the most important lifestyle factor for attaining and maintaining adequate bone mass [3]. Vitamin D increases intestinal absorption of calcium. Levels of vitamin D are depleted as we age, thus increasing the importance of vitamin D supplementation. The daily recommendations are currently 1200 mg calcium and vitamin D 400 IU for the patient 70 years of age or less. Older patients should increase vitamin D to 600 IU [3]. Numerous studies demonstrate the benefit of combination therapy of calcium and vitamin D for maintenance of BMD at the spine, femoral neck, and total body, and for reduction of fracture risk [3].

It is also important to appreciate external factors that influence bone mass. Elderly patients are more likely to be placed on medications that can deplete BMD by limiting calcium absorption. Medications such as diuretics, corticosteroids, antibiotics, anticonvulsants, nonsteroidal anti-inflammatory drugs (NSAIDS), and immunosuppressants may fill this role. In the high-risk patient these medications should be alternated for other classes of drugs if possible.

Current treatments

There are two main categories of agents used to treat osteoporosis. The majority of the treatment options are anti-resorptive agents designed to slow bone turnover, thus allowing bone formation to exceed bone resorption. The alternative way to treat osteoporosis depends upon direct stimulation of bone formation. The goal of either category of treatment is to increase BMD and to decrease fracture risk.

Most of the anti-resorptive pharmacologic approaches fail to restore the normal bone density. The anti-resorptive approach involves calcitonin, hormone replacement therapy, selective estrogen receptor modulators (SERMs) and bisphophonates. The anabolic approach to osteoporosis treatment involves PTH (Table 1).

Calcitonin is a hormone that regulates calcium metabolism via inhibition of osteoclast function. It has been shown to decrease bone-related pain after

Table 1
FDA approved pharmaceutical treatments of osteoporosis

Drug	Indication	Dosage
Dietary		
Calcium	Most men and women > 50 years old	1000 to 1500 mg/day
Vitamin D	Recommended for men and women > 50 taking calcium	51–70 years old = 400 IU/day > 70 years old = 600 IU/day
Bisphosphonates		
Alendronate	Prevention and treatment of postmenopausal osteoporosis	Prevention = 5 mg/day or 35 mg/week Treatment = 10 mg/day or 35 mg/week
Ibandronate	Prevention and treatment of postmenopausal osteoporosis	Prevention and treatment = 150 mg/month
Risedronate	Prevention and treatment of postmenopausal osteoporosis, Paget's disease, glucocorticoid-induced osteoporosis	Prevention and treatment = 5 mg/day and 35 mg/week
Raloxifene	Prevention and treatment of postmenopausal osteoporosis	60 mg/day
Teriparatide	Treatment of postmenopausal osteoporosis with high fracture risk	20 µg/day SQ injection
Calcitonin	Treatment of postmenopausal osteoporosis in women menopausal > 5 years	200 IU/day intranasally alternating nostrils daily

an injury, increase BMD, and decrease fracture risk [22]. Gass and Dawson-Hughes [3] reported a reduction in vertebral fracture risk by 33% to 36%.

Ishida and Kawai [24] compared the efficacy of various treatment options in a randomized study of 396 postmenopausal women ages 50 to 75 years who were diagnosed with osteoporosis. The calcitonin dose was 20 IU weekly via parenteral route, whereas the standard dose in the United States is 200 IU daily via intranasal route. This was done to decrease risk of developing antibodies to calcitonin, which may limit the effectiveness of the medication long term. Results showed a mild reduction of bone loss after 2 years in the vitamin K and the etidronate (bisphosphonate) groups. The control group sustained a 3.3% loss in BMD during the 2-year period, in comparison with a 1.6% increase for calcitonin and a 2.0% increase for hormone replacement therapy (HRT), which consisted of estrogen and progesterone. A significant reduction in risk of vertebral fractures was noted for HRT, etidronate, and calcitonin therapy.

HRT augments BMD because estrogen inhibits osteoclast function, whereas progestin stimulates osteoblast activity. Unfortunately, approximately 40% of women who start HRT cease taking the medication secondary to the numerous side effects [2]. These side effects are present in all forms of HRT, although most women are taking the hormones orally. Additionally, there is an increased risk of breast and ovarian cancer, stroke, thromboses, and cardiovascular disease [3].

SERMs function by binding to the estrogen receptors, acting as either an agonist or an antagonist on particular tissues. They may play a role in treating patients who are at risk of breast or uterine cancer, and are unable to take hormone replacement. Raloxifene is currently the only SERM that is approved by the Food and Drug Administration (FDA) to treat postmenopausal osteoporosis. It has no effect on breast or uterine tissue while up-regulating OPG production [7]. Studies on the efficacy of raloxifene have shown a 2.4% increase in BMD at the lumbar spine and the total hip after 2 years of treatment. In addition, markers of bone resorption were also decreased significantly [25]. In one study, osteoporotic women treated with Raloxifene for 3 years showed a 30% to 50% reduction in vertebral fractures [26].

Other SERMS that have been tested are the triphenylethylenes (tamoxifen, clomphene citrate). Tamoxifen has been shown to have similar properties to raloxifene on both breast tissue and bone, but it has agonist properties on uterine tissue causing proliferation of the endometrium; however, Powles and colleagues [27] reported a possible loss of bone in premenopausal women after 3 years of treatment.

Unlike the other SERMs, tibolone is more tissue-specific and is unlikely to effect breast or uterine tissue. Tibolone acts on the arterial wall endothelium triggering NO synthesis [28]. Clinically, it has been recognized to increase trabecular BMD and to reduce bone turnover. Although it is not approved in the United States for osteoporosis treatment, it is being used for treatment of vasomotor symptoms of menopause and osteoporosis prevention in Europe. Two other triphenylethylenes are in development. Both idoxifene and FC1271A are being researched and have shown early indications of being an agonist on bone and reducing markers of bone resorption, while lowering low-density lipoprotein (LDL) or cholesterol [29].

The efficacy of these medications has been debated. Wilkins and Biorge [30] report that calcitonin and raloxifene are probably no more effective than calcium and vitamin D supplementation in preventing bone loss. Calcitonin is usually reserved for those unable to tolerate bisphosphonates [31].

Bisphosphonates have also been approved for the prevention and treatment of osteoporosis. Oral and parenteral forms are currently available; however, only oral forms are FDA-approved for osteoporosis. This class of drugs accelerates osteoclast apoptosis and inhibits recruitment, maturation, and activity of osteoclasts [3,32].

Alendronate has been shown to be effective after 4 weeks of treatment, because a decrease in the number of osteoclasts appears at that time [33]. The efficacy of the therapeutic doses has been shown with reduction of fracture risk and increased BMD at the lumbar spine and hip [33]. A double-blinded a study of postmenopausal women ages 44 to 84 demonstrated increased BMD at the lumbar spine and greater trochanter with maintained BMD at the femoral neck, forearm, and total body BMD [3]. Bisphosphonate treatment with alendronate for a 7-year period showed a BMD increase of

11.4% at the lumbar spine, which increased to 13.7% after 10 years. The estimated drop in BMD over 1 year in postmenopausal patients is 0.5% to 1.0%, whereas the bisphosphonate group after 18 months had a 0.8% increase in lumbar spine BMD [34,35].

Ibandronate sodium reduces the incidence of vertebral fractures and risk of fracture, and maintains BMD. A double-blinded study of osteoporotic women who suffered one to four vertebral fractures before enrolling in the study [36] showed a 52% reduction of new vertebral fractures when taking a daily dose of ibandronate. BMD was increased for total body, lumbar spine, and femoral neck and trochanter; however, nonvertebral osteoporotic fractures were unaffected [36].

Risedronate is FDA-approved for glucocorticoid-induced osteoporosis and other more unique causes of secondary osteoporosis, in addition to reducing fracture risk and maintaining BMD in postmenopausal women. Daily administration in placebo-controlled studies showed a significant relative risk reduction of osteoporotic nonvertebral fractures over a 3-year period, and a decreased incidence of nonvertebral fractures [37].

The possible complications associated with bisphosphonates have been seen with alendronate. Suppression of both osteoblasts and osteoclasts has been observed with long-term treatment [3,33]. Additionally, mandibular osteonecrosis has been documented, but these cases involve patients on high-dose intravenous forms of bisphosphonates for diagnoses other than osteoporosis [3]. Lastly, bisphophonates have strict requirements for dosing to increase tolerability, thus making the medication harder on patient compliance.

Combination therapy of bisphosphonates and SERMs has been tested as well. Together, additive effects on BMD have been identified. Increased BMD of 5.3% in the lumbar spine and 3.7% in the femoral neck with 1 year of therapy has been observed; however, reduction of fracture risk was not assessed in this study [23].

The first drug recommended for anabolic treatment of postmenopausal osteoporosis was fluoride; however, the FDA withheld approval secondary to the high rate of side effects and the patients being intolerant of the high doses. In addition, it was found to increase the risk of nonvertebral fractures despite increasing BMD [38]. Since then, PTH has been approved by the FDA for use in osteoporosis.

Intermittent dosing of PTH is being used because it increases bone turnover via resorption and formation, increases BMD, and increases the architectural integrity and stability of the bone [3,22,30]. Rosen and Bilezikian [38] reported an up-regulation of TGF-β, IGF-I, and IGF-II. The mechanism of the anabolic effects of intermittent PTH dosing is as follows: (1) activation of resting osteoblasts, (2) stimulates osteoprogenitor cells to differentiation to osteoblasts, and (3) delays osteoblast apoptosis. Clinically, there are few side effects reported, including transient hypercalcemia, nausea, and headache [3].

Numerous studies have bee done to determine the efficacy of the recombinant PTH injections. Koester and Spindler [39] reported that PTH intermittent dosing may be more beneficial in cancellous bone, because an increased
efficacy is noted in the lumbar spine when compared with the calcaneus.
Some studies demonstrated a 10% increase in lumbar spine BMD and
a 65% risk reduction of new vertebral fractures [40]. The principal finding
amongst studies on intermittent PTH treatment in men and women is an
increase in BMD, especially in trabecular bone. There is an estimated benefit
of a 10% increase in BMD when tested by dual radiographic absorptiometry (DXA) and a 40% increase in BMD when measured by quantitative
computed tomography (QCT) [30,38]. Lin and Lane [22] have reported an
increased bone density, thickened trabecular and cortical bone, and an inhibition of apoptosis of osteocytes. Clinically, this was seen with an
increased total body bone mineral content and increased BMD of the
femoral neck, with a decrease in nonvertebral fractures by 54% after 10
months. Unfortunately, PTH injections require about 10 months before
there is clinical effectiveness, whereas bisphosphonates require only 3
months. Combination therapy of bisphosphonates and PTH has shown
a detrimental effect because there is attenuation of the effect of PTH on
bone density [22,30].

The future

Research on a number of treatments are currently being investigated and
designed to address the specific areas of the pathogenesis of osteoporosis
mentioned earlier in this article. Current investigation focuses on beta
blockers, L-arginine supplementation, and other medications designed to
block RANKL and leptin and enhance nitric oxide.

In addition to intermittent dosing of PTH, other anabolic means of
increasing BMD are being investigated because human studies have yet to
validate the benefits of the statins, recombinant growth hormone (rhGH),
and iIGF-1.

The hypercholesterolemia medications commonly used to reduce lipids
and cardiovascular risk have recently been shown to decrease glucose
resistance; however, in 1999 Mundy and his colleagues [41] discovered
that lovastatin and simvastatin caused a twofold to threefold increase in
bone formation in mice, increased bone morphogenic protein-2 (BMP-2)
concentrations, and prevented bone loss in ovariectomized rats.

The statins mechanism of action is similar to the mechanism of the
bisphosphonates, because they both act along the mevalonate pathway,
inhibiting prenylation of guanosine triphosphate (GTP) binding proteins.
These HMG-CoA reductase inhibitors are known to inhibit IL-6 and
TNF-α production and increase NO production [6,32]. McFarlane and
colleagues [42] reported on numerous studies illustrating that statins inhibit
bone resorption and stimulate bone formation in various animal models.

Unlike bisphosphonates, the statins do not have the capacity to bind bone. Despite functioning along the same biochemical pathway, the statins are anabolic, whereas bisphosphonates are anti-resorptive.

In an attempt to determine the clinical benefit of statins, after adjusting for other potential factors such as tobacco, body mass index, and steroid use, Meier and coworkers [43] demonstrated that women over 50 years of age currently taking statins had a significantly reduced risk of fracture, even with a short duration of 1 to 4 months of use; however, these findings have not been shown to be conclusive. McFarlane and colleagues [42] reported that clinical support of the beneficial effect of statins on BMD and fracture risk remains inconclusive. Analysis of 218,062 patients in the General Practice Research Database showed no relationship between statin use and nonvertebral fractures [42,44].

IGF-1 and rhGH have been studied in animals, with early human studies remaining inconclusive. Although rhGH has been shown to increase bone formation, it has also been shown to increase bone turnover. One trial of 132 elderly patients showed an increase in urinary N-telopeptide, and osteocalcin increased at the same rate as bone formation [38]. In another human trial consisting of elderly men with osteoporosis, rhGH stimulated only a small increase in BMD of the lumbar spine, with no benefit sustained at 1 year [45]. Like the previously attempted fluoride treatment, side effects of the rhGH have caused concern because there is a high incidence of weight gain, glucose intolerance, carpal tunnel syndrome, and edema.

IGF-1 has been deemed an important growth factor in bone metabolism, and thus may become one of the main treatments of osteoporosis, pending further research. IGF-1 stimulates chondrocyte and osteoblast differentiation and maturation. BMD is directly related to IGF-1 concentrations; low levels of IGF-1 are associated with an increased risk of hip and spine fractures [38]. Low serum levels of IGF-1 has also been implicated in the pathogenesis of male osteoporosis [46].

In comparison with rhGH, IGF-1 increased bone formation at a faster rate than resorption, whereas rhGH had equal rates of formation and resorption. IGF-1 also has fewer side effects then rhGH. Unfortunately, high levels of serum IGF-1 have been linked to neoplastic transformation, although the true clinical relevance of this finding is unknown [38].

NO donors, such as nitroglycerin, are currently being considered as potential treatment options as well. Nitroglycerin decreases osteoclastic activity and stimulates osteoblast activity [12,47]. Another NO donor, L-arginine, has been evaluated, but no benefit has been demonstrated on BMD, bone mass, bone structure, or IGF-I levels. L-arginine supplementation can increase serum NO levels and GH levels, but the clinical relevance of the increased growth hormone is unknown. Ultimately, L-arginine supplements are ineffective for improving bone mass [47].

Approaches involving nutritional medicine are also being studied. Flavonoids have been shown to have some estrogen like activity. Isoflavone, a phytoestrogen, has been studied in postmenopausal women. Those taking isoflavone had a higher BMD at Ward's triangle and the lumbar spine than those consuming low levels of isoflavone. The results also indicated that approximately 53.3 mg/day may have a greater effect on the cancellous bone than the cortical bone [48]. Mundy [49] reported that the flavonoids increase BMP-2 expression, whereas Mei and coworkers [48] reported isoflavone stimulates osteoblast formation and inhibits osteoclast formation.

Lastly, β-blockers have been evaluated because the central nervous system may have an effect on BMD. An increase in BMD of mice calvarium has been reported with β-blocker use [19]. The Geelong Osteoporosis Study of women over 50 years of age showed fewer fractures and a 30% reduction in fracture risk with use of β-blockers [18]. Although there may be evidence of reduced fracture risk in patients taking β-blockers or thiazides, Bhandari and Devereaux [50] concluded that there is insufficient evidence to recommend use of these medications to decrease fracture risk in osteoporotic patients.

A novel, nonpharmaceutical therapy for osteoporosis involves the growing field of vibrational medicine, where Juvent, Inc. (Somerset, New Jersey) continues to investigate the use of vibrational plates through numerous studies. The magnitude of the mechanical strain applied to the bone from the vibration signal is three orders of magnitude below strains that damage bone [51]. On the cellular level, strain on bone cells decreases RANKL and increases eNOS expression [52]. The number of osteoclasts decreases because of RANKL sensitivity to mechanical pressures on stromal cells [53]. These cellular changes on RANKL and eNOS suggest that low-level mechanical signals have anti-resorptive properties and anabolic properties on bone.

The anti-resorptive benefits were demonstrated by Rubin and coworkers [51], who showed that there was a 2.13% loss of BMD in the femoral neck in the placebo group, with a 0.04% gain in the active group after 1 year. The spine showed a 1.6% loss in the placebo group and only a 0.1% loss in the active group. Another study demonstrated the anabolic benefit, where 20 children with cerebral palsy received low level mechanical stimulation for 6 months [54]. Placebo controls lost 12% trabecular BMD while the active treatment group gained more than 6% trabecular BMD [54].

Judex and colleagues [55] reported that small, high frequency signals (90 Hz for 10 minutes/day) applied to bone at specific frequencies showed anabolic effects in trabecular and cortical bone formation in hormone-challenged rats. In a developing animal model, a 30% increase in the endocortical surface of metaphyseal tibia and a 30% lower osteoclast activity in tibial trabecular bone in the metaphysis and epiphysis was noted with small, high frequency signals [56]. High frequency vibrational plates have demonstrated increased bone and muscle mass in young women with low BMD (Gilsanz V., unpublished data). The effect on young women may indicate the potential benefit for prevention in high-risk patients. This increase not only may serve as a good method of prevention secondary to the anabolic effects on the bone, but with the increased muscle mass it is possible that fall risk is also decreased.

Elderly patients have also been studied with vibrational plates. The focus on the elderly stems from the safety profile, because vibrational stimulation is a nonpharmaceutical approach and elderly patients consume 30% of prescription medicine in the United States. This decreases the risk of adverse reactions, drug interactions, and decreasing compliance. In a comprehensive review of 34 studies of pharmaceutical osteoporosis treatments [57], over 50% of the studies had 20% of the patients stop their medication. Osteoporosis drug compliance usually ranges from 40% to 50%, and use of the vibrational plates for 10 minutes/day in elderly patients is 80% over a 6-month period [58].

Surgical implications

Osteoporosis potentially causes a number of considerations when dealing with the surgical patient. The decreased bone density may cause a delay in bone healing secondary to the possible causes of the osteoporosis. It may also loosen fixation or prevent rigid internal fixation. Lastly, there may be some changes necessary to managing the surgical patient postoperatively in regards to pharmaceutical choices, because some medications may effect BMD.

Fixation

The basic concept of fixation of bone with low BMD is to achieve a rigid construct for increased stability through concentric joint loading [59,60]; however, in the osteoporotic patient, fixation strength is affected because of an alteration of cortical and trabecular bone structural and material properties. Fixation failure rates of up to 50% has been reported in osteoporotic patients; fixation pull-out was determined to be the primary cause [61]. Multiple animal studies provide evidence of altered fracture healing in experimental osteoporosis, but aged patients with osteoporosis have not been reported [62]. With pull-out strength in mind, Seebeck and colleagues [63] studied tibia cadaveric specimens to determine that pull-out strength was dependent upon the cortical thickness. In cortical bone less than 1.5 mm, the holding strength is dependent on cancellous bone density, whereas in cortices greater than 1.5 mm, the pull-out strength depends exclusively upon the cortical bone. It was concluded that this may alter the surgeon's screw choice or orientation of the fixation.

When discussing the effects of decreased BMD on the use of fixation, there are a few approaches the surgeon can employ to help eliminate these potentially difficult factors. Typically the decrease in BMD may make obtaining rigid internal fixation difficult because the mechanical stability is affected, compromising the rigidity. The loosening of the fixation is a common problem, which may lead to backing out of pins, screws and plates. A few different approaches may eliminate the potential loss of rigid fixation at the bone-screw interface.

Polymethylmethacrylate (PMMA) has been used to fill bone holes before screw insertion. Unfortunately, the excess PMMA when filling the screw hole may cause thermal injury to the surrounding tissues because of the local exothermic reaction that occurs with PMMA use. Although pedicle screws augmented with PMMA in spinal surgery have a 49% increase in pull-out strength [64], the PMMA remains a foreign body because it is a biotolerant material with no affinity for bone [65]. Additionally, PMMA does not allow for altering the screw hole after the cement hardens.

Altering the bone-screw interface via changing the screw has also been attempted in numerous other ways. Augmentation with cancellous bone, hydroxyapetite grout (HA), and calcium phosphate cement (CPC) have been tried. HA-coated screws have been shown to decrease the incidence of fixation failure in osteoporotic trochanteric fractures. Moroni and colleagues [66] showed no cut-out of dynamic hip screw fixation with HA screws, whereas standard rate of cut-out occurred with AO screw fixation. Additionally, no fixation failure occurred even in the instances of suboptimal screw position in the HA group. HA-coated screws are stronger and have increased osteointegration when compared with uncoated screws of similar size in loaded and unloaded animal models [67].

CPC is a powdered material that is mixed with liquid before use, but unlike the reaction of PMMA, it occurs through a non-exothermic reaction. When compared with HA-coated screws, however, CPC is technically more demanding and time-consuming, with a higher cost. The CPC is an osteo-conductive agent that enhances osteogenesis and is eventually replaced by bone [68]. Increased pull-out strength when using pedicle screws in conjunction with CPC has been reported [69]. In a study done on ovariectomy-induced osteoporotic dogs, Taniwaki and coworkers [65] showed that the pull-out strength of screws used with CPC increased with time after surgery, and was greater than that of the screws not enhanced by CPC immediately following surgery and weeks later. They concluded that the initial increased pull-out strength is likely secondary to CPC hardening, and that the continued increase was secondary to the bonding of the CPC to the surrounding bone [65].

Ankle fractures in the diabetic patient are well-documented to have a host of potential complications, whether one undertakes conservative or surgical care. Osteoporotic bone typically further complicates this patient. Schon and coworkers [70] attributed poor outcome after open reduction and internal fixation (ORIF) of neuropathic displaced ankle fractures to inadequate reduction, suboptimal rigid fixation, or inadequate period of immobilization [70], all of which have potential associations to osteoporotic bone quality. Additional fixation in conjunction with traditional fixation techniques for ankle fractures has been employed in the complicated neuropathic diabetic patient. Koval and colleagues [71] achieved 81% increased stability in cadaveric models with axial fibular Kirschner wires to supplement plate fixation. Schon and Marks [60] incorporated additional syndesmotic screws. Intermedullary nails or pins and tension banding have also been recommended for elderly foot and ankle fracture management to limit stress shielding, which will further decrease the BMD secondary to disuse [72].

Certain types of plate fixation are advisable in the osteoporotic patient. The blade plate relies on a borad blade that is not dependent on thread-bone interface, so a more substantial amount of bone would need to be lost for fixation failure [73]. The Schuhli nut converts screws to screws that lock into the plate based on the spikes on the nut engaging the underlying bone. The nut is placed between the bone and the plate, and the screw then passes through the plate and nut. This is technically more difficult and requires more advanced preparation than a more conventional locking plate.

The standard locking plate construct allows for the screw-plate interface to function as a single unit, eliminating points of failure with the increased potential for loosening of the screw. Ring and coworkers [73] demonstrated good to excellent results in 22 of 24 osteoporotic nonunions in the humeral diaphysis using the locking compression plate. Thus they concluded that osteoporotic bone is no longer a contraindication to operative fixation in these patients.

An alternative to rigid internal fixation in osteoporotic bone relies on external fixation. Good compression can be achieved with minimal reliance on the bone density to maintain the fixation. External fixation is the least invasive means of adequate immobilization while maintaining the vascular status around the fracture. External fixation may allow for earlier weight-bearing with dynamization of the external fixator, thus allowing for some ambulation, albeit somewhat protected [74].

Bone healing

Bone healing in the osteoporotic patient is always something to consider before proceeding with the surgery. There are a number of options to help counter the bone metabolism equilibrium that favors degradation of the bone, thus increasing the potential for delayed healing. The options discussed below can be used exclusively or in any combination with the other methods.

First, there are bone stimulation methods of addressing the altered bone metabolism. This can be achieved with low-intensity pulsed ultrasound or electromagnetic fields. It has been well-documented that electrical fields around the bone can be altered to stimulate bone growth. Numerous studies on pulsed electromagnetic fields show up-regulation of BMP-2 and BMP-4 in osteoblasts, resulting in osteogenesis [75]. Direct currents reduce tissue oxygenation, inducing osteoblast differentiation [76].

Low intensity pulsed ultrasound (LIPUS) is another means of stimulating bone via an external mechanical source. LIPUS is based upon acoustic waves that are less than the intensity in therapeutic ultrasound for rehabilitation, thus resulting in a nonthermal signal. The ultrasound signal sends pressure waves to the cell surface, possibly similar to the low mechanical signals mentioned earlier. The chain of events at the cellular level occurs via integrin receptors on the cell surface. Through intracellular reorganization, up-regulation of various cytokines and various proteins involved in bone growth occurs. At the clinical level, this vibrational stimulation of bone growth has been shown to decrease nonunion rates and expedite fracture healing [77,78]. Although no study on osteoporotic bone has been done with either electromagnetic fields or LIPUS, one can extrapolate that the increased cytokines and growth factors have increased bone growth, which should be useful in healing osteoporotic bone.

The second option relies on local placement of orthobiologics around the surgical site. This realm of treatment involves both materials that are not osteoinductive and many new treatments that are osteoinductive. Numerous recent studies have shown that a variety of orthobiologics can be used to stimulate bone healing in instances of nonunions, particular fractures, and bone defects through regulation of cytokines and BMPs. In fact, Simpson and colleagues [79] recommended that growth factors and other related agents be considered in clinical situations such as osteoporotic fractures. Although a complete discussion of each agent is beyond the scope of this article, it can again be inferred that up-regulation of cytokines, growth factors, and BMPs that stimulate bone growth would be beneficial in osteoporotic bone with a low mineral density.

The remaining method is one of the ongoing research areas of osteoporosis. The pharmaceutical treatment options can be given preoperatively or postoperatively to enhance the healing potential. Bisphophonates, PTH injections, and SERMs can be used; however, there is no evidenced-based research to support the use of these medications to enhance bone healing. Bisphosphonates have been used to help improve the durability of total joint replacements. The role of the bisphosphonates is to increase bone ingrowth into the porous implant surface, thus preventing bone resorption. Decreased bone resorption reduces the occurrence of loosening of the implant. Hilding and colleagues [80] demonstrated that oral clodronate was effective in reducing migration of the tibial component in total knee arthroplasty in a double-blinded trial in which the bisphosphanates were taken 3 months preoperatively and for an additional 6 months postoperatively. Animal studies have also shown an increase in bone growth of cortical bone adjacent to titanium implants with alendronate and zoledronate, and a decrease in wear debris-induced osteolysis of the femoral components for total hip arthroplasty [81,82].

PTH has not been evaluated for its role in fracture healing beyond speculation from a few animal studies; however, mechanical strength in the femur and vertebrae has been shown to increase with intermittent PTH treatment [38]. It has also been suggested that PTH may be more effective on bone with increased vascularity, such as cancellous bone, and in areas of greater stress. This suggestion has been proposed secondary to the greater effects of PTH in the lumbar spine than the proximal femur, where a greater number of osteoblasts and osteoprogenitor cells are present in the vertebrae [39]. With the need for the presence of osteoblasts, Koester and Spindler [39] also proposed that PTH may benefit the healing of particular fractures but may not be effective in healing avascular nonunions.

Pain management

NSAIDs are commonly used after an injury or postoperatively to decrease inflammation and pain. The current literature is inconclusive with regard to the affect on bone healing and the increased risk of nonunions; however, animal studies demonstrate the need for normal cyclooxygenase-2 (COX-2) function for endochondral ossification during fracture healing. Simon and coworkers [83] found that celecoxib-treated rats had more incomplete unions than nonunions, whereas nonunions were more prevalent in rofecoxib treated rats; however, the dosing was continuous over 8 weeks [83]. In a Level I therapeutic study on the benefits of celecoxib in 80 patients undergoing spinal fusion, no increase in nonunion was observed. These patients received celecoxib for 5 days at therapeutic doses for acute pain. Currently, the authors of this study are prescribing less than 1 week of celecoxib. If long-term management is needed, it is resumed after 6 weeks to allow for bone healing to start without the potential of prostaglandin inhibition [84]. In contrast to the COX-2 selective NSAIDs, indomethacin has been shown to delay fracture healing, but not prevent it [85]. COX-2 selective NSAIDs may prove to be detrimental in the osteoporotic patient, because their use would possibly further complicate the healing process.

Narcotic pain medication alters normal physiologic function by affecting the CNS. Although there are no data to show any change in the BMD or the osseous metabolic equilibrium, the potential for an increase in falls is present, which may increase the risk of osteoporotic fractures in the high-risk patient.

Summary

Osteoporosis is a common process defined by a decreased bone mineral density. With the incidence increasing as the population ages, we need to be prepared to understand the new medications being used for preventative and therapeutic solutions to this sometimes complicated problem. As surgeons, we also need to understand the variety of modalities that may effect the BMD and the outcomes of our surgery and rehabilitation.

References

[1] Lane N. Epidemiology, etiology and diagnosis of osteoporosis. Am J Obstr Gyn 2006;194: S3–11.

[2] Friedlander AH, Jones LJ. The biology, medical management, and podiatric implications of menopause. J Am Podiatr Med Assoc 2002;92(8):437–43.

[3] Gass M, Dawson-Hughes B. Preventing osteoporosis-related fractures: an overview. Am J Med 2006;119(4A):3S–11S.

[4] Pogoda P, Priemel M, Rueger JM. Bone remodeling: new aspects of a key process that controls skeletal maintenance and repair. Osteoporos Int 2005;16(Suppl 2): S18–24.

[5] Holstead Jones D, Kong YY, Penninger JM. Role of RANKL and RANK in bone loss and arthritis. Ann Rheum Dis 2002;61:32–9.

[6] Das U. Nitiric oxide as the mediator of the anti-osteoporotic actions of estrogen, statins, and essential fatty acids. Exp Biol Med 2002;227(2):88–93.

[7] Hofbauer LC, Kuhne CA, Viereck V. The OPG/RANKL/RANK systems in metabolic bone diseases. J Musculoskel Neuron Interact 2004;4(3):268–75.

[8] Rogers A, Saleh G, Hannon RA, et al. Circulating estradiol and osteoprotegerin as determinants of bone turnover and bone density in post-menopausal women. J Clin Endocrinol Metab 2002;87:4470–5.

[9] Fan X, Roy E, Zhu L, et al. Nitric oxide regulates receptor activity of nuclear factor-kappa B ligand and osteoprotegrin expression in bone marrow stromal cells. Endocrinology 2004; 145(2):751–9.

[10] Seck T, Diel I, Bismar H, et al. Serum parathyroid hormone, but not menopausal status, is associated with the expression of osteoprotegrin and RANKL mRNA in human bone samples. Eur J Endocrinol 2001;145:199–205.

[11] Das UN. Essential fatty acids and osteoporosis. Nutrition 2000;16:386–390.

[12] Wimalawansa SJ. Nitorglycerin therapy is as efficacious as standard estrogen therapy (premarin) in prevention of oopherectomy-induced bone loss: a human pilot clinical study. J Bone Miner Res 2000;15:2240–4.

[13] Van't Hof R, Macphee J, Libouban H, et al. Regulation of bone mass and turnover by neuronal nitric oxide synthase. Endocrinology 2004;145(11):5068–74.

[14] Levy R, Prince J, Billiar T. Nitric oxide: a clinical primer. Crit Care Med 2005;33(12): S492–5.

[15] Afzal F, Polak J, Buttery L. Endothelial nitric oxide synthase in the control of osteoblastic mineralizing activity and bone integrity. J Pathol 2004;202:503–10.

[16] Li F, Muhlbauer RC. Food fractionation is a powerful tool to increase bone mass in growing rats and decrease bone loss in aged rats: modulation of the effect by dietary phosphate. J Bone Miner Res 1999;14:1457–65.

[17] Clowes JA, Khosla S, Eastell R. Perspective: potential role of pancreatic and enteric hormones in regulating bone turnover. J Bone Miner Res 2005;20(9):1497–506.

[18] Pasco J, Henry M, Sanders K, et al. Beta-androgenic blockers reduce the risk of fracture partly by increasing bone mineral density: Geelong Osteoporosis Study. J Bone Miner Res 2004;19(1):19–24.

[19] Takeda S, Elefteriou F, Levasseur R, et al. Leptin regulates bone formation via the sympathetic nervous system. Cell 2002;111:305–17.

[20] Kinjo M, Setoguchi S, Schneeweiss S, et al. Bone mineral density subjects using central nervous system-active medications. Am J Med 2005;118(12):7–12.

[21] Lang T, LeBlanc A, Evans H, et al. Cortical and trabecular bone mineral loss from the spine and hip in long-duration spaceflight. J Bone Miner Res 2004;19:1006–12.

[22] Lin J, Lane J. Osteoporosis: a review. Clin Orthop Rel Res 2004;425:126–34.

[23] Delaney M. Strategies for the prevention and treatment of osteoporosis during early post-menopause. Am J Obstet Gynecol 2006;194(2):S12–23.

[24] Ishida Y, Kawai S. Comparative efficacy of hormone replacement therapy, etidronate, calcitonin, alfacalcidol, and vitamin K in postmenopausal women with osteoporosis: the Yamaguchi Osteoporosis Prevention Study. Am J Med 2004;117:549–55.

[25] Delmas PD, Bjarnason NH, Mitlak BH, et al. Effects of raloxifene on bone mineral density, serum cholesterol concentrations, and uterine endometrium in postmenopausal women. N Engl J Med 1997;337:1641–7.

[26] Ettinger B, Black DM, Mitlak BH, et al. Reduction in vertebral fracture risk in postmenopausal women with osteoporosis treated with raloxifene: results from a 3-year randomized clinical trial. JAMA 1999;282:637–45.

[27] Powles TJ, Hickish T, Kanis JA, et al. Effect of tamoxifen on bone mineral density measured by dual-energy x-ray absorptiometry in healthy premenopausal and postmenopausal women. J Clin Oncol 1996;14:78–84.

[28] Simoncini T, Mannellea P, Fornari L, et al. Tobulone activates nitric oxide synthesis in human endothelial cells. J Clin Endocrinol Metab 2004;89(9):4594–600.

[29] Haskell S. Selective estrogen receptor modulators. South Med J 2003;96(5):469–76.

[30] Wilkins C, Birge S. Prevention of osteoporosis fractures in the elderly. Am J Med 2005;118: 1190–5.

[31] Zizic T. Pharmacological prevention of osteoporotic fractures. Am Fam Physician 2004; 70(7):1293–300.

[32] MacFarlane S, Muniyappa R, Shin J, et al. Osteoporosis and cardiovascular disease. Endocrine 2004;23(1):1–10.

[33] Sama A, Khan S, Myers E, et al. High-dose alendronate uncouples osteoclast and osteoblast function: a study in rat spine pseudoarthritis model. Clin Ortho Rel Res 2004; 425:135–42.

[34] Tonino RP, Meunier PJ, Emkey R, et al. Skeletal benefits of alendronate: 7-year treatment of postemenopausal osteporotic women: Phase III Osteoporosis Treatment Study Group. J Clin Endocrinol Metab 2000;85:3109–15.

[35] Emkey R, Reid I, Mulloy A, et al. Ten-year efficacy and safety of alendronate in the treatment of osteoporosis in postmenopausal women. J Bone Miner Res 2002;S1059.

[36] Boniva (ibandronate sodium) [prescribing information]. Nutley, NJ: Roche Laboratories Inc.; 2005.

[37] Actonel (risedronate sodium) [prescribing information]. Kansas City, MO: Aventis Pharmaceuticals Inc.; 2004.

[38] Rosen C, Bilezikian J. Anabolic therapy for osteoporosis. J Clin Endocrinol Metab 2001; 86(3):957–64.

[39] Koester M, Spindler K. Pharmacologic agents in fracture healing. Clin Sports Med 2006;25: 63–73.

[40] Neer RM, Arnaud CD, Zanchetta JR, et al. Effect of parathyroid hormone (1-34) on fractures and bone mineral density in post-menopausal women with osteoporosis. N Engl J Med 2001;344:1434–41.

[41] Mundy G, Garrett R, Harris S, et al. Stimulation of bone formation in vitro and in rodents by statins. Science 1999;286:1946–9.

[42] McFarlane S, Muniyappa R, Francisco R, et al. Pleiotropic effects of statins: lipid reduction and beyond. J Clin Endocrinol Metab 2002;87(4):1451–8.

[43] Meier C, Schlienger R, Kraenzlin M, et al. HMG-CoA reductase inhibitors and the risk of fractures. JAMA 2000;283(24):3205–10.

[44] VanStaa TP, Wegman S, deVries F, et al. Use of statins and risk of fractures. JAMA 2001; 285:1850–5.

[45] Rudman DV, Feller AG, Nagrog HS, et al. Effect of human growth hormone in men over age 60. N Engl J Med 1990;323:52–4.

[46] Kurland ES, Cosman F, McMahon DJ, et al. Therapy of idiopathic osteoporosis in men with parathyroid hormone: effects on bone mineral density and bone markers. J Clin Endocrinol Metab 2000;85:3069–76.

[47] Baecker N, Boese A, Schoenau E, et al. L-arginine, the natural precursor of NO, is not effective for preventing bone loss in postmenopausal women. J Bone Miner Res 2005;20: 471–9.

[48] Mei J, Yeung S, Kung A. High dietary phytoestrogen intake is associated with higher bone mineral density in postmenopausal but not premenopausal women. J Clin Endocrinol Metab 2001;86(11):5217–21.

[49] Mundy G. Nutritional modulators of bone remodeling during aging. Am J Clin Nutr 2006; 83(Suppl):427S–30S.

[50] Bhandari M, Devereaux PJ. Do beta blockers and thiazides reduce fracture risk? Can Med Assoc J 2005;172(1):37.

[51] Rubin C, Recker R, Callen D, et al. Prevention of postmenopausal bone loss by a low magnitude, high frequency mechanical stimuli: a clinical trial assessing compliance, efficacy, and safety. J Bone Miner Res 2004;19(3):343–51.

[52] Rubin J, Murphy TC, Zhu L, et al. Mechanical strain differentially regulates endothelial nitric-oxide synthase and receptor activator of nuclear kappa B ligand expression via ERK $\frac{1}{2}$ MAPK . J Biol Chem 2003;278:34018–25.

[53] Rubin J, Murphy T, Fan X, et al. Mechanical strain inhibits RANKL expression through activation of ERK $\frac{1}{2}$ in bone marrow stromal cells. J Bone Miner Res 2002;17:1452–60.

[54] Ward K, Alsop C, Caulton J, et al. Low magnitude mechanical loading is osteogenic in children with disabling conditions. J Bone Miner Res 2004;19:360–9.

[55] Judex S, Garman R, Squire M, et al. Genetically based influences on the site-specific regulation of tranecular and cortical bone morphology. J Bone Miner Res 2004;19:600–6.

[56] Xie L. Bone, in press.

[57] Hauselmann HJ, Rizzoli R. A comprehensive review of treatments for post-menopusal osteoporosis. Osteoporos Int 2003;14:2–12.

[58] Hannan MT, Cheng DM, Green E, et al. Establishing the compliance in elderly women for use of a low level mechanical stress device in a clinical osteoporosis study. Osteoporos Int 2004;15:918–26.

[59] Holmes GB, Hill N. Fractures and dislocations of the foot and ankle in diabetics associated with Charcot joint changes. Foot Ankle Int 1994;4:182–5.

[60] Schon LC, Marks RM. The management of neuropathic fracture dislocation in the diabetic patient. Orthop Clin North Am 1995;26:375–92.

[61] Cornell CN. Internal fracture fixation in patients with osteoporosis. J Am Acad Orthop Surg 2003;11:109–19.

[62] Egermann M, Schneider E, Evans CH, et al. The potential for gene therapy for fracture healing in osteoporosis. Osteoporos Int 2005;16:S120–8.

[63] Seebeck J, Goldham J, Morlock MM, et al. Mechanical behavior of screws in normal and osteoporotic bone. Osteoporos Int 2005;16:S107–11.

[64] Pfiefer BA, Krag MH, Johnson C. Repair of failed transpedicle screw fixation. Spine 1994; 19:350–3.

[65] Taniwaki Y, Takemasa R, Tani T, et al. Enhancement of pedicle screw stability using calcium phosphate cement in osteoporotic vertebrae: in vivo biomechanical study. J Orthop Sci 2003;8:408–14.

[66] Moroni A, Faldini C, Pegreffi F, et al. HA-coated screws decrease the incidence of fixation failure in osteoporotic trochanteric fractures. Clin Orthop Rel Res 2004;425:87–92.

[67] Moroni A, Faldini C, Rocca M, et al. Improvement of the bone-screw interface with hydroxyapetite coated AO/ASIF cortical screws. J Orthop Trauma 2002;16:257–63.

[68] Yamamoto H, Niwa S, Hori M, et al. Mechanical strength on calcium phosphate cement in vivo and in vitro. Biomaterials 1998;19:1587–91.

[69] Iai H, Yamamoto H, Kamioka Y, et al. An experimental study on the biomechanical effect of TCP cement for the vertebra with osteoporosis. Orthop Ceramic Implants 1991;11:43–6.

[70] Schon LC, Easley ME, Weinfeld SB. Charcot neuroarthropathy of the foot and ankle. Clin Orthop 1998;349:116–31.

[71] Koval KJ, Petraco DM, Kumer FJ, et al. A new technique for complex fibula fracture fixation in the elderly: a clinical and biomechanical evaluation. J Orthop Trauma 1997;11: 28–33.

[72] Kettunen J, Kroger H. Surgical treatment of ankle and foot fractures in the elderly. Osteoporos Int 2005;16(Suppl 2):S103–6.

[73] Ring D, Kloen P, Kadzielski J, et al. Locking compression plates for osteoporotic nonunions of the diaphyseal humerus. Clin Orthop Rel Res 2004;425:50–4.

[74] Chao EYS, Inoue N, Koo TKK, et al. Biomechanical considerations of fracture treatment and bone quality maintenance in elderly patient and patients with osteoporosis. Clin Orthop Res Res 2004;425:12–25.

[75] Bodamyali T, Kanczler SM, Simon B, et al. PEMF simultaneously induce osteogenesis and upregulate transcription BMP-2 and BMP-4 in rat osteoblasts in vitro. Biochem Biophys Res Commun 1998;250:458–61.

[76] Brighton CT, Hunt RM. Ultrastructure of electrical induced osteogenesis in the rabbit medullary canal. J Orthop Res 1986;4:27–36.

[77] Heckman JD, Ryaby JP, McCabe J, et al. Acceleration of tibial fracture-healing by non-invasive low-intensity pulsed ultrasound. J Bone Joint Surg 1994;76-A:26–34.

[78] Kristiansen TK, Ryaby JP, McCabe J, et al. Accelerated healing of distal radial fractures with the use of specific, low-intensity ultrasound. A multi-center, prospective, randomized, double-blind, placebo-controlled study. J Bone Joint Surg 1997;79-A:961–73.

[79] Simpson AHRW, Mills L, Noble B. The role of growth factors and related agents in accelerating fracture healing. J Bone Joint Surg Br 2006;88-B(6):701–5.

[80] Hilding M, Ryd L, Toksvig-Larsen S, et al. Clodronate prevents prosthetic migration: a randomized radiostereometric study of 50 total knee patients. Acta Orthop Scand 2000; 71:553–7.

[81] Von Knoch F, Cho MR, Garrigues GE, et al. Effects of bisphosphonates (alendronate and zoledronate) on bone ingrowth in a rabbit model: a radiographic and histomorphometric analysis. Trans Orthop Res Soc 2003;27:1375.

[82] Shanbhag AS, Hasselman CT, Rubash HE. The John Charnley Award. Inhibition of wear debris mediated osteolysis in a canine total hip arthroplasty model. Clin Orthop Rel Res 1997;344:33–43.

[83] Simon AM, Manigrasso MB, O'Connor JP. Cyclo-oxygenase 2 function is essential for bone fracture healing. J Bone Miner Res 2002;17:963–76.

[84] Reuben SS, Ekman EF. The effect of cyclooxygenase-2 inhibition on analgesia and spinal fusion. J Bone Joint Surg Am 2005;87:536–42.

[85] Ro J, Sudmann E, Marton PF. Effect of indomethacin on fracture healing in rats. Acta Orthop Scand 1976;47:588–99.

ELSEVIER
SAUNDERS

Clin Podiatr Med Surg
24 (2007) 333–351

CLINICS IN
PODIATRIC
MEDICINE AND
SURGERY

Concepts in Pain Management

Padma Gulur, MD[a,*],
Simon Maurice Soldinger, MD[b],
Martin A. Acquadro, MD, DMD, FACP, FACPM[c,d,e]

[a]Harvard Medical School, Massachusetts General Hospital Pain Center,
15 Parkman Street, WACC 333, Boston, MA 02114, USA
[b]University of California Los Angeles, 15300 Ventura Boulevard, #502,
Sherman Oaks, CA 91403, USA
[c]Tufts University School of Medicine 2100 Dorchester Avenue, Dorchester, MA 02124, USA
[d]Department of Anesthesiology and Pain Services 2100 Dorchester Avenue,
Dorchester, MA 02124, USA
[e]Caritas Carney Hospital, 2100 Dorchester Avenue, Dorchester, MA 02124, USA

Pain is the most common symptom for which patients seek medical care. The International Association for the Study of Pain defines pain as "an unpleasant sensory and emotional experience associated with actual or potential tissue damage" [1]. Untreated pain is a common cause of disability. Foot pain is a common symptom that patients and physicians confront. Frequently, it remains a challenging problem to treat. Foot pain may result from a number of pathologic processes ranging from local factors such as fractures and neuromas to systemic conditions such as gout and diabetes.

Our understanding of pain mechanisms has progressed over the years. Pain management has evolved as a specialty encompassing many disciplines; however, the role of primary care physicians and surgeons continues to be vital in managing painful states early on. There is a national drive to adequately recognize pain and to provide appropriate treatment. The Joint Commission on Accreditation of Healthcare Organizations declared "pain" as the fifth vital sign and issued standards for its management [2].

Classification of pain syndromes

A classification based on pathophysiology broadly divides pain syndromes into nociceptive, neuropathic, psychogenic, mixed, or idiopathic.

* Corresponding author. Harvard Medical School, Massachusetts General Hospital Pain Center, 15 Parkman Street, WACC 333, Boston, MA 02114.
E-mail address: pgulur@partners.org (P. Gulur).

Nociceptive pain involves the normal activation of the nociceptive system by noxious stimuli and usually involves tissue injury. It is further stratified into superficial, deep, and visceral. Visceral pain is characterized by its diffuse nonlocalizing nature as opposed to superficial and deep nociceptive pain, which are more easily localized. Neuropathic pain is thought to result from direct injury or from dysfunction of the sensory axons in the peripheral or central nervous system [3,4]. It is widely recognized that the patient's psychologic state contributes significantly to pain perception and associated suffering, especially in chronic pain states. When the pathophysiology of a pain state is primarily influenced by psychologic factors, the term "psychogenic pain state" is applied [5,6]. When no clear pathophysiology can be identified, it is classified as an "idiopathic pain state."

Pain can also be classified in terms of etiology, such as postoperative or cancer pain. Other classifications can be based on location; for example, low back pain, neck pain, facial pain, and headaches. Specialized terms commonly used in pain management to describe pain states are summarized in Box 1.

Classification based on duration (ie, acute versus chronic pain) is also widely used. Acute pain is pain that does not last beyond the usual course of an acute illness or the time required for an injury to heal. Pain is usually considered chronic if it persists more than 3 to 6 months. Management strategies are very different for the two classifications; initiating timely pain management interventions is essential for the management of chronic pain (Table 1).

Mechanisms of pain

Although the exact mechanisms underlying the generation of pain are not well understood, recent advances in basic and clinical neuroscience have

---

Box 1. Terms commonly used in pain management

Allodynia: perception of non-noxious stimuli as pain
Analgesia: absence of any perception of pain
Anesthesia: absence of any perception of sensation
Anesthesia dolorosa: perception of pain in an area that lacks
   a perception of sensation
Hypoalgesia: decreased sensation to noxious stimuli
Hyperalgesia: increased sensation to noxious stimuli
Hyperesthesia: increased response to mild stimulation
Neuralgia: pain in the distribution of nerve groups
Paresthesia: abnormal sensation in the absence of stimulus
Radiculopathy: pain in the distribution of one or more nerve roots

Table 1
Differences between acute and chronic pain

Characteristics	Acute pain	Chronic pain
Temporal features	Recent onset and expected to last no longer than days or weeks	Remote, often ill-defined onset; duration unknown
Intensity	Variable	Variable
Associated affect	Anxiety may be prominent when pain is severe or cause is unknown; sometimes irritability	Irritability or depression
Associated pain-related behaviors	Pain behaviors (eg, moaning, rubbing, splinting) may be prominent when pain is severe	May or may not give any indication of pain; specific behaviors (eg, assuming a comfortable position) may occur
Associated features	May have signs of sympathetic hyperactivity when pain is severe (eg, tachycardia, hypertension, sweating, mydriasis)	May or may not have vegetative signs such as lassitude, anorexia, weight loss, insomnia, or loss of libido; these signs may be difficult to distinguish from other disease-related effects

From Portenoy RK, Kanner RM. Definition and assessment of pain. In: Portenoy RK, Kanner RM, editors. Pain management: theory and practice. New York: Oxford University Press; 1998, with permission.

provided insights into a few potential pathways. Although the pathophysiology of acute and chronic pain syndromes differs, the fundamental pain transmission pathways are characterized by peripheral receptors that transduce energy from noxious stimuli and transmit to the central nervous system what is finally perceived as "pain" in the brain. The primary afferent neurons whose free nerve endings have receptors for pain transduction are located in the dorsal root ganglion. The primary sensory neurons synapse on the second-order neurons in the dorsal horn of the spinal cord that transmit noxious signals higher up to the thalamus and then to several cortical and subcortical centers account for the emotional-affective and sensory-discriminative components of the pain experience. It is believed that substantial modulation of pain signals occurs at the dorsal horn region, resulting from excitatory and inhibitory neuromediators and descending inhibitory systems that originate at supraspinal levels.

Persistent or repeated peripheral stimulation of nociceptors can result in increased sensitivity at the peripheral and central levels due to reduction in the thresholds of pain stimulation. Injury to the nervous system can lead to persistent dysfunction of pain processing, leading to neuropathic pain that is clinically reflected by phenomena such as "allodynia," whereby innocuous stimuli lead to pain, and "hyperalgesia," whereby painful stimuli are perceived as exaggerated pain.

The pain state involves three main components (Box 2): a sensory-discriminative component (eg, location, intensity, quality), a motivational-affective component (eg, depression, anxiety), and a cognitive-evaluative component (eg, thoughts concerning the cause and significance of the pain) [7].

Woolf and DeCosterd [8] advocate the recognition that reorganization at a molecular and structural level of pain pathways produces chronic pain, not the primary disease factors that initiate these pain mechanisms. Because a particular disease may initiate several distinct pain mechanisms, a disease-based classification, although useful for disease-modifying therapy, is not as useful for pain therapy, which should primarily focus on the mechanisms. Similarly, symptoms are not equivalent to mechanisms, although they may reflect them. The same symptom may be produced by different mechanisms; similarly, a single mechanism may elicit multiple symptoms.

Fundamental pain mechanisms include the response to acute painful stimuli, which is mediated by the high-threshold nociceptors and their afferents, the unmyelinated C fibers, and lightly myelinated A delta fibers. Nociceptor transduction mechanisms involve activation of temperature ion channel transducers of the transient receptor potential family, in addition to sodium and potassium channels, chemosensitive ion channels, or metabotropic receptors (eg, acid-sensing ionic channels, among others). This activation of nociceptors through transduction leads to transmission of the nociceptive stimulus through glutamate release. Glutamate generates fast synaptic potentials in the dorsal horn neurons, which are boosted and prolonged by the N-methyl-D-aspartate (NMDA) receptor ion channel. The inputs generated are then integrated in the higher centers in the cortex into an acute pain sensation. Such nociceptive pain (normal pain) has an adaptive protective role, warning of potential tissue damage and instituting strong reflex and behavioral avoidance responses.

Box 2. Components of pain

Sensory-discriminative component
   Location
   Intensity
   Quality

Motivation-affective component
   Depression
   Anxiety

Cognitive-evaluation component
   Thought concerning the cause and significance of the pain

Another fundamental pain mechanism is peripheral sensitization. The sensitivity of the peripheral terminal nociceptors is not fixed, and activation by repeated peripheral stimulation or by changes in the chemical milieu of the terminal can sensitize the primary sensory neuron. This pheneomenon represents peripheral sensitization.

Central sensitization and modulation refer to an augmentation of nociceptive synaptic transmission in the dorsal horn of the spinal cord that contributes to increased pain sensitivity. After peripheral nerve injury, central sensitization is driven by ectopic activity in injured nerve fibers resulting from changes in the expression, distribution, or activity of voltage-gated ion channels. Changes or switches in the phenotype of the primary sensory neurons contribute to these central functional changes in synaptic transmission.

Disinhibiton is the phenomenon of a decrease in phasic and tonic inhibition, which can produce changes in dorsal horn excitability. This disinhibition may result from a down-regulation of inhibitory neurotransmitters or from a disruption of descending inhibitory pathways (Fig. 1).

Common pain conditions in podiatry

Patients present with pain that is mostly described by anatomic location (Box 3). Broadly, pain is described in the forefoot, arch, heel, or ankle. Pain in the forefoot could be caused by ingrown toenails, bunions, hammertoes,

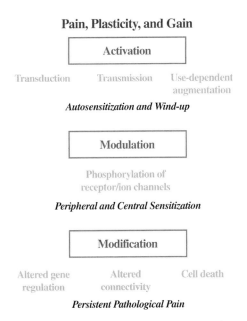

Fig. 1. Summary of the three forms of neural plasticity that can produce pain hypersensitivity. (*From* Woolf CJ, Salter MW. Neuronal plasticity: increasing the gain in pain. Science 2000; 288:1766; with permission).

Box 3. Pain described by anatomic location

Forefoot pain
  Ingrown nail
  Hammertoes
  Bunions
  Metatarsalgia
  Neuroma
  Gout
  Rheumatoid arthritis

Arch pain
  Plantar fasciitis
  Flat foot

Heel pain
  Calcaneal apophysitis
  Cracked heels
  Retrocalcaneal bursitis
  Achilles tendonitis

Ankle pain
  Tarsal tunnel syndrome
  Ankle sprain

Whole foot
  Claudication
  Peripheral neuropathy
  Diabetic neuropathy

---

metatarsalgia, or systemic causes such as gout or rheumatoid arthritis. Pain in the arch of the foot could be due to plantar fasciitis or flat foot. Pain in the heel could be secondary to cracked heels, calcaneal apophysitis, retrocalcneal bursitis, or Achilles tendonitis. Pain in the ankle could be due to pathology such as tarsal tunnel syndrome or sprained ankle. Pain involving the entire foot could be secondary to claudication or peripheral neuropathy. In the paragraphs that follow, the authors take a brief look at the more common conditions.

Plantar fasciitis

The plantar fascia is a band of connective tissue on the plantar aspect of the foot, from the medial plantar tuberosity of the calcaneus to the base of the digits. It helps support the medial longitudinal arch of the foot. It is frequently a site of chronic pain [9,10]. Patients typically complain of pain that starts on waking in the morning or after prolonged sitting. Pain onset is usually insidious and of unknown etiology but also may commence after a traumatic injury. Diagnosis is made by eliciting pain with palpation in the region of the origin of the plantar fascia or sometimes into the arch along the medial band of the plantar fascia. Pain may be worsened by passive dorsiflexion of the foot or hallux.

Therapies for this condition include active stretching, use of nonsteroidal anti-inflammatory drugs (NSAIDs), cushioning heel cups, nighttime plantar fascia splints, and foot orthotics [11,12]. As a later stage of therapy, corticosteroid injection effectively provides pain relief [13], although it carries the risk of plantar fascia rupture [14] and fat pad atrophy.

Tarsal tunnel syndrome

The tarsal tunnel is formed by the medial malleolus and a fibrous ligament, the flexor retinaculum. The posterior tibial nerve passes through the tunnel, which is a common site for compression. The medial plantar, lateral plantar, and calcaneal branches of the posterior tibial nerve innervate the base of the foot.

Patients who have symptoms of tarsal tunnel syndrome may complain of a burning sensation, pain, and paresthesias over the distribution of the posterior tibial nerve and its branches that worsen with weight bearing [11]. Symptoms are often related to chronic conditions such as impingement syndromes and hyperpronation or may be secondary to acute trauma [12]. Eliciting a positive Tinel's sign by tapping over the tarsal tunnel typically causes discomfort in the medial one third of the distal plantar foot, although the entire plantar foot surface may be affected.

Treatment for tarsal tunnel includes stretching, rest, use of shoe inserts or orthotics, medications such as NSAIDs. Neuropathic pain medications have also shown efficacy (see the Pharmacologic therapies section). Corticosteroid injections have limited benefit.

Morton's neuroma

The interdigital spaces of the foot are common sites for the occurrence of painful Morton's neuromas. The second and third common digital branches of the medial plantar nerve are the most frequent sites for development of interdigital neuromas. They develop secondary to chronic trauma and repetitive stress [15]. Pain and paresthesias are usually insidious at onset and located in the interdigital space of the affected nerve. In some cases, the interdigital space between the affected toes may be widened as a result of the neuroma or another space-occupying lesion such as a ganglion or synovial cyst. Pain is elicited in the affected interdigital space when the metatarsal heads of the foot are squeezed together. A diagnostic injection with lidocaine can be used to confirm the diagnosis.

Treatment for Morton's neuroma can include the use of NSAIDs, neuro-pathic pain medications as described in the next section, metatarsal pads, or-thotics, and corticosteroid injections. Injection may be considered as an early therapeutic option [16]. Surgery is usually a last resort.

Management

Pharmacologic therapies

Analgesics act at different sites. Some act at the site of injury and decrease the pain associated with an inflammatory reaction (eg, NSAIDs). Others al-ter nerve conduction (eg, local anesthetics). They may modify transmission in the dorsal horn or they may affect the central component and the emo-tional aspects of pain (eg, opioids and some antidepressants). The common underlying mechanism of action for neuropathic pain medications is periph-eral or central reduction of neuronal hyperexcitability.

Analgesic drugs can be broadly divided into nonopioid, opioid, and ad-juvant analgesics. Nonopioid analgesics include acetaminophen and non-selective and selective NSAIDs, which include salicylates. The main characteristics of this class of medications are that they have a ceiling effect to analgesia, they do not produce tolerance or physical dependence, they are not associated with abuse or addiction, and their primary mechanism of ac-tion is inhibition of prostaglandin formation. Per the World Health Organi-zation guidelines, this is the standard of care for mild to moderate pain, or the "first step" in their ladder [17]. The American Pain Society recommends that a nonopioid drug be considered for all analgesic regimens (unless the risk is high or the drugs are ineffective), even when pain is intense enough to require the addition of an opioid analgesic [18].

Opioids produce analgesia by acting on centrally and peripherally located opioid receptors (μ, κ, and δ) to inhibit the transmission of nociceptive input from the periphery to the spinal cord, activate descending inhibitory path-ways that modulate transmission in the spinal cord, and alter limbic system activity [19]. Opioids can be classified by their action (full agonist, partial agonist, antagonist, or mixed agonist-antagonist) at various opioid recep-tors. Commonly used opioids such as morphine, oxycodone, and fentanyl are full agonists. Partial agonists (eg, buprenorphine) have low intrinsic ac-tivity at the opioid receptor. Agonist-antagonists have a ceiling effect com-pared with full agonists. Opioid-induced respiratory depression, sedation, mental clouding, impaired psychomotor function, and constipation are some of the adverse effects, which limit their use. Addiction and dependence are serious concerns with this class of drugs. Of special note, methadone is gaining popularity because in addition to its opioid receptor activity, it has NMDA antagonistic activity.

Opioids in the treatment of acute pain or postoperative pain are usually short acting and are commonly delivered by means of oral or intravenous routes. Intravenously administered opioids have a quicker onset of action, but this benefit is offset by their shorter duration. One popular mode of delivery is patient controlled analgesia. The benefit of this delivery system is that as long as a basal rate is not used, it has little to no risk of overdose. The patient's control over this modality also provides better satisfaction.

Opioids in the control of chronic pain are more challenging. Issues such as tolerance, dependence, and opioid-induced hyperalgesia are common concerns and need to be monitored carefully. Most practitioners agree that the use of longer-acting preparations is preferable to short-acting medications, to which tolerance is developed more quickly. There is, however, an abuse potential with long-acting preparations that needs to be monitored carefully by the prescribing practitioner. The treatment of chronic pain with opioids should always be undertaken with an opioid contract between the prescriber and patient at the outset. Random urine toxicology screens should be performed regularly to ensure there is no diversion or abuse of other illicit substances while the patient is on prescription opioids.

The term "adjuvant analgesics" traditionally refers to a large and diverse group of drugs, most of which have demonstrated analgesic effects in specific circumstances but do not have Food and Drug Administration (FDA)-approved labeling for pain (Table 2). This situation is changing, however, because some of the drugs traditionally included in this class, like the anticonvulsants and antidepressants, are now FDA approved for the treatment of neuropathic pain [20].

Neuropathic pain, in particular, has shown good response to the anticonvulsant class of medications (eg, gabapentin, pregablin, carbamazepine, oxycarbazepine) [21] and the antidepressant class of medications (especially the tricyclics and the combined norepinephrine and serotonin reuptake inhibitors such as duloxetine and venlafaxine).

Anticonvulsants

Anticonvulsant drugs act by a variety of known mechanisms, including effects on sodium or calcium conductance, increases in γ-aminobutyric acid (GABA) levels, and decreases in glutamate levels, and by other unknown mechanisms. These agents have been used in the management of neuropathic pain for many years, but only limited evidence exists for the efficacy of phenytoin and carbamazepine.

Gabapentin is now widely used for neuropathic symptoms. This agent is structurally similar to the neurotransmitter GABA and was introduced some years ago as an anticonvulsant for complex partial seizures. The efficacy of gabapentin has been confirmed in two placebo-controlled clinical trials. The precise mechanism of action of gabapentin for pain relief is unknown; however, a specific calcium channel binding site has been identified, and regulation of calcium may play a role. Reported side effects include sedation, dizziness, headache, pedal edema, and weight gain. Slow dose titration may reduce the incidence of side effects.

Table 2
Adjuvant analgesics for persistent nonmalignant pain conditions

Drug class	Starting dose	Titration	Maximum dose	Comments
Tricyclic antidepressants (TCAs)				
Amitriptyline	10–25 mg qd	10–25 mg qd, 3–5 d	100–150 mg/d	TCAs are multipurpose analgesics and may be considered for a trial in any type of persistent pain. The analgesic effect of TCAs is separate from their antidepressant effects. Depression also may be a target, and doses sometimes require escalation to achieve this effect. The use of amitriptyline may be limited in many patients due to its side effects; desipramine and nortriptyline are preferred. A therapeutic response is usually seen within 3–10 d for neuropathic pain. TCA dosage should depend on the degree of pain relief balanced against the emergence of adverse effects. An adequate trial with a TCA needs to be given before determining treatment failure; some patients require higher dosages and several weeks of treatment before efficacy is evident. Failure of one TCA agent does not preclude a response to another, and two or more agents should be tried sequentially before selecting another class of adjuvant analgesic agents
Desipramine	10–25 mg qd	10–25 mg qd	100–150 mg/d	
Nortriptyline	10–25 mg qd	10–25 mg qd, 3–5 d	100–150 mg/d	
Norepinephrine/serotonin reuptake inhibitors (SNRIs)				
Venlafaxine	25 mg tid[a]	25 mg tid q > 4 d[a]	225 mg/d[a]	The newer SNRIs (eg, duloxetine, venlafaxine) also may be considered multipurpose analgesics. Duloxetine has FDA-approved labeling for the management of pain caused by diabetic neuropathy. Side effects are usually less than those caused by the TCAs.
Duloxetine	60 mg qd		120 mg/d	

Selective serotonin reuptake inhibitors (SSRIs)				
Paroxetine	20 mg/d[a]	10 mg/d q 7 d[a]	50 mg/d[a]	The SSRIs have been used as adjunctive therapy for patients who are depressed. There is some evidence of analgesic efficacy (eg, paroxetine, citalopram), but it is limited. SSRIs have fewer side effects than TCAs and are generally considered safer. In patients who have depression and persistent pain and cannot tolerate TCAs, a trial with an SSRI is reasonable. Experience is greatest with paroxetine and citalopram.
Citalopram	20 mg/d[a]	20 mg/d q 7 d[a]	40 mg/d[a]	
Antiepileptics				Antiepileptics are used in the management of neuropathic pain and are similar to TCAs in producing a graded analgesic effect.
Gabapentin	300 mg/d	300 mg bid, d 2; 300 mg tid, d 3	1800–3600 mg/d or higher	Gabapentin and pregabalin have FDA-approved labeling for PHN. Most who respond to gabapentin do so at total daily doses of 900–1800 mg/d, but some patients require higher doses. Dose-related sedation is a limiting factor with gabapentin.
Pregabalin (for PHN)	50 mg tid; 75 mg bid or 50 mg tid	100 tid after 1 wk; 100 tid after 1 wk	300 mg/d; 300 mg/d	Pregabalin has FDA-approved labeling for neuropathic pain associated with diabetic peripheral neuropathy.
Carbamazepine	200 mg/d	200 mg/d q 12 h	1200 mg/d	Carbamazepine has FDA-approved labeling for trigeminal neuralgia. Oxcarbazine, topiramate, lamotrigine, tiagabine, and valproate have been reported to have effect against neuropathic pain based on case studies. These agents are typically used at their antiepileptic dosages.
γ-Aminobutyric acid agonists				
Baclofen	5–10 mg bid or tid	5–10 mg/d q 2–3 d prn	80 mg/d	The analgesic effect of baclofen in trigeminal neuralgia has led to wider use in neuropathic pain of other types. Although less effective than carbamazepine, the adverse-reaction profile for baclofen is more favorable, making it an attractive initial drug to treat trigeminal neuralgia in select patients. The reported effective dose range is 50–60 mg/d.

(continued on next page)

Table 2 (*continued*)

Drug class	Starting dose	Titration	Maximum dose	Comments
Oral sodium channel blockers				
Mexiletine	150–200 mg bid	150 mg q 2–3 d prn	1200 mg/d	Mexiletine, an oral analog of intravenous lidocaine has been used to treat difficult-to-control neuropathic pain secondary to diabetic neuropathy, spinal cord injury, and persistent pain syndromes secondary to peripheral nerve injury.
α_2-Adrenergic agonists				Sympatholytic agents are first- or second-line drugs for the intervals prn treatment of CRPS.
Clonidine	0.1 mg bid	0.1 mg/d at weekly intervals prn	2.4 mg/d	Most analgesic data support the effectiveness of intrathecal and epidural administration of clonidine. The usual effective dosage is 0.3 mg/d. Transdermal clonidine may decrease swelling and pain in CRPS areas with hyperalgesia.
Tizanidine	4 mg initially	2 mg q 6–8 h	36 mg/d	Tizanidine is a muscle relaxant with centrally acting α_2-adrenergic agonist activity. It can produce hypotension, but this occurs less than with clonidine. Tizanidine may have some inherent analgesic activity.
NMDA receptor antagonists				NMDA receptor antagonists can be useful in intractable neuropathic pain. The experience with dextromethorphan for persistent pain syndromes has been mixed. One study has shown that dextromethorphan treatment improved pain assessment scores in patients who had diabetic neuropathy but not PHN. The optimal dose is unknown. The dose is likely to exceed the antitussive dose of 10–20 mg qid by a factor of 10. Doses in this range are inconsistently reported to be helpful and are reported to produce significant adverse reactions.
Ketamine	See comments	See comments	See comments	Ketamine, a dissociative anesthetic, has been used by pain specialists in some cases of intractable neuropathic pain. Even with low (subanesthetic) doses, however, psychotomimetic side effects may limit its utility and safety, thus requiring careful patient selection.
Dextro-methorphan	See comments	See comments	See comments	

Topical agents				
Capsaicin	0.025%– 0.075% qid	See comments	See comments	Topical capsaicin has been used to treat a number of persistent pain conditions including diabetic neuropathy, PHN, osteoarthritis, rheumatoid arthritis, and postmastectomy pain. One study concluded that topical capsaicin therapy for 22 wk reduced pain in patients who had diabetic neuropathy. Patients should be instructed to use the lower strength concentration qid before attempting to use the higher strength concentration. Initial burning is common, but most patients become tolerant within a few days. Optimal effects are typically seen after about 4 wk of qid application. Patients should be advised to wash hands thoroughly after using capsaicin and avoid contact with eyes and mucous membranes.
Lidocaine patch	Lidocaine 5%	Up to 3 patches applied at once, for up to 12 h in 24-h period	See comments	Topical local anesthetics are commonly used. Lidocaine patch (5%) is available with labeled indications for PHN, but it is also used for other conditions. Up to 3 patches per day can be used.
Miscellaneous agents				
Calcitonin, IM or SC	50–100 IU/d	Maintenance dose 50–100 IU q 1–3 d	100 IU/d	Calcitonin has been reported to reduce persistent pain associated with osteoporotic fractures, bone metastases, CRPS, and phantom limb pain. Although the long-term efficacy has not been established, a trial of calcitonin may be considered in patients who have refractory pain.

Abbreviations: CRPS, complex regional pain syndrome; IM, intramuscularly; PHN, postherpetic neuralgia; prn, as needed; SC, subcutaneously.
[a] Antidepressant dose.

From the American Medical Association. Pain management: assessing and treating persistent nonmalignant pain. Available at: http://www.ama-cmeonline.com/pain_mgmt/module07/index.htm. Accessed April 2, 2007; with permission.

A newer drug, pregabalin, which is a central nervous system active compound and an analog of GABA, has recently been introduced. Pregabalin shares gabapentin's binding site on a subunit of voltage-dependent calcium channels. Pregabalin has been marketed for its higher bioavailability and ease of titration. Its side effect profile is similar to gabapentin. A number of other anticonvulsant agents including lamotrogine and sodium valproate have confirmed efficacy in randomized, controlled trials.

Antidepressants

Tricyclic antidepressants (TCAs) and serotonin and norepinephrine reuptake inhibitors have proven efficacy in the treatment of neuropathic pain. Numerous clinical trials demonstrate the safety and efficacy of TCAs when used to treat diabetic neuropathy or postherpetic neuralgia. Amitriptyline was the first tricyclic used to treat neuropathy, and is still widely prescribed. Because amitriptyline also has a high incidence of anticholinergic side effects and can lead to delirium in elderly patients, it should be avoided in that population. Desipramine and nortriptyline, which have the least anticholinergic activity of the TCAs, are equally efficacious substitutes. The pain-relieving properties of TCAs occur independently of their effect on mood.

TCAs have proarrhythmic effects, including an increased risk for torsades de pointes. Patients should have a baseline ECG, with a repeat ECG after achieving a therapeutic dose. The greatest risk for developing arrhythmias occurs with a QRS greater than 100 milliseconds (ms) or a prolonged QTC ($\geq$440–470 ms). Other risk factors include congestive heart failure with an ejection fraction less than 35%, active ischemic heart disease, and bundle branch block. TCAs should also be avoided in patients who have closed-angle glaucoma, benign prostatic hypertrophy, uncontrolled seizure disorder, and bipolar disorder.

Selective serotonin reuptake inhibitors (SSRIs) have less consistent effects on neuropathic pain and have fallen into disfavor.

Duloxetine and venlafaxine have gained interest as a potential treatment for neuropathic pain because they combine the norepinephrine-reuptake inhibiting effects of TCAs with the serotonin-reuptake inhibiting effects of the SSRIs, without the anticholinergic side effects. Duloxetine has FDA approval for the treatment of diabetic neuropathy. The most common side effects of venlafaxine include increased blood pressure with or without hypertension, irritability, insomnia, nausea, vomiting, and constipation. NMDA receptor antagonists such as ketamine and dexmetomidine also have shown efficacy in neuropathic pain states, as have sodium channel blockers such as mexiletine [22].

For complex regional pain syndrome (CRPS), drugs such as clonidine and prazosin have also been used. For bone pain from cancer, calcitonin and the bisphosphonates have been used. Muscle relaxants such as tizanidine have gained popularity to treat the myofascial components of pain.

Interventional therapies

These techniques include injection therapies (eg, joint injection and epidural injection), neural blockade (eg, sympathetic blocks), and implant therapies (eg, dorsal column stimulation and neuraxial infusion by way of an implanted pump), depending on indications [23].

Patients who have moderate to severe pain and signs of joint inflammation may benefit from intra-articular injections of corticosteroids [14]. Intra-articular corticosteroid injections can provide pain relief from 6 months to 1 year. Some data support the use of fluoroscopic guidance when performing these blocks [24].

Also of interest is the injection of hyaluronic acid into the ankle joint. There is evidence to support its use in the knee joint for osteoarthritis. Although its use in the ankle joint has also been studied [25], hyaluronic acid is not FDA approved for use in the ankle.

Corticosteroids have also been injected for plantar fasciitis, tarsal tunnel, interdigital space, and first metatarsophalangeal joint. Techniques for the specific injection points are beyond the scope of this article.

Patients who have CRPS with moderate to severe pain and do not respond to medication and physical modalities, patients who have signs and symptoms of severe sympathetic dysfunction, and patients who experience marked improvement after a diagnostic sympathetic nerve block are candidates for regional anesthetic blocks [26]. Spinal cord stimulation (dorsal column) has also shown efficacy in the management of CRPS. Also called neurostimulation, it delivers low-voltage electrical stimulation to the spinal cord or targeted peripheral nerve to block the sensation of pain.

The Gate Control Theory of pain, developed by researchers Ronald Melzack and Patrick Wall, proposes that neurostimulation activates the body's pain inhibitory system. The neurostimulation system, implanted in the epidural space, stimulates these pain-inhibiting nerve fibers, masking the sensation of pain with a tingling sensation (paresthesia) [27]. Another therapy that has shown some benefit in the management of CRPS is intrathecal or epidural clonidine [24].

Rehabilitative therapies

Physical therapy has quickly become the mainstay in the treatment of many persistent pain conditions. Therapy can include gait analysis, ergonomics assessment, posture training, stretching, and exercises. Physical therapy alters physiologic responses, improves physical function, and prevents deconditioning.

Plantar fascia stretch exercises have shown improved outcomes for chronic plantar fasciitis [28]. CRPS of the lower extremity has also been shown to respond well to physical therapy [29].

Cognitive behavioral therapy

Psychologic interventions usually include cognitive and behavioral therapies. These therapies include strategies that may lessen pain intensity or improve pain coping. Cognitive behavioral therapy has been shown to lessen the morbidity associated with chronic pain (eg, coping skills, absenteeism from work, and healthcare costs) [13]. Therapy includes biofeedback, relaxation, and imagery. Psychologic interventions are most appropriate for patients who have a high degree of anxiety associated with pain or a psychiatric comorbidity, have a relatively high level of pain-related disability, have inadequate relief after pharmacologic intervention, or who experience persistent or recurrent pain and may benefit from a multimodal approach [30].

Cognitive behavioral therapy is aimed at helping patients understand that their thoughts and behaviors can affect their pain experience. Patients are trained in effective coping skills and how to apply and maintain their coping skills [31]. These therapies are aimed at the emotional and psychosocial distress caused by persistent pain [32]. Therapy may be one-on-one or in small group sessions of four to eight patients. In several clinical trials of pain patients, group programs were found to be effective in helping patients manage their persistent pain and increase their ability to function, including return to the workplace [33]. Biofeedback, relaxation techniques, and hypnotherapy are other components that are used from a behavioral perspective.

These modalities can best be summarized under the following approaches.

Functional restoration or "operant" approach

This approach primarily revolves around realistic goal setting. It is not uncommon for patients who have chronic pain to set global and, at times, overwhelming goals. For instance, a disabled person has only "return to work" as his goal and forms an all-or-nothing approach. The therapist works with the patient to set initial, small, achievable goals revolving around activities of daily living, with a plan for graded increase of such activity. This technique is formally known as graded behavior change. Formal functional restoration programs usually occur in a multidisciplinary setting and convey the consistent message of pain acceptance versus pain relief.

Cognitive approaches

Cognitive traits associated with negative outcomes in chronic pain include "catastrophizing," fear avoidance, and helplessness. Catastrophizing is the belief that the situation is out of control and outcomes are negative. The patient believes that the pain indicates progressing injury and that something is being missed medically. Fear avoidance is the patient's avoidance of many activities completely due to the misconception that this is leading to further pain and injury. The clinician works with the patient to address these dysfunctional beliefs and to allow resumption of activities.

Cognitive interventions target the patient's perception of pain, whereby operant approaches target return of function and perception of pain is not given importance.

Relaxation training and biofeedback

Relaxation training has been supported by evidence-based reviews. Anxiety, pain, and functional sleep disorders are conditions that benefit from this training. Diaphragmatic breathing, progressive muscle relaxation, and passive relaxation are techniques commonly employed. Passive relaxation depends more on the use of guided imagery than on isometric muscle exercises. Self-hypnosis procedures are a variant of the imagery approach.

Biofeedback-assisted relaxation provides immediate physiologic input to the patient on their responses to pain. Surface electromyography and temperature biofeedback are the modalities most commonly used for pain. There are possible contraindications to this technique in patients who have a somatic focus. These patients are already acutely aware of their bodily functions and additional close monitoring can result in an aggravation of their somatization and distress. These patients are better served by operant approaches or distraction techniques.

Summary

Pain has become an increasingly recognized symptom that plays a major role in the treatment of many podiatric patients. Management of this now accepted fifth vital sign can be accomplished through many avenues. NSAIDs and short- and long-acting opioids are typically used by many podiatric physicians; however, the benefits and potential hazards of other pharmaceutic approaches using antidepressants, anticonvulsants, topical medications, and other centrally acting medications must also be recognized. In addition, the role of the psychiatrist or therapist should not be neglected because many types of cognitive therapies are available to aid in treating these patients.

Acknowledgments

The authors would like to acknowledge Tina Toland for her support in preparing this manuscript.

References

[1] The International Association for the Study of Pain. IASP pain terminology. In: Classification of chronic pain. 2nd edition. IASP Task Force on Taxonomy. Merskey H, Bogduk N, editors. Seattle (WA): IASP Press; 1994.

[2] Joint Commission on Accreditation of Healthcare Organizations. Jt Comm Perspect 1999.
[3] Gracely RH, Kwilosz DM. The descriptor differential scale: applying psychophysical principles to clinical pain assessment. Pain 1988;35:279–88.
[4] Portenoy RK. Issues in the management of neuropathic pain. In: Basbaum AI, Besson JM, editors. Towards a new pharmacotherapy of pain. Chichester (UK): John Wiley & Sons; 1991. p. 393–416.
[5] Gamsa A. The role of psychological factors in chronic pain. I. A half century of study. Pain 1994;57:5–15.
[6] Frances A, Pincus HA, First MB, et al, editors. Pain disorder. In: Diagnostic and statistical manual of mental disorders. 4th edition. Washington, DC: American Psychiatric Association; 2000. p. 498–503.
[7] Melzack R. Neurophysiological foundation of pain. In: Sternbach RA, editor. The psychology of pain. New York: Raven Press; 1986. p. 1–12.
[8] Woolf CJ, Decosterd I. Implication for recent advances in the understanding of pain pathophysiology for the assessment of pain in patients. Pain 1999;6:S141–7.
[9] Silko GJ, Cullen PT. Indoor racquet sports injuries. Am Fam Physician 1994;50:374–80, 383–4.
[10] Barrett SJ, O'Malley R. Plantar fasciitis and other causes of heel pain. Am Fam Physician 1999;59:2200–6.
[11] Lau JT, Daniels TR. Tarsal tunnel syndrome: a review of the literature. Foot Ankle Int 1999; 20:201–9.
[12] Oh SJ, Meyer RD. Entrapment neuropathies of the tibial (posterior tibial) nerve. Neurol Clin 1999;17:593–615, vii.
[13] Linton SJ, Andersson T. Can chronic disability be prevented? A randomized trial of a cognitive-behavior intervention and two forms of information for patients with spinal pain. Spine 2000;25:2825–31.
[14] Simon LS, Lipman AG, Jacox A, et al, editors. Guideline for the management of pain. In: Osteoarthritis, rheumatoid arthritis, and juvenile chronic arthritis. 2nd edition. Glenview (IL): American Pain Society; 2002. p. 179.
[15] Wu KK. Morton's interdigital neuroma: a clinical review of its etiology, treatment, and results. J Foot Ankle Surg 1996;35:112–9.
[16] Greenfield J, Rea J, Ilfeld FW. Morton's interdigital neuroma. Indications for treatment by local injections versus surgery. Clin Orthop 1984;185:142–4.
[17] World Health Organization. Who's pain ladder. Available at: http://www.Who.Int/Cancer/Palliative/Painladder/En/. Accessed November 7, 2006.
[18] Max MB, Payne R, Edwards WT, et al, editors. Principles of analgesic use in the treatment of acute pain and cancer pain. 4th edition. Glenview (IL): American Pain Society; 1999.
[19] Stein C. The control of pain in peripheral tissue by opioids. N Engl J Med 1995;332: 1685–90.
[20] Backonja M, Beydoun A, Edwards KR, et al. Gabapentin for the symptomatic treatment of painful neuropathy in patients with diabetes mellitus: a randomized controlled trial. JAMA 1998;280:1831–6.
[21] Rowbotham M, Harden N, Stacey B, et al. Gabapentin for the treatment of postherpetic neuralgia: a randomized controlled trial. JAMA 1998;280:1837–42.
[22] Carter GT, Galer BS. Advances in the management of neuropathic pain. Phys Med Rehabil Clin N Am 2001;12:447–59.
[23] Manchikanti L, Singh V, Kloth D, et al. Interventional techniques in the management of chronic pain part 2. Pain Physician 2001;4:24–96.
[24] Beukelman T, Arabshahi B, Cahill AM, et al. Benefit of intraarticular corticosteroid injection under fluoroscopic guidance for subtalar arthritis in juvenile idiopathic arthritis. J Rheumatol 2006;33(11):2330–6.
[25] Sun S-F, Chou Y-J, Hsu C-W, et al. Efficacy of intraarticular hyaluronic acid in patients with osteoarthritis of the ankle—a prospective study. Osteoarthritis Cartilage 2006;14(9):867–74.

[26] Rho RH, Brewer RP, Lamer TJ, et al. Complex regional pain syndrome. Mayo Clin Proc 2002;77:174–80.
[27] Kemler MA, Barendse GA, van Kleef M, et al. Spinal cord stimulation in patients with chronic reflex sympathetic dystrophy. N Engl J Med 2000;343:618–24.
[28] Digiovanni BF, Nawoczenski DA, Malay DP, et al. Plantar fascia-specific stretching exercise improves outcomes in patienst with chronic plantar fasciitis. A prospective clinical trial with two-year follow-up. J Bone Joint Surg Am 2006;88(8):1775–81.
[29] Lee KJ, Kirchner JS. Complex regional pain syndrome and chronic pain management in the lower extremity. Foot Ankle 2002;7(2):409–19.
[30] Gordon DB, Dahl JL, Miaskowski C, et al. American Pain Society recommendations for improving the quality of acute and cancer pain management. American Pain Society Quality of Care Task Force. Arch Intern Med 2005;165:1574–80.
[31] Keefe FJ, Gil KM. Behavioral concepts in the analysis of chronic pain syndromes. J Consult Clin Psychol 1986;54:776–83.
[32] Leo RJ. Concise guide to pain management for psychiatrists. Arlington (VA): American Psychiatric Publishing, Inc.; 2003.
[33] Sullivan MJ, Stanish WD. Psychologically based occupational rehabilitation: the pain-disability prevention program. Clin J Pain 2003;19:97–104.

ELSEVIER
SAUNDERS

Clin Podiatr Med Surg
24 (2007) 353–363

CLINICS IN
PODIATRIC
MEDICINE AND
SURGERY

Index

Note: Page numbers of article titles are in **boldface** type.

A

Acarbose, for diabetes mellitus, 166

Adalimumab, 239

Alcohol use, 239–240, 269

Alendronate, for osteoporosis, 318–320

Alpha-2 blockers
for cardiac risk reduction, 275
for hypertension, 229–230
for pain, 344

Alpha-glycosidase inhibitors, for diabetes mellitus, 166

Alternative therapies, nutritional supplements as. *See* Nutritional supplements.

Amenorrhea, in female athletes, 142–144

American Academy of Neurology, concussion guidelines of, 132, 136

American Association of Clinical Endocrinologists, glycemic control goals of, 160–161

American College of Cardiology, cardiovascular evaluation guidelines of, 261–266, 271–273

American College of Endocrinology, glycemic control goals of, 160–162

American Diabetes Association, glycemic control goals of, 160–162

American Heart Association, cardiovascular evaluation guidelines of, 261–266, 271–273

Amikacin, 298, 303–304

Aminoglycosides, 298, 303–304

Amitriptyline, for pain, 342, 346

Amnesia, in concussion, 136

Amoxicillin, 294

Amoxicillin/clavulanate, 295

Ampicillin, 294

Ampicillin/sulbactam, 295

Amylin analogs, for diabetes mellitus, 182

Anakinra, 239

Analgesics, 340–346

Anastomotic leak, after bariatric surgery, 216

Anesthesia, for bariatric surgery, 211–212

Angiography, in cardiac risk evaluation, 275–276

Angioplasty, for cardiac risk reduction, 275–277

Angiotensin receptor blockers, for hypertension, 231

Angiotensin-converting enzyme inhibitors, for hypertension, 230–231

Anomalous origin of the left main coronary artery, sudden death in, 129–130

Anorexia, in female athletes, 141–142

Antacid drugs, 236

Antibiotics. *See also specific antibiotics.*
for endocarditis prophylaxis, 231, 279–280
for methicillin-resistant *Staphylococcus aureus* infections, 139–140
resistance to
in aminoglycosides, 304
in carbapenems, 302
in daptomycin, 299, 305–306
in glycopeptides, 300, 306
in glycylcyclines, 300, 304
in linezolid, 299
in macrolides, 304
in monobactams, 303
in penicillins, 302
in rifampin, 305
in streptogramin, 299
in sulfonamides, 298, 304

Rheumatic disease, drugs for, 236–238

Rifampin, 301, 305

Rimonabant, for diabetes mellitus, 182–183

Risedronate, for osteoporosis, 318, 320

Rosiglitazone, for diabetes mellitus, 165

Roux-en Y gastric bypass, for morbid obesity, 207–208

S

St. John's wort, discontinuation of, 247–248

Screw fixation, osteoporosis effects on, 324–326

Selective estrogen receptor modulators, 227, 319–320

Selective serotonin reuptake inhibitors, for pain, 343, 346

Selenium supplementation, 250

Simvastatin
for cardiac risk reduction, 275
for osteoporosis, 321

Sitagliptin, for diabetes mellitus, 182

Skin, excess, after bariatric surgery, 219

Sleep apnea, in morbid obesity, 198

Smoking, 239, 269

Social history, in cardiac risk evaluation, 269

Socioeconomic impact, of morbid obesity, 199–200

Sodium channel blockers, for pain, 344, 346

Spinal cord stimulation, for pain, 347

Sports participants. See Athletes.

Standardized Assessment of Concussion tool, 133–135

Staphylococcus aureus infections, methicillin-resistant, 138–140

Stapling, gastric, for morbid obesity, 202, 205

Statins, 227
for cardiac risk reduction, 275
for osteoporosis, 321–322

Stents, coronary, for cardiac risk reduction, 276

Streptogramin, 299, 305

Stroke, in cardiac risk evaluation, 268

Sudden cardiac death, in athletes, 127–130

Sulfasalazine, 237

Sulfonamides, 298, 304

Sulfonylureas, for diabetes mellitus, 165

Superoxide dismutase, 256

Swelling, reduction of, nutritional supplements for, 254–255

Sympathetic blocks, for pain, 347

Sympathetic nervous system, in bone metabolism, 315–316

Sympatholytics, 229–230

Syncope, in hypertrophic cardiomyopathy, 128

T

Tamoxifen, 227, 319

Tarsal tunnel syndrome, pain management in, 339

Teicoplanin, 300, 306

Teriparatide, for osteoporosis, 318

Tetanus prophylaxis, 306

Tetracyclines, 299, 304

Theophylline, 238

Thiazolidinediones, for diabetes mellitus, 164–165

Thrombosis, deep venous. See Deep venous thrombosis.

Thyroid disease, drugs for, 228

Tibolone, for osteoporosis, 319

Ticlopidine, 233

Tigecycline, 300, 304

Tizanidine, for pain, 344, 346

Tobacco use, 239, 269

Tobramycin, 298, 303–304

Topical agents, for pain, 345

Transforming growth factor-β, in osteoporosis, 313–315

Tricyclic antidepressants, for pain, 342, 346

Trimethoprim-sulfamethoxazole, 298, 304

Tumor necrosis factor-a, in osteoporosis, 313–315

Moving?

Make sure your subscription moves with you!

To notify us of your new address, find your **Clinics Account Number** (located on your mailing label above your name), and contact customer service at:

E-mail: elspcs@elsevier.com

800-654-2452 (subscribers in the U.S. & Canada)
407-345-4000 (subscribers outside of the U.S. & Canada)

Fax number: 407-363-9661

Elsevier Periodicals Customer Service
6277 Sea Harbor Drive
Orlando, FL 32887-4800

*To ensure uninterrupted delivery of your subscription, please notify us at least 4 weeks in advance of move.